Atlas of Chest Imaging in COVID-19 Patients

Jinxin Liu • Xiaoping Tang • Chunliang Lei
Editors

Atlas of Chest Imaging in COVID-19 Patients

清华大学出版社
TSINGHUA UNIVERSITY PRESS

Springer

Editors
Jinxin Liu
Department of Radiology
Guangzhou Eighth People's Hospital,
Guangzhou Medical University
Guangzhou, China

Xiaoping Tang
Department of Infectious Diseases
Guangzhou Eighth People's Hospital,
Guangzhou Medical University
Guangzhou, China

Chunliang Lei
Department of Infectious Diseases
Guangzhou Eighth People's Hospital,
Guangzhou Medical University
Guangzhou, China

ISBN 978-981-16-1084-4 ISBN 978-981-16-1082-0 (eBook)
https://doi.org/10.1007/978-981-16-1082-0

Jointly published with Tsinghua University Press

This Springer imprint is published by the registered company Springer Nature Singapore Pte Ltd.
The registered company address is: 152 Beach Road, #21-01/04 Gateway East, Singapore 189721, Singapore

Foreword

The first glimpse of this book *Atlas of Chest Imaging in COVID-19 Patient*, which is edited by Jinxin Liu, Xiaoping Tang, and Chunliang Lei from the Guangzhou Eighth People's Hospital, sent my thoughts back to early 2003, when a comprehensive book named Chest *Imaging Diagnostic Altas of SARS* was published in which I wrote the preface and contributed as the chief reviewer. Now, 17 years after the 2003 SARS outbreak, I am very delighted to know that the same three anti-SARS heroes in 2003 accomplished such a comprehensive book with high-resolution images about COVID-19 in such a short time. This book embodies the hard work of all medical personnel, especially imaging medical workers, in the Guangzhou Eighth People's Hospital. This book summarized their hard-won, precious, and encyclopedic imaging data about COVID-19 patients in different conditions. It was also a testimony of their dedication to the development of science. I express my sincere gratitude to them for their scientific attitude in seeking truth from facts.

The book has the following features:

Firstly, chest CT and X-ray data which are extensively collected from COVID-19 patients at different stages (including early stage, progressive stage, peak stage, and absorption stage) provide an imaging reference covering the entire disease course to the readers and will help readers to establish a better understanding of how the disease evolves and will guide the clinical diagnosis and treatment as well.

Secondly, the chest CT images of some cases finally confirmed by multiple nucleic acid tests and of different cases occurred in one family were presented, which strongly confirmed the important role of chest CT in the diagnosis of COVID-19 pneumonia.

Thirdly, the follow-up CT examinations of COVID-19 patients who were CT normal during the first examination recorded their lung imaging changes over the whole disease course and emphasized the necessity and importance of multiple CT reexaminations for early patient identification and diagnosis, isolation, and treatment for suspected and confirmed patients. In addition, chest CT images of confirmed COVID-19 patients during the follow-up stage revealed that over 90% lung lesions could be completely absorbed (or only a slight focal linear opacity remained), which demonstrates that COVID-19 pneumonia is not only preventable and controllable but curable.

I believe that this book can provide an important reference for medical workers and researchers in the clinical diagnosis, assessment of disease changes, and prognosis about COVID-19 pneumonia.

I would like to express my gratitude to the medical workers who have worked hard and contributed to this book.

Nanshan Zhong
State Key Laboratory of Respiratory Disease
National Clinical Research Center for Respiratory Disease
Guangzhou Institute of Respiratory Health
First Affiliated Hospital of Guangzhou Medical University
Guangzhou, China

Preface

Life is like a dream. A scene like the SARS outbreak in 2003 which reoccurs countless times in my dream now occurred 17 years later in reality at almost the same season in early 2020. For us who once witnessed the SARS outbreak, and experienced and survived the hard and warlike times in 2003, our first reaction after we realized that an infectious "unknown pneumonia" extremely similar to SARS, named as COVID-19 now, emerged was that of anxiety and concern. We clearly know that the disease would cause severe social consequences once out of control. What we could do was to reallocate and train personnel, to prepare enough medicines and medical supplies, and to empty the occupied beds and backup isolation wards. We aimed to maximally protect the whole Guangzhou population from suffering the COVID-19 disease by admitting and treating the patients and by curing their diseases. With no delay, the Guangzhou Eighth People's Hospital arranged an emergency meeting which was called "preparatory meeting for admission and treatment of pneumonia of unknown cause" on January 6, 2020. Right after the meeting, the whole hospital immediately entered a state of preparation. On January 20, 2020, the hospital issued an emergency notice that required all staff to cancel their coming festival holidays and to stand by on call in Guangzhou. On the same day, the wards started to accept confirmed and suspected COVID-19 patients. The first batch of CT examinations were conducted on January 22. Seven of all eight patients who received CT examinations had typical imaging manifestations. By March 2, a total of 402 confirmed and suspected patients had been admitted, 295 (including 46 cases of severe illness, 15 cases of critical illness, and 1 case of death) were confirmed, and 232 cases were cured and discharged from hospital; no medical personnel were infected.

No one can escape by sheer luck when in front of a pandemic. I had the same feeling and agreed that "COVID-19 is still raging, we don't know how many people will die or how many families will never see the light of tomorrow from now on" in a news report when I knew that professor Shunfang Wang, the wife of my supervisor, who once worked in Renmin Hospital of Wuhan University, died of COVID-19 on February 26. She died only 5 days from confirmed diagnosis. May there be no novel coronavirus and no pain in heaven.

Just as professor Nanshan Zhong, one academician of the Chinese Engineering Academy, said, our understanding of COVID-19 is "just a preliminary understanding" and there are still many unknowns to be explored and studied. Here, I would like to mention the other two elder seniors who deserve our respect. One is professor Jincheng Chen from Jinan University; the other is professor Xuelin Zhang from Southern Medical University. In order to understand the imaging characteristics of SARS patients, they, regardless of their own safety, made a special trip to the Eighth People's Hospital of Guangzhou to check right after the SARS outbreak in 2003. They read the chest radiographs of all confirmed patients and gave us a lot of suggestions. Their rigorousness in science and truth-seeking spirit are worthy of our learning and inheritance.

This book is compiled on the basis of our consistent principles: data authenticity and completeness. We also provide our comments, insights, and interpretations after we have studied the images and the disease evolution.

We collected the image data of 295 confirmed COVID-19 cases in our Guangzhou Eighth People's Hospital and included 922 images from 82 selected and typical cases in this atlas.

This book covered the imaging manifestations of the confirmed COVID-19 cases in the onset of the early stage, early stage, progression, and absorption stage. In particular, special chest imaging data from first viral RNA test negative patients, from first CT test negative patients, and from family gathering history confirmed patients are included in the atlas. They can serve as references for our medical peers and aid their diagnosis and research.

We really wish to express our gratitude to Prof. Nanshan Zhong, academician of the Chinese Engineering Academy, who wrote the preface for the atlas for his chief reviewing and detailed suggestions.

Guangzhou, China Jinxin Liu

Contents

List of Contributors

Shuijiang Cai Guangzhou Eighth People's Hospital, Guangzhou Medical University, Guangzhou, China

Weiping Cai Guangzhou Eighth People's Hospital, Guangzhou Medical University, Guangzhou, China

Bihua Chen Guangzhou Eighth People's Hospital, Guangzhou Medical University, Guangzhou, China

Fengjuan Chen Guangzhou Eighth People's Hospital, Guangzhou Medical University, Guangzhou, China

Xilong Deng Guangzhou Eighth People's Hospital, Guangzhou Medical University, Guangzhou, China

Yan Ding Guangzhou Eighth People's Hospital, Guangzhou Medical University, Guangzhou, China

Yanqing Ding Nanfang Hospital, Southern Medical University, Guangzhou, China

Qingxin Gan Guangzhou Eighth People's Hospital, Guangzhou Medical University, Guangzhou, China

Wanhua Guan Guangzhou Eighth People's Hospital, Guangzhou Medical University, Guangzhou, China

Tianli Hu Guangzhou Eighth People's Hospital, Guangzhou Medical University, Guangzhou, China

Deyang Huang Guangzhou Eighth People's Hospital, Guangzhou Medical University, Guangzhou, China

Rui Jiang Guangzhou Eighth People's Hospital, Guangzhou Medical University, Guangzhou, China

Songfeng Jiang Guangzhou Eighth People's Hospital, Guangzhou Medical University, Guangzhou, China

Chunliang Lei Guangzhou Eighth People's Hospital, Guangzhou Medical University, Guangzhou, China

Feng Li Guangzhou Eighth People's Hospital, Guangzhou Medical University, Guangzhou, China

Yueping Li Guangzhou Eighth People's Hospital, Guangzhou Medical University, Guangzhou, China

Li Liang Nanfang Hospital, Southern Medical University, Guangzhou, China

Meiyan Liao Zhongnan Hospital of Wuhan University, Wuhan, China

Lin Lin Guangzhou Eighth People's Hospital, Guangzhou Medical University, Wuhan, China

Zhoukun Ling Guangzhou Eighth People's Hospital, Guangzhou Medical University, Guangzhou, China

Jinxin Liu Guangzhou Eighth People's Hospital, Guangzhou Medical University, Guangzhou, China

Ying Liu Guangzhou Eighth People's Hospital, Guangzhou Medical University, Guangzhou, China

Xiaoneng Mo Guangzhou Eighth People's Hospital, Guangzhou Medical University, Guangzhou, China

Jing Qu Guangzhou Eighth People's Hospital, Guangzhou Medical University, Guangzhou, China

Fei Shan Shanghai Public Health Clinical Center, Fudan University, Shanghai, China

Haiyan Shi Guangzhou Eighth People's Hospital, Guangzhou Medical University, Guangzhou, China

Xiaoping Tang Guangzhou Eighth People's Hospital, Guangzhou Medical University, Guangzhou, China

Sufang Tian Zhongnan Hospital of Wuhan University, Wuhan, China

Peixu Wang Guangzhou Eighth People's Hospital, Guangzhou Medical University, Guangzhou, China

Shuyi Xie Guangzhou Eighth People's Hospital, Guangzhou Medical University, Guangzhou, China

Xi Xu The First Affiliated Hospital, Jinan University, Guangzhou, China

Yanhong Yang Guangzhou Eighth People's Hospital, Guangzhou Medical University, Guangzhou, China

Chengcheng Yu Guangzhou Eighth People's Hospital, Guangzhou Medical University, Guangzhou, China

Lieguang Zhang Guangzhou Eighth People's Hospital, Guangzhou Medical University, Guangzhou, China

Zhiping Zhang Guangzhou Eighth People's Hospital, Guangzhou Medical University, Guangzhou, China

Overview

1

Jing Qu, Lin Lin, Shuyi Xie, Feng Li, Jinxin Liu, Wanhua Guan, Zhiping Zhang, Qingxin Gan, Chengcheng Yu, Rui Jiang, Zhoukun Ling, Yanhong Yang, and Xiaoping Tang

1.1 Introduction

Coronavirus disease 19 (COVID-19), caused by severe acute respiratory syndrome coronavirus 2 (SARS-CoV-2) infection, has spread around the world with no sign of ceasing. Over 40 million COVID-19 cases and more than 1 million fatal cases were reported by the end of October 2020, and the number is still increasing. The diagnosis of COVID-19 mainly relied on the laboratory viral RNA detection in upper respiratory samples, such as throat and nasal swabs, because of their ease of access. SARS-CoV-2 appears to be transmitted via respiratory droplets and aerosols and contact with contaminated surface. Because the viral receptor ACE2 is expressed abundantly in the lung epithelial cells, SARS-CoV-2 will easily establish infection in the lung if inhaled in after a deep breath and then spread gradually from the bottom to the other part of the upper respiratory tract. When throat and nasal samples are collected in this time window, viral RNA detection will fail and present a negative result. For a certain percentage of COVID-19 patients, the time window is so wide that the virus has caused lung damage long before it is detected in the throat samples. To overcome this limitation, computed tomography (CT) of the chest is definitely required as an alternative and complementary approach to diagnose and confirm virus infection through checking typical lung lesions when combined with a clear and close contact history with a confirmed or highly suspected SARS-CoV-2 infectee.

1.2 Epidemiological Characteristics [1–4]

Over 500 COVID-19 patients (over 90% of all COVID-19 patients in Guangzhou City) were admitted in Guangzhou Eighth People's Hospital on August 2020. Epidemiological analysis revealed that COVID-19 patients were middle-aged and older adults with no gender difference and that most COVID-19 patients had a clear disease-related exposure history. Similar to transmission of other respiratory viruses through respiratory droplets and close contact, SARS-CoV-2 infection also exhibits a pattern of clustering distribution, such as among familial members and relatives, in communities including neighborhoods, schools, and shared working space; and in public areas including malls, restaurants, and transportation vehicles.

1. Source of Infection

The SARS-CoV-2-infected patients are the main source of infection, and they usually shed higher concentrations of virus within 5 days after onset. Notably, COVID-19 patients in the incubation period start to excrete virus before obvious symptom onset and without seeking medical help, and some patients are completely asymptomatic infectees, serving unidentified viral reservoirs for rapid virus spreading.

2. Means of Transmission

The main routes of SARS-CoV-2 transmission are reported to be through respiratory droplets, person-to-person close contact, and contaminated items.

It is possible that the virus may spread through aerosols under prolonged exposure to high concentrations of aerosols in a relatively closed environment.

In addition, the live SARS-CoV-2 virus can be isolated from feces or urine samples, and thus, viral contaminated environment might also be a natural infection resource.

3. Susceptible Population

The whole population is generally susceptible since the virus originated from nature. Protective immunity may be obtained through natural SARS-CoV-2 infection or through

J. Qu · L. Lin · S. Xie · F. Li · J. Liu (✉) · W. Guan · Z. Zhang · Q. Gan · C. Yu · R. Jiang · Z. Ling · Y. Yang · X. Tang
Guangzhou Eighth People's Hospital, Guangzhou Medical University, Guangzhou, China

J. Liu et al. (eds.), *Atlas of Chest Imaging in COVID-19 Patients*, https://doi.org/10.1007/978-981-16-1082-0_1

vaccination. However, how long this protection lasts is still under observation.

1.3 Pathological Characteristics [1, 5–8]

Although COVID-19 is mainly a pulmonary disease, it can cause cardiac, dermatologic, hematological, hepatic, neurological, renal, and other complications [9–17]. Thromboembolic events were often observed in COVID-19 patients and were reported to significantly increase the risk for critical COVID-19 patients.

The imaging changes of COVID-19 pathogenesis in major organs (excluding underlying disease lesions) were discussed as follows.

1. Lungs

The lungs showed varying degrees of consolidation. The consolidation area mainly presented diffuse alveolar injury and exudative alveolitis. Pulmonary disease in different areas had become complex and varied, with old and new lesions interlaced. Serous exudate, fibrinous exudate, and hyaline membrane were found in the alveolar cavity. The exudate cells were mainly mononuclear, macrophages, and multinucleated giant cells. Type II alveolar epithelial cells proliferate, and some cells were exfoliated. There were occasional inclusions in type II alveolar epithelial cells and macrophages. Hyperemia, edema, and infiltration of monocytes and lymphocytes could be seen in the alveolar septa. A few alveoli were overfilled, alveolar compartments ruptured, and cysts formed. The bronchial epithelium of each level in the lung partly fell off, while exudate and mucus could be seen in the cavity. Pulmonary vasculitis and thrombotic formation (mixed thrombus, hyaline thrombus) appeared, and thrombotic lung tissue tended to demonstrate focal pulmonary hemorrhage.In some patients with long-term disease, fibrinogen exuded in the alveoli formed cellulose, and the organized cellulose caused diffuse thickening and fibrosis of the alveolar walls.

SARS-CoV-2 particles could be seen in the cytoplasm of the bronchial mucosal epithelium and type II alveolar epithelial cells under electron microscopy. Immunohistochemical staining revealed that some bronchial mucosal epithelium, alveolar epithelial cells, and macrophages were SARS-CoV-2 antigen immunostaining and nucleic acid test positive.

2. Lymphatic and Hematopoietic Systems

Immunohistochemical staining revealed a decreased CD4+ and CD8+ T cells in the spleen and lymph nodes. In lymph nodes, viral RNA were detected by in situ RNA staining, and macrophage was found by immunostaining. In bone marrow, hematopoietic cells were found to actively proliferate in some individuals, while they were decreasing in other individuals, and the ratio of granulocyte and erythrocyte was found to increase. Hemophagocytosis was also occasionally observed.

3. Cardiovascular System

The disease could cause degeneration and necrosis in cardiomyocytes, along with interstitial congestion and edema. There was a slight infiltration of monocytes, lymphocytes, and/or neutrophils.

In the small vessels of major organs, endothelial cell shedding and intimal or full-thickness inflammation could be seen. Mixed thrombosis, thromboembolism, and infarction occurred in the corresponding part. Obvious thrombosis was observed in the capillaries of the main organs.

1.4 General Clinical Manifestations [1, 18]

The general clinical symptoms of COVID-19 include fever, dry cough, fatigue, muscle soreness, headache, diarrhea etc. COVID-19 patients are classified as asymptomatic, mild, moderate, severe, and critical patients based on clinical symptoms.

The asymptomatic patients are only SARS-CoV-2 RNA positive but has no sign of clinical symptoms. Only a small percentage of COVID-19 patients are asymptomatic.

Mild patients may present with low fever, slight fatigue, smell and taste disorders, but no pneumonia. When patients have pneumonia, they are diagnosed as moderate COVID-19. Mild and moderate patients account for the majority of all COVID-19 patients.

Some patients progressed to severe and even critical stage at approximately 1–2 weeks after symptom onset. They manifested as acute respiratory distress syndrome, septic shock, hard-to-correct metabolic acidosis, blood coagulation dysfunction, etc. [1]. Those critical COVID-19 patients are elderly, people with chronic basic diseases, women in the third trimester and perinatal period, and obese people.

Symptoms in children were relatively mild. Some children and newborns had atypical symptoms, such as vomiting, diarrhea, and other gastrointestinal symptoms or only lack of alertness and shortness of breath.

COVID-19 children occasionally will have multisystem inflammatory syndrome (MIS-C), similar to Kawasaki disease, atypical Kawasaki disease, toxic shock syndrome, macrophage activation syndrome, etc., mostly during their recovery period. The main symptoms are fever with rash, nonsuppurative conjunctivitis, mucosal inflammation, hypotension or shock, coagulation disorders, acute gastrointestinal symptoms, etc. Once it happens, the disease can deteriorate rapidly in a short time.

1.5 Laboratory Examinations

1.5.1 Routine Blood Cell Examination and Biochemical Examinations

In the early stages of infection, the peripheral white blood cell counts and lymphocyte counts in most COVID-19 patients were in normal range or slightly decreased. C-reactive protein (CRP) and erythrocyte sedimentation rate were elevated in most patients, and procalcitonin was usually normal. Patients in the severe stage usually had substantially elevated D-dimer and progressively declining peripheral blood lymphocytes. Liver enzymes, lactate dehydrogenase, muscle enzymes, and myoglobin in some patients increased; some critically ill patients had increased troponin.

1.5.2 Serological Examination

1.5.2.1 Serological Diagnosis of SARS-CoV-2 Infection

Serological Examination: Detecting SARS-CoV-2 specific IgM and IgG antibodies was an easy and helpful test for clinical diagnosis in the early phase of SARS-CoV-2 pandemic. Because viral specific IgM and IgG generation requires several days after viral infection, antibody testing could not provide a reliable early diagnosis for those patients right after they are infected, typically within 1 week of onset.

The specificity and sensitivity of IgM and IgG test itself constrained their wide application. Endogenous interfering factors such as the presence of interfering substances (such as rheumatoid factor, heterophile antibodies, complement, and lysozyme) from the host, specimen contamination (such as hemolysis of specimens and environment pollutants) caused by bacteria, and improper handling procedures (such as longer sample storage and incomplete coagulation) could affect the detection specificity. Importantly, SARS-CoV-2 infection in a certain percentage of COVID-19 patients fails to evoke viral specific IgM and IgG antibodies. Therefore, IgM and IgG tests have not been taken as a confirmed diagnosis alone but are very beneficial for diagnosis when combined with other factors, especially a clear epidemiological history.

SARS-CoV-2 infection could be diagnosed by antibody tests for (1) highly suspected COVID-19 patients based on clinical symptoms but with negative viral RNA results and for (2) convalesced COVID-19 patients with negative viral RNA results.

1.5.2.2 Serologic Testing Protection Prediction

The expert panel recommended that serological testing could not be used to determine whether a person obtains protective immunity against SARS-CoV-2 infection. When antibodies were detected, the results should be interpreted carefully for the following reasons.

Not all SARS-CoV-2 antibodies are protective. SARS-CoV-2 expresses multiple proteins, and all secreted proteins can evoke antibodies. But antibodies against the receptor binding domain (RBD) of S proteins which can prevent SARS-CoV-2 from binding to an entry receptor are generally regarded as protective.

How long the protective antibodies can last after discharge is still unknown. Until now, it is too early to claim that one individual acquires long-term sterile immunity when antibodies are detected. Indeed, reinfection cases have been reported recently.

1.5.3 Etiological Examination

SARS-CoV-2 RNA is detected in the lung, upper respiratory and lower respiratory tracts, mouth, blood (occasional in severe/critical patients), feces (seldom), and urine (rare). However, because of easy access and availability, naso- and oropharyngeal swabs are widely used for SARS-CoV-2 viral RNA detection by real-time fluorescent reverse transcription polymerase chain reaction (RT-PCR) and/or next-generation sequencing (NGS). Viral detection in the lower respiratory tract specimens (sputum or airway extracts) where high concentrations of virus exist is much easily and thus more accurate.

Viral RNA nucleic acid testing would be affected by the course of disease and specimen collection procedure. Reliable detection reagent and standardized sample collection and process procedures will safeguard the detection accuracy.

1.6 Chest Imaging Examinations

Imaging examination is a critical alternative for early diagnosis, for monitoring disease process, for assessing the severity of the disease, and for evaluating the patient recovery after viral RNA becomes negative [19].

1.6.1 Chest Radiographs

In the early stage, some patients showed negative chest X-ray signs. In some patients, the chest radiographs showed scattered high-density shadows in the lateral field of the lung, and a few patients showed diffuse distribution of ground-glass opacities. The progress of the disease course in some patients was relatively rapid, and the consolidation was mainly seen in bilateral lower lobes. In a few patients, the lungs were "white lung" or similar to "white lung." Pleural effusion was rare.

1.6.2 Chest CT [20–22]

Early Period: The main CT findings were ground-glass opacification with or without thickening of the interlobular septum and dilated blood vessel crossing the lesion. Considering that the pathological changes were mainly acute inflammation, the virus mainly invaded the epithelial cells of bronchiole mucosa and type II alveolar epithelial cells (because the lesion was mainly distributed under the pleura of the bilateral lung field), causing epithelial shedding and inflammatory injury of the alveolar septal vessels and finally resulting in serous fibrinous exudation and lymphocyte infiltration in the alveolar cavity. And there had been some progress in developing artificial intelligence (AI) computer-aided systems for CT-based COVID-19 diagnosis [23].

Progression Period: The mainly manifestations were ground-glass opacities with consolidation and the change of interstitium of the lungs, including interlobular septal thickening, intralobular septal thickening, and subpleural line; moreover, "crazy-paving sign" was visible. The pathological changes included diffuse intra-alveolar hemorrhage, fibrinous exudation, and interstitial inflammatory cell infiltration. With the aggravation of lesions, mucus blockage occurred in the bronchioles and terminal bronchioles, resulting in alveolar collapse.

Severe Period: The most common manifestations were diffuse multiple patchy consolidation; some cases manifest as "white lung." The pathological changes included diffuse alveolar damage, intra-alveolar edema, and hyaline membrane formation.

Absorption Period: After treatment, the lesions were cleared in most patients. In addition, few fibrous lesions remain in the lungs of some patients.

The Distribution of Lesions: The lesions of two lungs were mainly multiple, especially in the bilateral lower lobes. The lesions were mainly distributed in the periphery of the lung, and the development trend of the lesion was generally from the periphery of the lung to the center of the bronchi. In the course of the disease, the lesions in the lungs manifested as "growing and disappearing," showing the coexistence of multiple manifestations.

Others: Pleural effusion and lymphadenopathy were rare.

1.7 Clinical Classification [1, 24]

1. Mild type

The clinical symptoms were mild, and no manifestations of pneumonia were found on imaging.

2. Moderate type

The clinical manifestations included fever and respiratory symptoms, accompanied with imaging manifestations of pneumonia.

3. Severe type

Adults meet any of the following criteria:

(a) Onset of shortness of breath, RR $\geq$ 30 times/min
(b) In the resting state, SpO_2 (oxygen saturation) $\leq$93% when inhaling air
(c) Partial pressure of blood oxygen (PaO_2)/oxygen absorption (FiO_2) $\leq$300 mmHg
(d) Patients with progressive clinical symptoms and whose pulmonary imaging showed lung infiltrates >50% within 24–48 h

A child meets any of the following criteria:

(a) Sustained high fever for more than 3 days
(b) Onset of shortness of breath (<2 months old, RR $\geq$ 60 times/min; 2–12 months old, RR $\geq$ 50 times/min; 1–5 years old, RR $\geq$ 40 times/min; >5 years old, RR $\geq$ 30 times/min), excluding the effects of fever and crying
(c) In resting state, oxygen saturation $\leq$93% when inhaling air
(d) Assisted ventilation (alar flap, three-concave sign)
(e) Lethargy and convulsions
(f) Refusal of food or difficulty in feeding and signs of dehydration

4. Critical type

One of the following conditions:

(a) Respiratory failure and requiring mechanical ventilation
(b) Septic shock
(c) Patients with multiple organ dysfunction or failure who should be monitored in the intensive care unit (ICU)

1.8 Differential Diagnosis

1. Mild COVID-19 symptoms should be distinguished from upper respiratory tract infection caused by other viruses.
2. COVID-19 was mainly differentiated from influenza virus, adenovirus, respiratory syncytial virus, and other known viral pneumonia and mycoplasma pneumoniae infection. Especially for suspected cases, rapid antigen detection and multiple PCR nucleic acid detection should

be adopted to detect common respiratory pathogens as far as possible.

3. It was necessary to distinguish from noninfectious diseases, such as vasculitis, dermatomyositis, and organized pneumonia.
4. When a rash or mucosal damage occurred in a child patient, it was necessary to differentiate from Kawasaki disease.

1.9 Treatment and Outcome

1.9.1 Treatment

According to the condition to determine the treatment site:

1. Suspected and confirmed cases should be isolated and treated in designated hospitals with effective isolation and protective conditions. Suspected cases should be isolated in a single room.
2. Critical cases should be admitted to ICU as soon as possible.

1.9.1.1 General Treatment

1. Maintain internal environmental stability with supportive treatment, and closely monitor vital signs, blood oxygen saturation of the pinched fingers, etc.
2. Monitor blood cells, urine, C-reactive protein (CRP), biochemical indicators (liver enzymes, cardiac enzymes, kidney function, etc.), and coagulation function. Perform arterial blood gas analysis, and repeat chest imaging if necessary.
3. Take effective oxygen therapy measures in time according to the changes in blood oxygen saturation.
4. Antimicrobial therapy: Avoid inappropriate use of antimicrobial drugs, especially combinations of broad-spectrum antibacterial drugs.

1.9.1.2 Antiviral Therapy

Although antiviral drugs had not been found to be effective after a rigorous "randomized, double-blind, placebo-controlled study," there was relatively consensus that the drugs with potential antiviral effect should be used in the early stage of the disease, and it was recommended to focus on the patients with severe risk factors and the tendency of severe disease, such as interferon-alpha nebulized inhalation, lopinavir/ritonavir, ribavirin, chloroquine phosphate, and Abidol.

1.9.1.3 Immunotherapy

1. Convalescent plasma from individuals who had recovered from SARS-CoV-2 infection [25, 26]: it was suitable for severe and critical patients with rapid disease progression.
2. Intravenous injection of COVID-19 human immunoglobulin: it could be applied to ordinary and severe patients with rapid disease progression in an emergency.
3. Tozumab: It could be used in patients with extensive bilateral lung diseases and severe patients, and the level of IL-6 will increase in laboratory tests. Pay attention to allergic reactions. Tuberculosis and other active infection were prohibited to use tozumab.

1.9.1.4 Glucocorticoid Therapy

For patients with gradual deterioration of oxygenation index, rapid imaging progress, and excessive activation of the body's inflammatory response, short-term glucocorticoid therapy should be given (generally recommended 3–5 days, no more than 10 days). The recommended dose of glucocorticoid was prednisolone 0.5–1 mg/kg/day. Due to immunosuppressive effects, we should pay attention to the use of high-dose glucocorticoids, which may delay the removal of the virus.

1.9.1.5 Treatment of Severe, Critical Cases

1. Treatment principle: Actively symptomatic treatment to prevent complications and secondary infections. Support organ functions in time.
2. Respiratory support includes oxygen inhalation by a nasal catheter or mask; transnasal high-flow oxygen therapy or noninvasive ventilation; invasive mechanical ventilation; airway management; extracorporeal membrane oxygenation (ECMO).
3. Circulatory support.
4. Anticoagulation therapy.
5. Acute kidney injury and renal replacement therapy.
6. Blood purification treatment.
7. Other treatment measures may be considered, such as antiendotoxin medicine like Xuebijing. Intestinal microecological regulator could be used to maintain intestinal microecological balance and prevent secondary bacterial infection. IVIG may be considered as appropriate in severe or critical children cases. Patients with severe or critical pregnancy should be actively terminated; C-section is the first choice.

1.9.1.6 Traditional Chinese Medical Treatment

Traditional Chinese Medical Treatment (TCM) may be effective in treating COVID-19. Jinhua Qinggan (JHQG) granules and Lianhua Qingwen (LHQW) capsules are recommended during medical observation; Lung Cleansing and Detoxifying Decoction (LCDD) is recommended for the treatment of both severe and non-severe patients; Xuanfeibaidu (XFBD) granules are recommended for treating moderate cases;

while Huashibaidu (HSBD) and Xuebijing (XBJ) have been used in managing severe cases effectively [27].

1.9.2 Prognosis and Outcomes

Over 500 COVID-19 patients were admitted to Guangzhou Eighth People's Hospital; after comprehensive treatment, most of the patients improved or were clinically cured and discharged. One patient died. The mortality rate was 0.3%.

1.9.3 Analysis of Death Cases

One fatal case of an 82-year-old male with COVID-19 was reported in Guangzhou Eighth People's Hospital. He had a history of chronic obstructive pulmonary disease (COPD). SARS-CoV-2 infection caused him a rapid disease progression to systemic multiorgan dysfunction. During his later hospitalization, his condition was deteriorated by complications of severe bacterial and fungal infection, which resulted in further severe acute respiratory distress syndrome, multiorgan failure, and disseminated intravascular coagulation. Despite attempts at resuscitation, he died in the hospital.

In Chap. 10, the imaging, we analyzed the imaging, autopsy, and pathology of clinical death cases.

1.10 Problems and Perspectives

So far, most of the data on the epidemiology, clinical course, prevention, and treatment of COVID-19 comes from research on nonpregnant adults. As described in the following sections of this book, there is an urgent need for more information about COVID-19 in other patient populations (such as children, pregnant women, and immunocompromised patients).

The overall disease severity of children with COVID-19 is generally less severe compared to COVID-19 adults. However, the recently reported occurrence of multisystem inflammatory syndrome in children (MIS-C) in COVID-19 children requires a systematic review. For pregnant women infected with SARS-CoV-2, concerns about their clinical characteristics and pregnancy outcome and existence of the vertical transmission from mother to child are also emerging. For those immunocompromised patients, such as transplant recipients, cancer patients, and HIV-infected patients, special consideration is needed because of the increased risk of serious complications due to COVID-19.

In addition, the long-term prognosis of COVID-19 patients is still unclear, which may require meticulous and lasting follow-up.

References

1. General Office of National Health Committee. Office of State Administration of Traditional Chinese Medicine. Notice on the issuance of a program for the diagnosis and treatment of novel coronavirus (2019-nCoV) infected pneumonia (trial eighth edition). China Med. 2020;15(10) https://doi.org/10.3760/j.issn.1673-4777.2020.10.002.
2. Chan JF, Yuan S, Kok KH, et al. A familial cluster of pneumonia associated with the 2019 novel coronavirus indicating person-to-person transmission: a study of a family cluster. Lancet (London). 2020;395(10223):514–23.
3. Chen N, Zhou M, Dong X, et al. Epidemiological and clinical characteristics of 99 cases of 2019 novel coronavirus pneumonia in Wuhan, China: a descriptive study. Lancet (London). 2020;395(10223):507–13.
4. Xu X, Chen P, Wang J, et al. Evolution of the novel coronavirus from the ongoing Wuhan outbreak and modeling of its spike protein for risk of human transmission. Sci China Life Sci. 2020;63(3):457–60.
5. Chong S, Kim TS, Cho EY. Herpes simplex virus pneumonia: high-resolution CT findings. Br J Radiol. 2010;83(991):585–9.
6. Tian S, Hu W, Niu L, Liu H, Xu H, Xiao SY. Pulmonary pathology of early-phase 2019 novel coronavirus (COVID-19) pneumonia in two patients with lung cancer. J Thoracic Oncol. 2020;15(5):700–4.
7. Xu Z, Shi L, Wang Y, et al. Pathological findings of COVID-19 associated with acute respiratory distress syndrome. Lancet Respir Med. 2020;8(4):420–2.
8. D'Errico S, Zanon M, Montanaro M, et al. More than pneumonia: distinctive features of SARS-Cov-2 infection. From autopsy findings to clinical implications: a systematic review. Microorganisms. 2020;8(11)
9. Liu PP, Blet A, Smyth D, Li H. The science underlying COVID-19: implications for the cardiovascular system. Circulation. 2020;142(1):68–78.
10. Madjid M, Safavi-Naeini P, Solomon SD, Vardeny O. Potential effects of coronaviruses on the cardiovascular system: a review. JAMA Cardiol. 2020;5(7):831–40.
11. Sachdeva M, Gianotti R, Shah M, et al. Cutaneous manifestations of COVID-19: report of three cases and a review of literature. J Dermatol Sci. 2020;98(2):75–81.
12. Henry BM, de Oliveira MHS, Benoit S, Plebani M, Lippi G. Hematologic, biochemical and immune biomarker abnormalities associated with severe illness and mortality in coronavirus disease 2019 (COVID-19): a meta-analysis. Clin Chem Lab Med. 2020;58(7):1021–8.
13. Agarwal A, Chen A, Ravindran N, To C, Thuluvath PJ. Gastrointestinal and liver manifestations of COVID-19. J Clin Exp Hepatol. 2020;10(3):263–5.
14. Whittaker A, Anson M, Harky A. Neurological manifestations of COVID-19: a systematic review and current update. Acta Neurol Scand. 2020;142(1):14–22.
15. Paniz-Mondolfi A, Bryce C, Grimes Z, et al. Central nervous system involvement by severe acute respiratory syndrome coronavirus-2 (SARS-CoV-2). J Med Virol. 2020;92(7):699–702.
16. Pei G, Zhang Z, Peng J, et al. Renal involvement and early prognosis in patients with COVID-19 pneumonia. J Am Soc Nephrol. 2020;31(6):1157–65.
17. Su H, Yang M, Wan C, et al. Renal histopathological analysis of 26 postmortem findings of patients with COVID-19 in China. Kidney Int. 2020;98(1):219–27.
18. Huang C, Wang Y, Li X, et al. Clinical features of patients infected with 2019 novel coronavirus in Wuhan, China. Lancet (London). 2020;395(10223):497–506.

19. Yang W, Sirajuddin A, Zhang X, et al. The role of imaging in 2019 novel coronavirus pneumonia (COVID-19). Eur Radiol. 2020;30(9):4874–82.
20. Ooi GC, Daqing M. SARS: radiological features. Respirology (Carlton, Vic). 2003;8(Suppl 1):S15–9.
21. Das KM, Lee EY, Langer RD, Larsson SG. Middle east respiratory syndrome coronavirus: what does a radiologist need to know? AJR Am J Roentgenol. 2016;206(6):1193–201.
22. Chung M, Bernheim A, Mei X, et al. CT imaging features of 2019 novel coronavirus (2019-nCoV). Radiology. 2020;295(1):202–7.
23. Zhou L, Li Z, Zhou J, et al. A rapid, accurate and machine-agnostic segmentation and quantification method for CT-based COVID-19 diagnosis. IEEE Trans Med Imaging. 2020;39(8):2638–52.
24. Wu Z, McGoogan JM. Characteristics of and important lessons from the coronavirus disease 2019 (COVID-19) outbreak in China: summary of a report of 72 314 cases from the Chinese Center for Disease Control and Prevention. JAMA. 2020;323(13):1239–42.
25. Wang X, Guo X, Xin Q, et al. Neutralizing antibodies responses to SARS-CoV-2 in COVID-19 inpatients and convalescent patients. Clin Infect Dis. 2020;
26. Mair-Jenkins J, Saavedra-Campos M, Baillie JK, et al. The effectiveness of convalescent plasma and hyperimmune immunoglobulin for the treatment of severe acute respiratory infections of viral etiology: a systematic review and exploratory meta-analysis. J Infect Dis. 2015;211(1):80–90.
27. Huang K, Zhang P, Zhang Z, Youn JY, Zhang H, Cai HL. Traditional Chinese Medicine (TCM) in the treatment of viral infections: Efficacies and mechanisms. Pharmacol Ther. 2021:107843.

2 Common CT Features of COVID-19 Pneumonia

Chengcheng Yu, Wanhua Guan, Shuijiang Cai, and Fei Shan

2.1 Introduction

Since the outbreak of coronavirus disease (COVID-19) pneumonia in January 2020, collections of imaging features from COVID-19 patients have been documented. Diagnosis of COVID-19 pneumonia is usually made by a combination of epidemiology of close contact history, clinical symptoms, and imaging features. In this chapter, we described the typical features of computed tomography (CT) imaging from COVID-19 pneumonia, and we hope they can be helpful in improving the diagnostic accuracy.

1. Ground-glass opacity. Ground-glass density was the most common feature of COVID-19 pneumonia which can be presented as single, multiple nodular, or patchy shadows on chest CT. Besides, the unclear boundary and thickened blood vessels can be seen [1]. Most lesions are mainly distributed in the subpleural area and/or the periphery of both lung fields. The reasons for above features may be the thickening of the alveolar interval due to infiltration of inflammatory cells, alveolar collapse, and the increase of local capillary blood volume. At this time, the patients were in the early course of disease, and the symptoms of patients were mostly mild [2]. When the density of lung lesions increased, it indicated that the course of disease was at an advanced stage, the alveolar exudation increased more than before, and some lesions merged with each other.
2. Consolidation. Consolidation refers to the replacement of air in the alveoli by pathological fluids, cells, or tissues, presented as the increase of pulmonary parenchymal density and multifocal, patchy, or segmental consolidation shadows distributed in subpleural areas or along bronchovascular bundles [3]. "Air bronchial sign" can be seen in some lesions. The appearance of consolidation indicated the progression of COVID-19 pneumonia.
3. Interstitial changes. Thickening of the lobular interstitia, interlobular interstitia, and subpleural interstitium can be seen in both lungs, which manifested as reticular or linear opacities in the background of ground-glass opacities on chest CT. The appearance of these features may be associated with interstitial lymphocyte infiltration [4]; "crazy-paving sign" and "honeycomb-like" shadow can be seen in few patients.
4. Pleura thickening. The thickening of the pleura adjacent to the lesion was commonly observed.
5. Pleural effusion and lymphadenopathy occurred rarely.

2.2 Ground-Glass Opacity

At the early stage of COVID-19 pneumonia, CT scans show ground-glass opacity mainly distributing in the periphery of lung field or around the bronchial vascular bundle with unclear boundary, which implies inflammatory exudation in alveolar cavity and alveolar septum in pathological. The CT findings show nodule (Fig. 2.1a, b), patchy shadows (Fig. 2.1c–f). With the progression of disease, the focal lesion may develop into consolidation (Fig. 2.1g, h).

2.3 Consolidation

Consolidation refers to the alveolar air being replaced by pathological fluids, cells, or tissues, manifested by an increase in pulmonary parenchymal density that obscures the margins of underlying vessels and airway walls. Multifocal, patchy, or segmental consolidation are mainly distributed in subpleural areas or along bronchovascular bundles.

Air bronchogram is a pattern of air-filled (tree branch-shape low-attenuation) bronchi on a background of pulmonary consolidation (Fig. 2.2a, b).

C. Yu (✉) · W. Guan · S. Cai
Guangzhou Eighth People's Hospital, Guangzhou Medical University, Guangzhou, China

F. Shan
Shanghai Public Health Clinical Center, Fudan University, Shanghai, China

J. Liu et al. (eds.), *Atlas of Chest Imaging in COVID-19 Patients*, https://doi.org/10.1007/978-981-16-1082-0_2

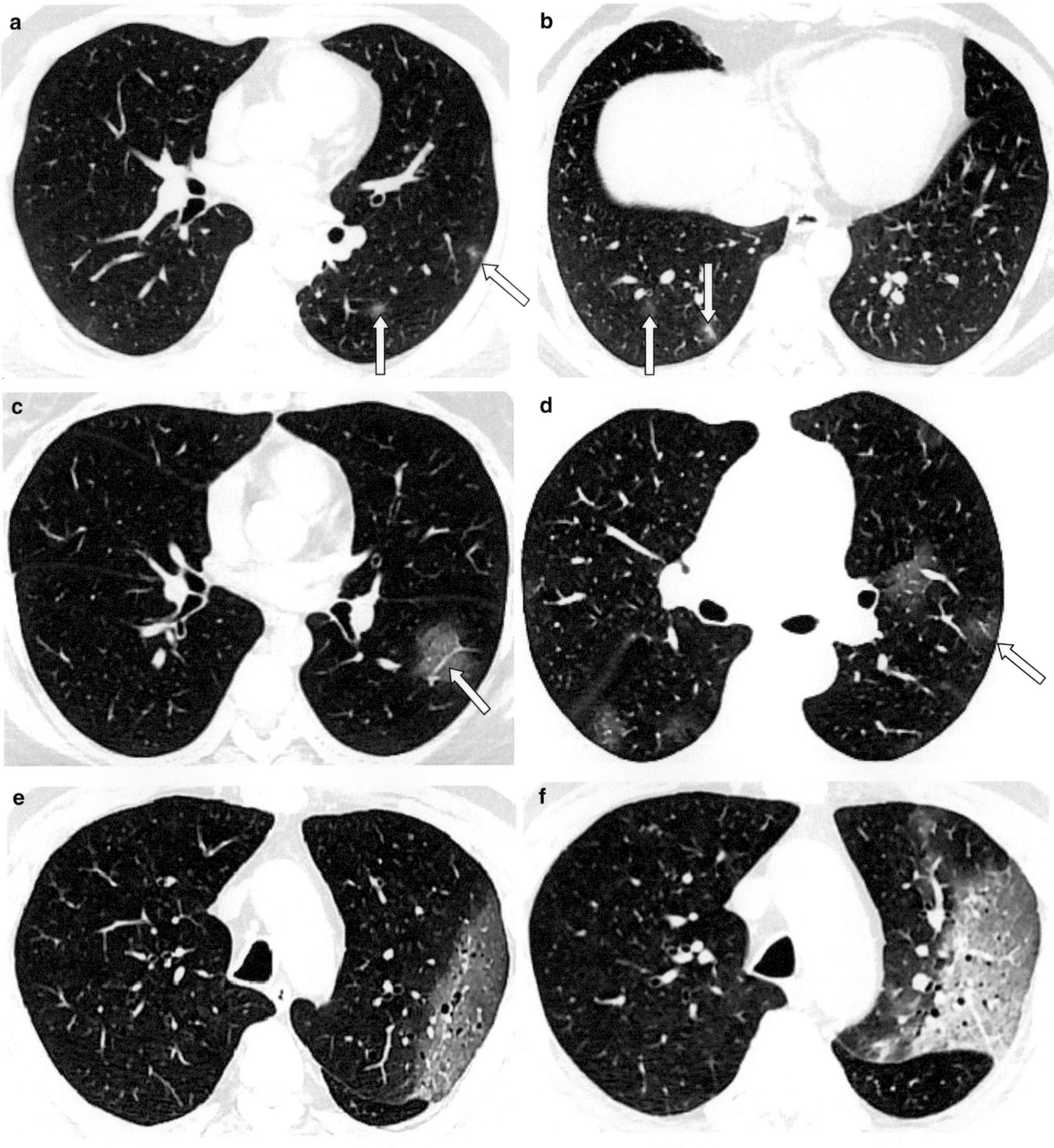

Fig. 2.1 (**a**) A 33-year-old male patient. CT scan shows two ground-glass nodules in the left lower lobe, with unclear boundary. (**b**) A 26-year-old male patient. CT scan shows two ground-glass nodules in the right lower lobe, with unclear boundary. (**c**) A 32-year-old female patient. CT scan shows ground-glass opacity in the left lower lobe, with thickened vascular shadow (empty arrow). (**d**) A 55-year-old female patient. CT scan shows multiple ground-glass opacities in bilateral lungs, with thickened vascular shadow (empty arrow). (**e**) A 63-year-old male patient. CT scan shows patchy ground-glass opacity in the left upper lobe, with unclear boundary and bronchiectasis. (**f**) Follow-up CT scans after 3 days; the lung involvement and density of lesion increased, with larger patchy ground-glass opacity and focal consolidation. (**g**, **h**) A 65-year-old male patient. CT scans show diffuse ground-glass opacity in both lungs, with focal consolidation

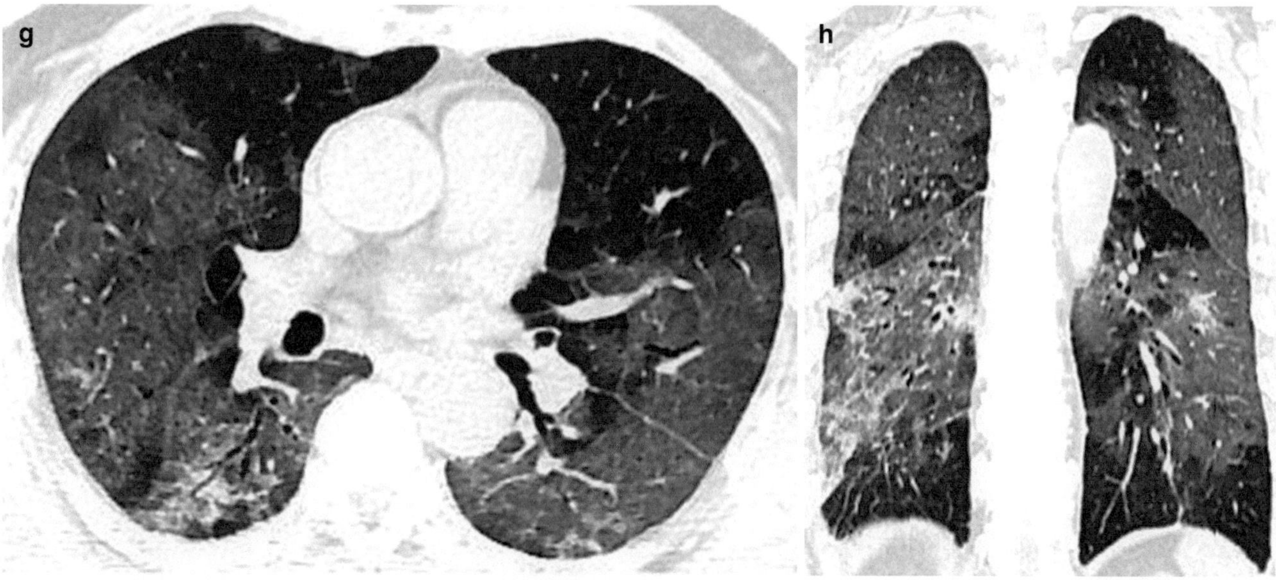

Fig. 2.1 (continued)

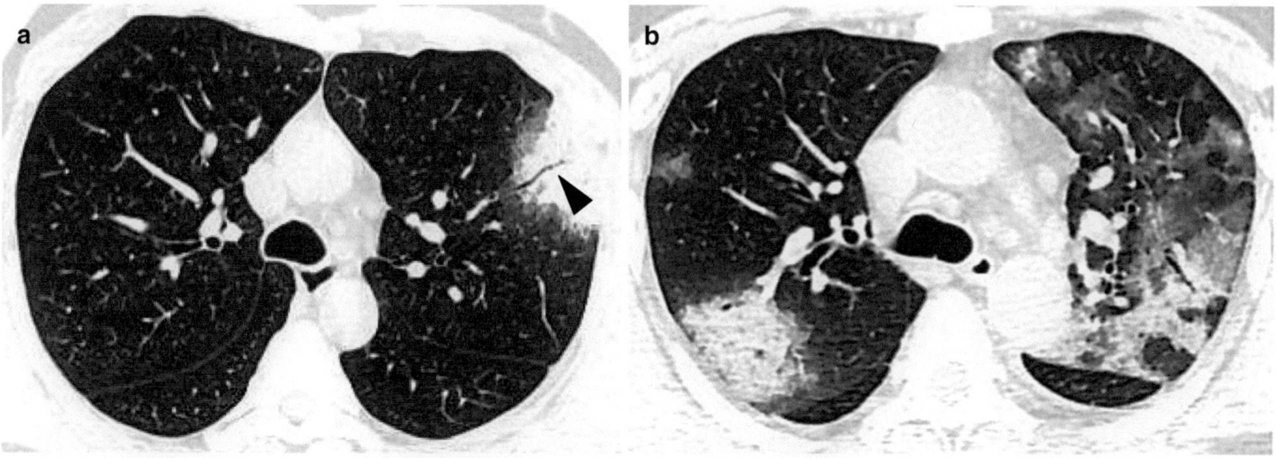

Fig. 2.2 (**a**) A 39-year-old male patient. CT scan shows patchy consolidation in the left upper lobe, with "air bronchogram" sign inside (black arrow). (**b**) A 43-year-old male patient. CT scan shows multiple ground-glass opacities and consolidation in bilateral lungs

2.4 Interstitial Changes

1. Interlobular Septa and Lobular Interstitium Thickening

Thickened interlobular septa can delineate the edge of the lung lobule; when it is located on the periphery of the lung, it often extends to the surface of the pleura, perpendicular to the pleural surface (Fig. 2.3a, b). Its appearance often suggests interstitial exudation, cell infiltration, or fibrosis.

Crazy-paving sign demonstrates thickened interlobular septa and intralobular lines as a slight reticular pattern with superimposition on a ground-glass opacity background, resembling irregular paving stone (Fig. 2.3c, d).

Honeycomb-like shadow refers to a cystic translucent shadow located in the center of the leaflet, demonstrating "honeycomb" change, on the background of ground glass-like density shadow accompanied by thickened interlobular septal. On the formation basis, on the basis of "paving stone sign," the change of emphysema appears in the lobule center; or on the basis of emphysema of the lobe center, a "paving stone sign" appears (Fig. 2.3e, f).

2. Subpleural Curvilinear Line

Subpleural curvilinear line is defined as a thin curvilinear opacity, lying less than 1 cm from and parallel to the pleu-

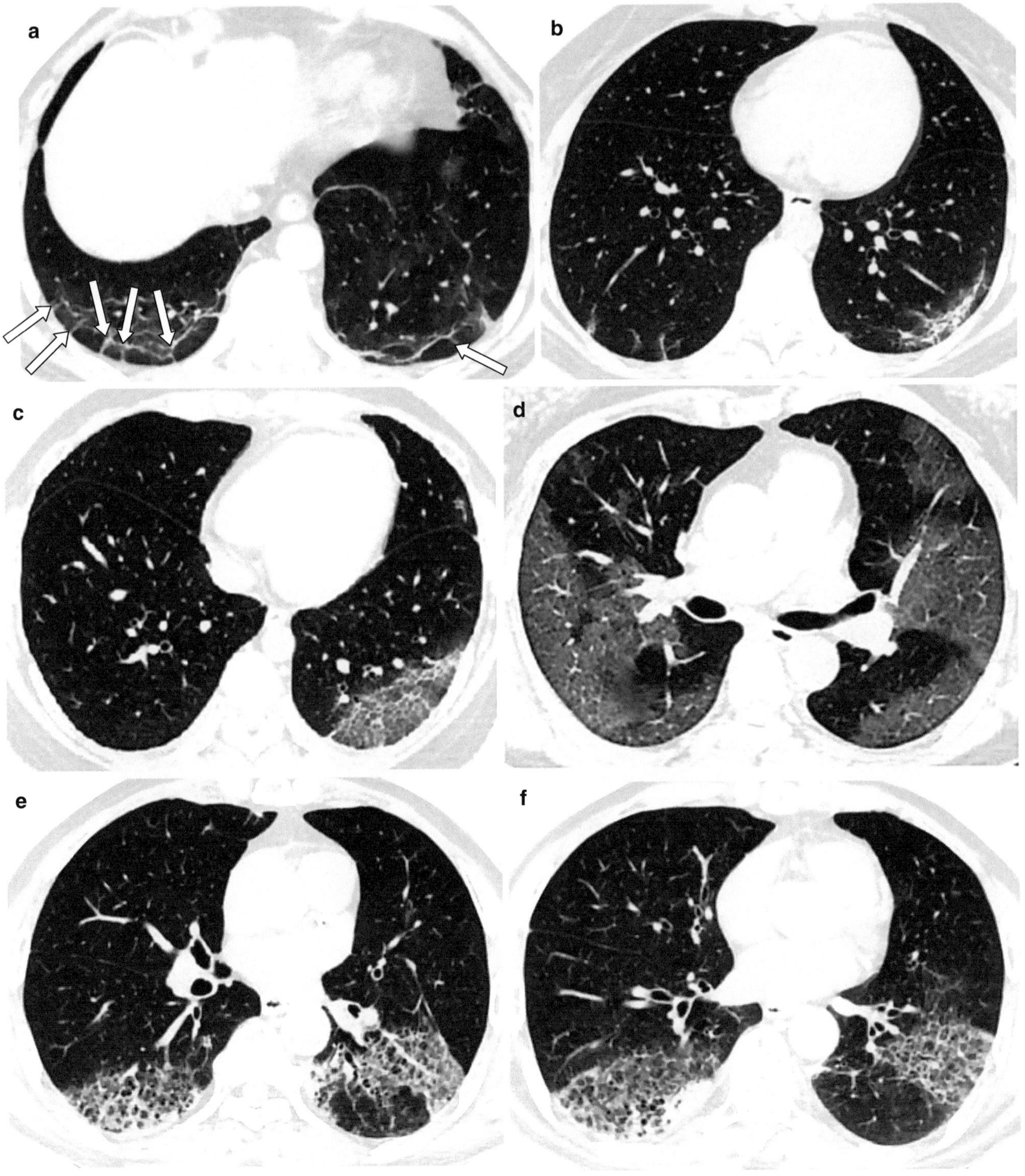

Fig. 2.3 (**a**) A 54-year-old male patient. CT scan shows multiple ground-glass opacities and stripe shadows in the bilateral lower lobes, and the thickened interlobular septa can be seen, which is obviously in the right lower lobe, perpendicular to the pleura (empty arrow). (**b**) A 55-year-old female patient. An arc-shaped band of increased density was seen in the lower lobe of the left lung adjacent to the dorsal pleura. The interlobular septum in the lesion of the right lower lobe is thickened and perpendicular to the pleura. (**c**) A 32-year-old female patient. CT scan shows ground-glass opacity in the left lower lobe, presenting reticular pattern as "crazy-paving sign." (**d**) A 55-year-old female patient. CT scan shows extensive ground-glass opacities in bilateral lungs, with peripheral and subpleural distribution; part of the lesion presents reticular pattern and "crazy-paving sign." (**e**, **f**) A 62-year-old male patient. CT scans show multiple patchy ground-glass opacities in the lower lobes of both lungs. Increased grid-like density was observed in the lesion, with mixed small saccular lucent areas in it, resembling a "honeycomb"-like change. (**g**–**j**) A 37-year-old male patient. (**g**) CT scan shows subpleural curvilinear line in the bilateral lower lobes (empty arrow). The lesion gradually disappeared after 4 and 7 days of treatment (**h**)–(**j**)

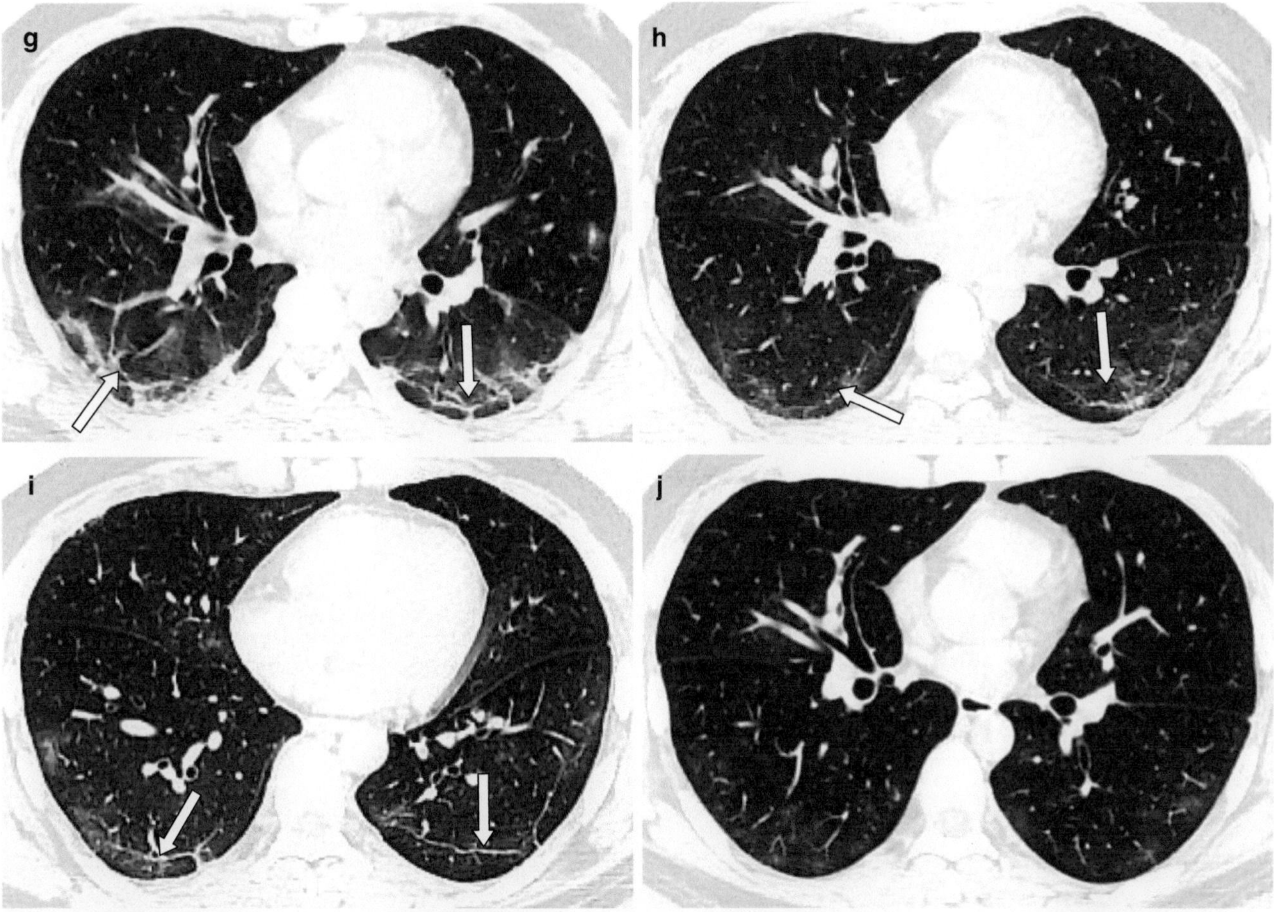

Fig. 2.3 (continued)

ral surface, most commonly seen in the posterior of lower lobes, suggesting alveolar collapse or fibrosis. With effective treatment, the subpleural curvilinear line of early stage could disappear gradually (Fig. 2.3g–j).

2.5 Pleural Thickening

The thickening of the pleura is the dense shadow of the band-like soft tissue along the chest wall, the thickness is uneven, the surface is not smooth, and the interface with the lung is mostly visible with small adhesions. It is more common in COVID-19 pneumonia (Fig. 2.4a, b).

2.6 Pleural Effusion

Pleural effusion is uncommon in patients with COVID-19 pneumonia; some patients may have little pleural effusion and pleural thickening (Fig. 2.5a, b).

2.7 Halo Sign

The "halo sign" can be found in some nodules, surrounded by ground-glass opacity, suggesting inflammatory exudation and edema of the alveolar compartment (Fig. 2.6a, b).

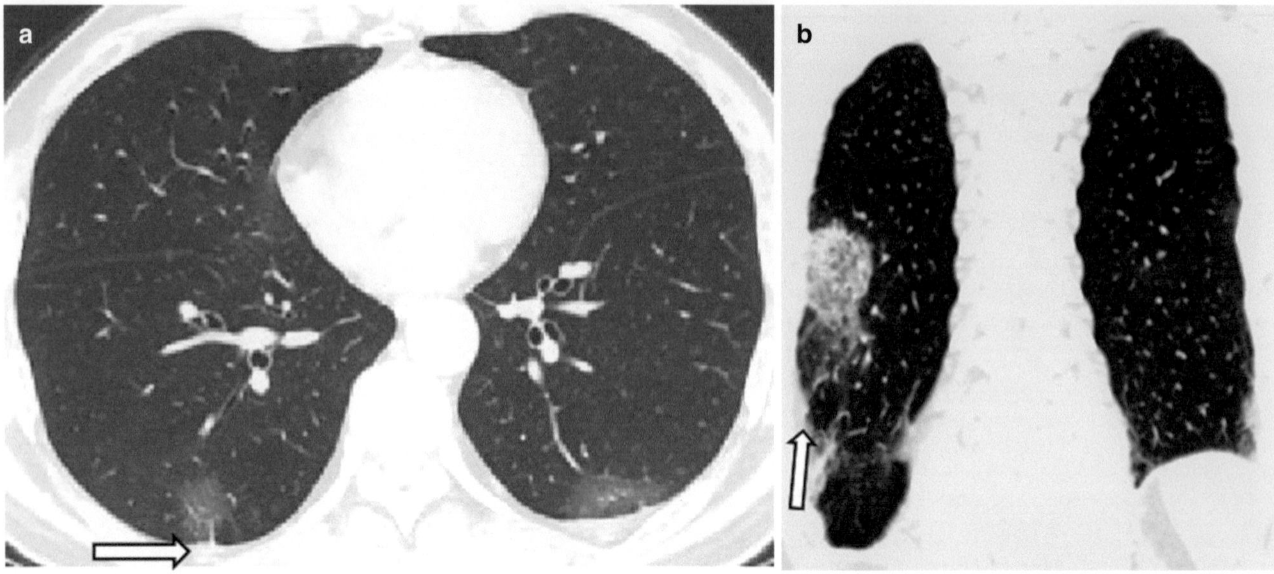

Fig. 2.4 (**a**) A 56-year-old male patient. CT scan shows ground-glass opacity in both lungs, with unclear boundary. Some lesions were pulled near the pleura. The stripe shadow can be seen (empty arrow). The lesions are mainly distributed in the pleura. (**b**) A 56-year-old male patient. CT scan shows ground-glass opacities in both lungs with unclear boundary. The thickened interlobular septum of the lesion and the "paving stone sign" can be seen. Some lesions were adjacent to pleural traction (empty arrow)

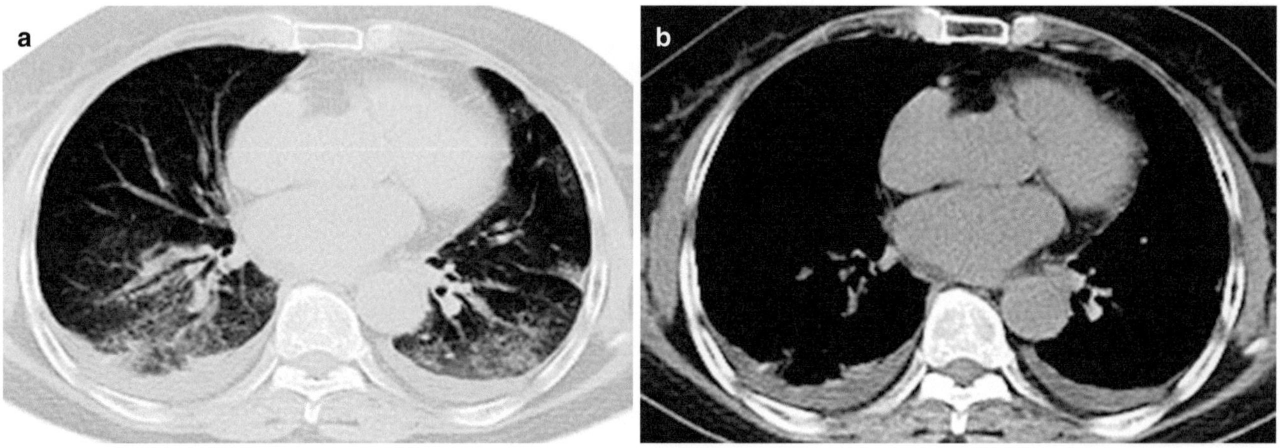

Fig. 2.5 (**a**, **b**) A 71-year-old female patient. CT scans show multiple ground-glass opacities and reticular pattern, accompanied by pleural effusions

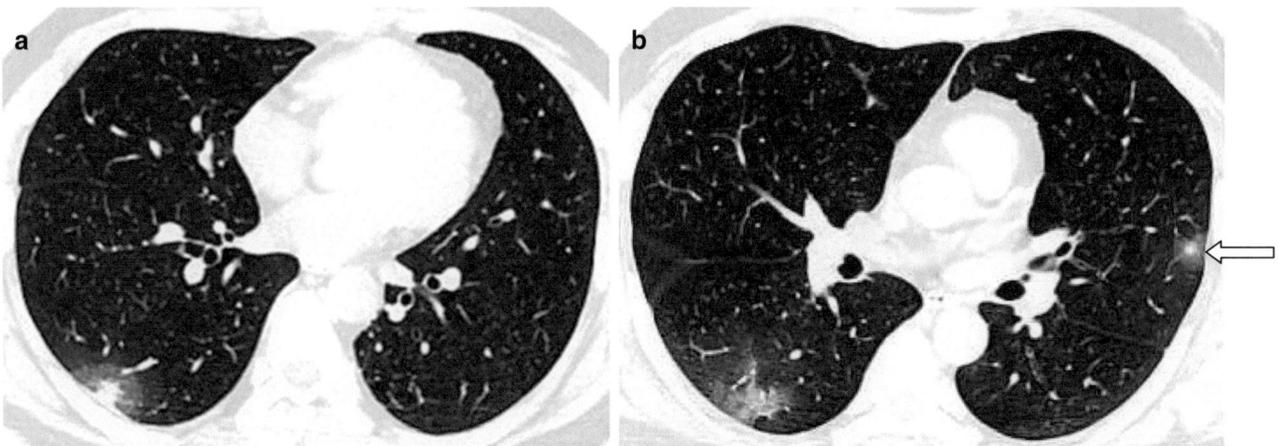

Fig. 2.6 (**a**) A 33-year-old male patient. CT scan shows a nodule surrounded by ground-glass opacity in the right lower lobe, which manifests as "halo sign." (**b**) A 43-year-old male patient. CT scan shows multiple ground-glass opacities in bilateral lungs. A nodule of the left upper lobe is surrounded by ground-glass opacity and presents as "halo sign" (empty arrow)

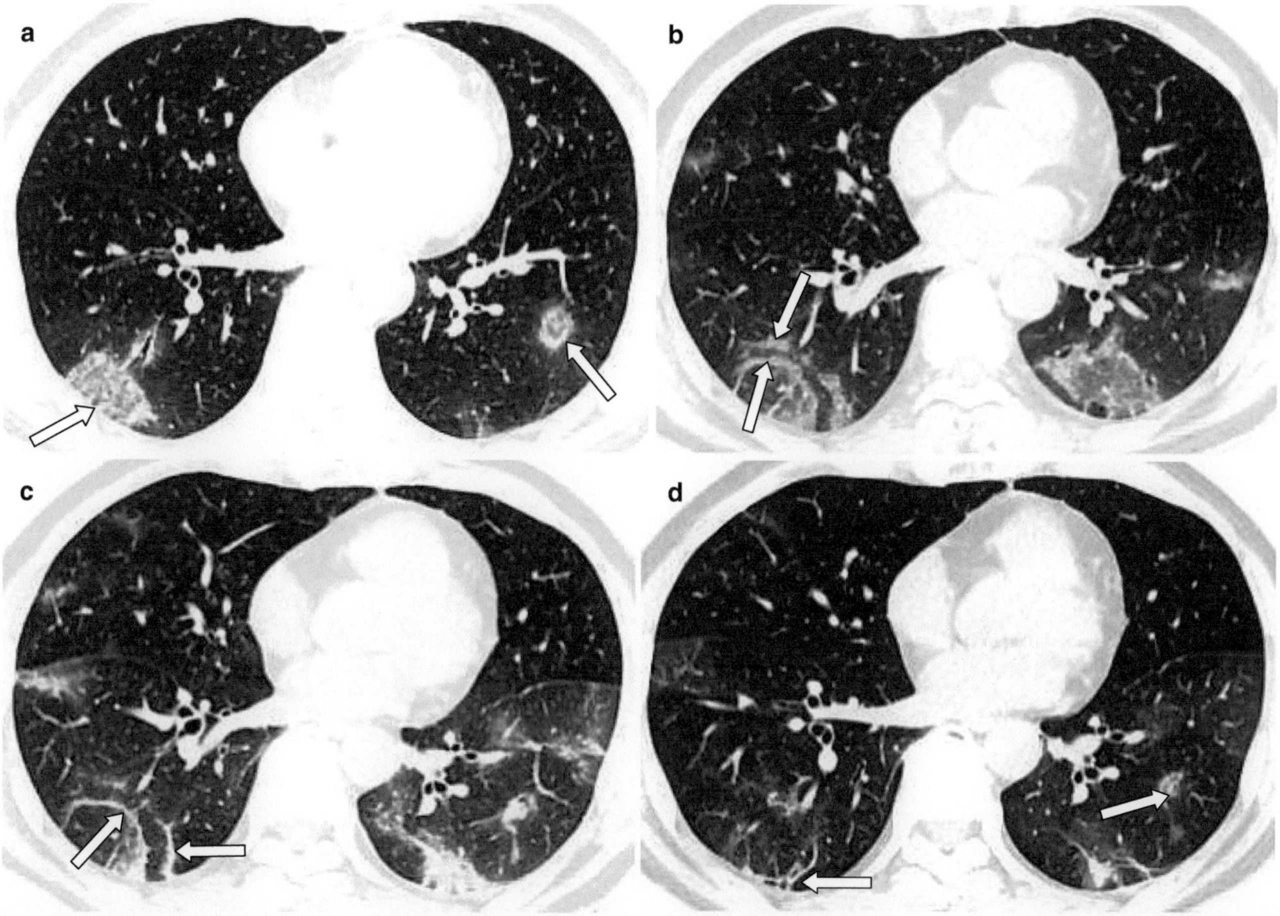

Fig. 2.7 (**a–d**) A 53-year-old male patient. CT scans show reversed halo signs in bilateral lower lobes (empty arrows) and focal rounded ground-glass opacity with ring-like consolidation margin (**a**). Follow-up CT scans on days 7, 13, and 18 of admission (**b–d**) show the decreased interior density of reversed halo sign in the right lower lobe. After effective treatment, the lesions shrunk and disappeared gradually.

2.8 Reversed Halo Sign

Also called "atoll sign," it is defined as a focal rounded ground-glass opacity surrounded by annular or crescent-shaped consolidation. After effective treatment, the "reversed halo sign" could disappear gradually (Fig. 2.7a–d).

References

1. Xu X, Yu C, Qu J, et al. Imaging and clinical features of patients with 2019 novel coronavirus SARS-CoV-2. Eur J Nucl Med Mol Imaging. 2020;47(5):1275–80. https://doi.org/10.1007/s00259-020-04735-9.
2. Chung M, Bernheim A, Mei X, et al. CT imaging features of 2019 novel coronavirus (2019-nCoV). Radiology. 2020;295(1):202–7. https://doi.org/10.1148/radiol.2020200230.
3. Hansell DM, Bankier AA, MacMahon H, McLoud TC, Müller NL, Remy J. Fleischner Society: glossary of terms for thoracic imaging. Radiology. 2008;246(3):697–722. https://doi.org/10.1148/radiol.2462070712.
4. Xu Z, Shi L, Wang Y, et al. Pathological findings of COVID-19 associated with acute respiratory distress syndrome [published correction appears in Lancet Respir Med. 2020 Feb 25]. Lancet Respir Med. 2020;8(4):420–2. https://doi.org/10.1016/S2213-2600(20)30076-X.

CT Features of Early COVID-19 Pneumonia (PCR-Positive)

3

Zhiping Zhang, Yan Ding, and Bihua Chen

3.1 Introduction

Coronavirus disease (COVID-19) pneumonia is caused by severe acute respiratory syndrome coronavirus 2 (SARS-CoV-2) [1, 2]. It is highly infectious and spreads through respiratory droplets, contact, and the fecal-oral route. It is characterized by acute onset and severe symptoms and is a serious threat to human health and safety. According to the latest diagnosis and treatment scheme for COVID-19 pneumonia issued by the National Health Commission of the People's Republic of China (trial version 8), the diagnosis of COVID-19 pneumonia is mainly based on epidemiologic factors, clinical manifestations, computed tomography (CT) findings, and nucleic acid detection of SARS-CoV-2.

At the early stage of COVID-19 pneumonia, most lesions are multiple and distribute in the periphery of the lung or subpleural regions, especially in the lower lobe of the lung. An investigation of initial chest CT imagings from 21 viral RNA-confirmed COVID-19 patients found that 18 of 21 (86%) patients had abnormal findings in the lung and the majority of them (16/18) had bilateral lung involvement [3]. The common CT imaging features of COVID-19 pneumonia include nodular or patchy ground-glass opacities with or without interlobular septal thickening and consolidative opacities. Besides, halo sign, vascular thickening, crazy paving pattern, or air bronchogram sign was reported [4]. On the contrary, pleural effusion, cavitation, and mediastinum and hilar lymphadenopathy in COVID-19 are not commonly detected.

The clinical role of chest CT examination should be emphasized. High-resolution CT is able to detect millimeter-size lesions and plays an important role in the early diagnosis of viral pneumonia [5], including COVID-19 pneumonia [4, 6]. The reported imaging features in COVID-19 are variable and nonspecific and have significant overlap with those of SARS and MERS. In this chapter, we aim to describe the early chest CT manifestations of COVID-19 to provide important reference values for early diagnosis, early prevention, and early treatment of COVID-19 pneumonia.

Z. Zhang (✉) · Y. Ding · B. Chen
Guangzhou Eighth People's Hospital, Guangzhou Medical University, Guangzhou, China

3.2 **Case 1** (Fig. 3.1a–l)

A 30-year-old male patient presented with fever for 3 days. The body temperature peaked at 38 °C, accompanied by chills, cough, and throat discomfort, without expectoration. He was exposed in the epidemic area. At admission, the body temperature was 36 °C, the pulse rate was 80 beats per minute, the respiratory rate was 18 breaths per minute, and the blood oxygen saturation was 98.2%. Blood routine examination: white-cell count, lymphocyte count, and C-reactive protein were 5.26×10^9/L, 1.64×10^9/L, and <10 mg/L, respectively.

Chest CT scan taken 4 days after symptom onset showed multiple patchy ground-glass opacities in the lower lobe of both lungs with blurred edge and "halo sign," mainly located in the peripheral area of the bilateral lung (Fig. 3.1a–l, white arrow). A ground-glass nodule was found in the posterior basal segment of the left lower lobe (Fig. 3.1i, j, black arrowhead).

3.3 **Case 2** (Fig. 3.2a–l)

A 29-year-old male patient presented with pharyngeal discomfort, cough, and expectoration for 3 days. He was exposed in the epidemic area. At admission, his body temperature was 37.8 °C, the pulse rate was 97 beats per minute, the respiratory rate was 18 breaths per minute, and the blood oxygen saturation was 96%. Blood routine examination: white-cell count, lymphocyte count, and C-reactive protein were 5.25×10^9/L, 2.64×10^9/L, and <10 mg/L, respectively.

J. Liu et al. (eds.), *Atlas of Chest Imaging in COVID-19 Patients*, https://doi.org/10.1007/978-981-16-1082-0_3

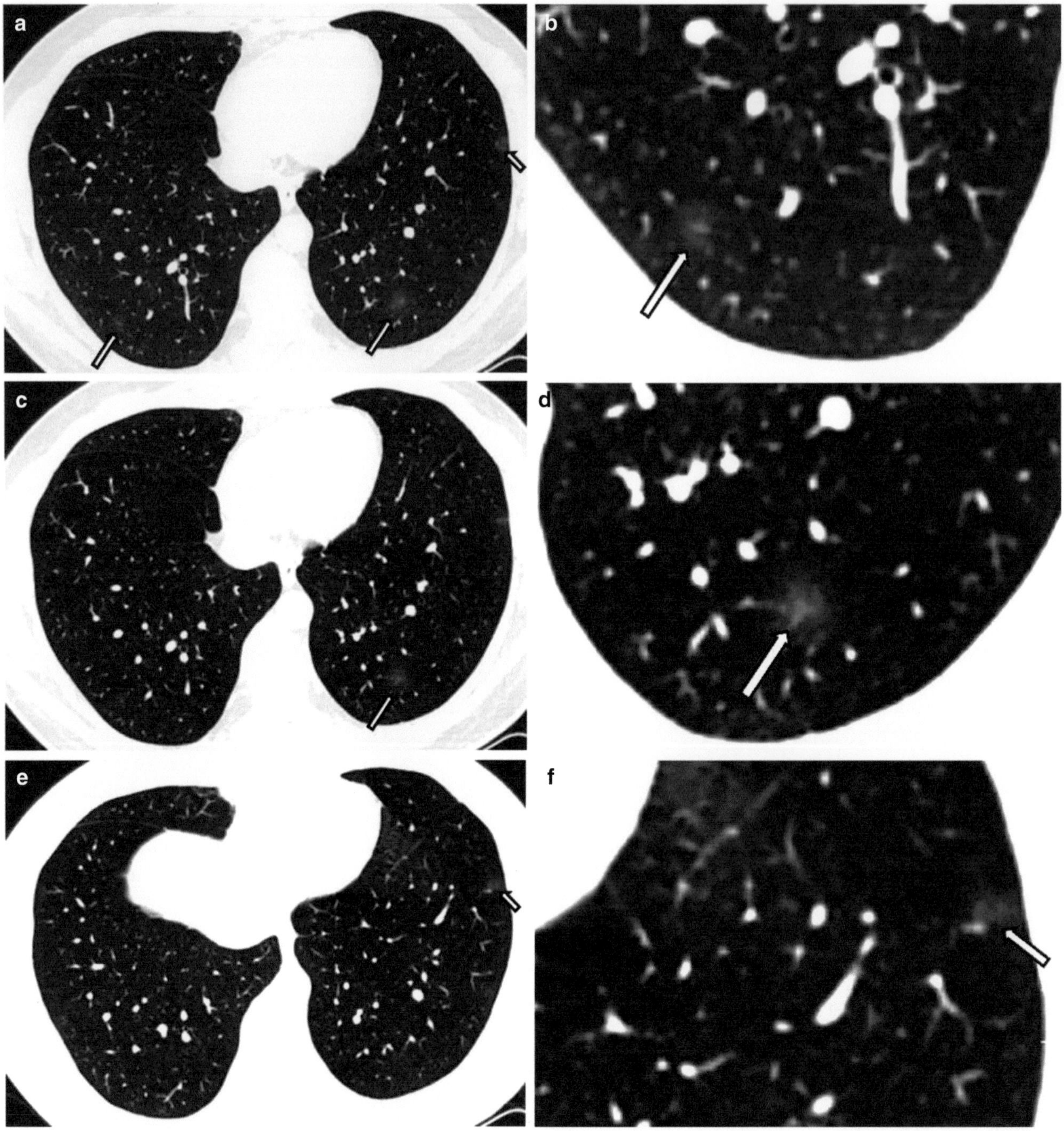

Fig. 3.1 Chest CT scan taken 4 days after symptom onset showed multiple patchy ground-glass opacities in the lower lobe of both lungs with blurred edge and "halo sign," mainly located in the peripheral area of the bilateral lung (**a**–**l**, white arrow). A ground-glass nodule was found in the posterior basal segment of the left lower lobe (**i**, **j**, black arrowhead)

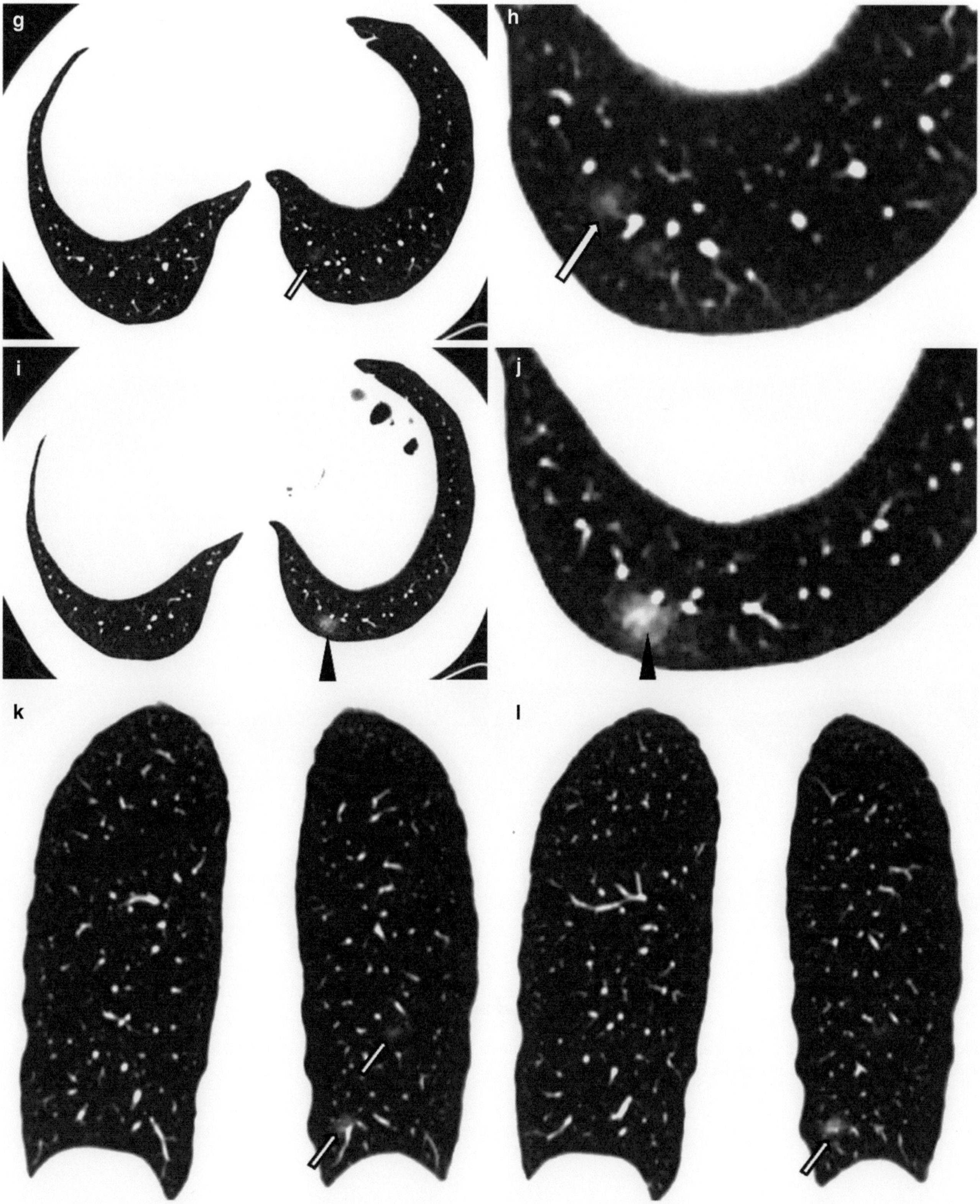

Fig. 3.1 (continued)

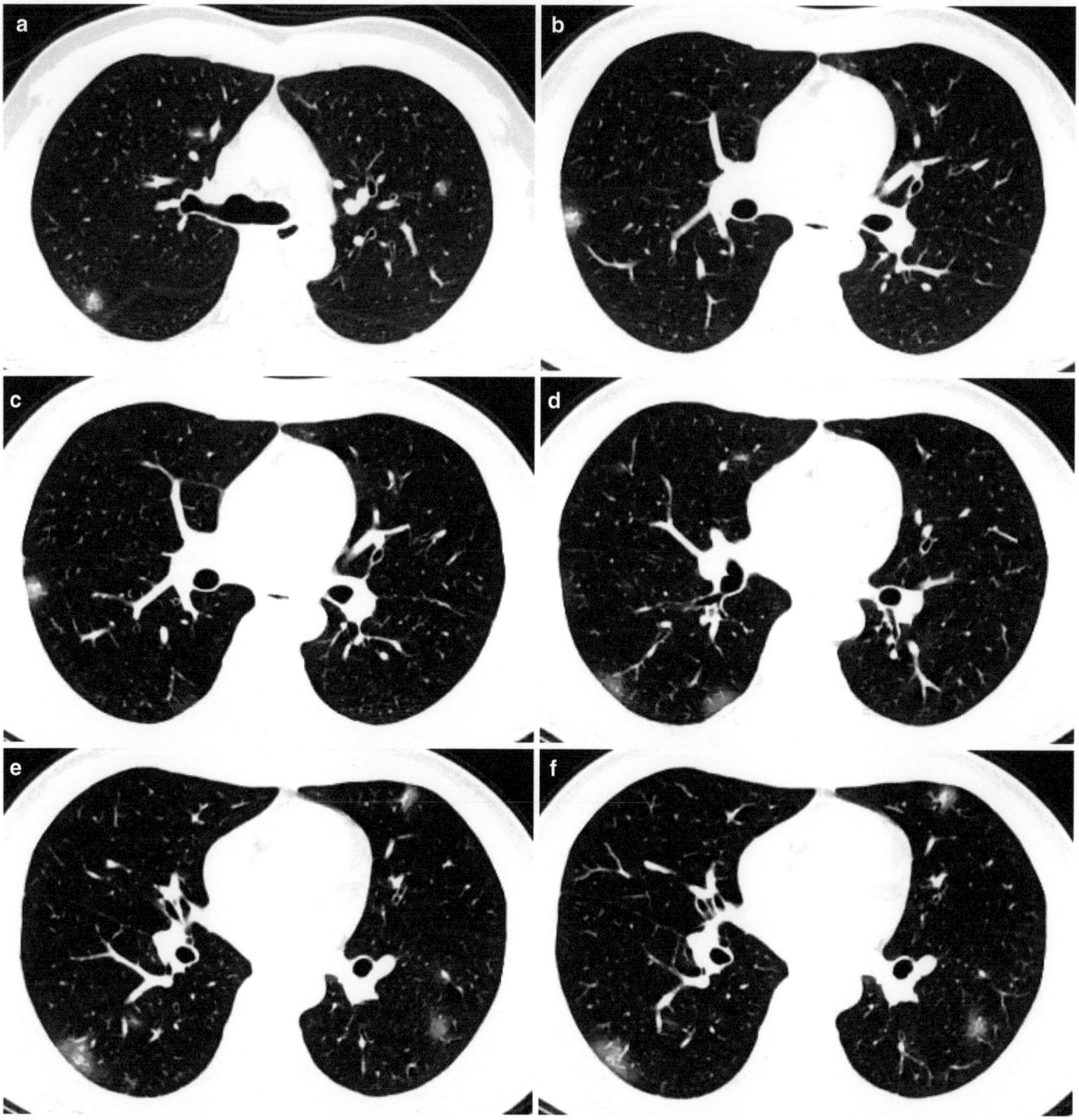

Fig. 3.2 Chest CT scan taken 4 days after symptom onset showed multiple patchy ground-glass opacities in both lungs with blurring edge, mainly distributed in the subpleural area of bilateral lower lobes (**a–l**)

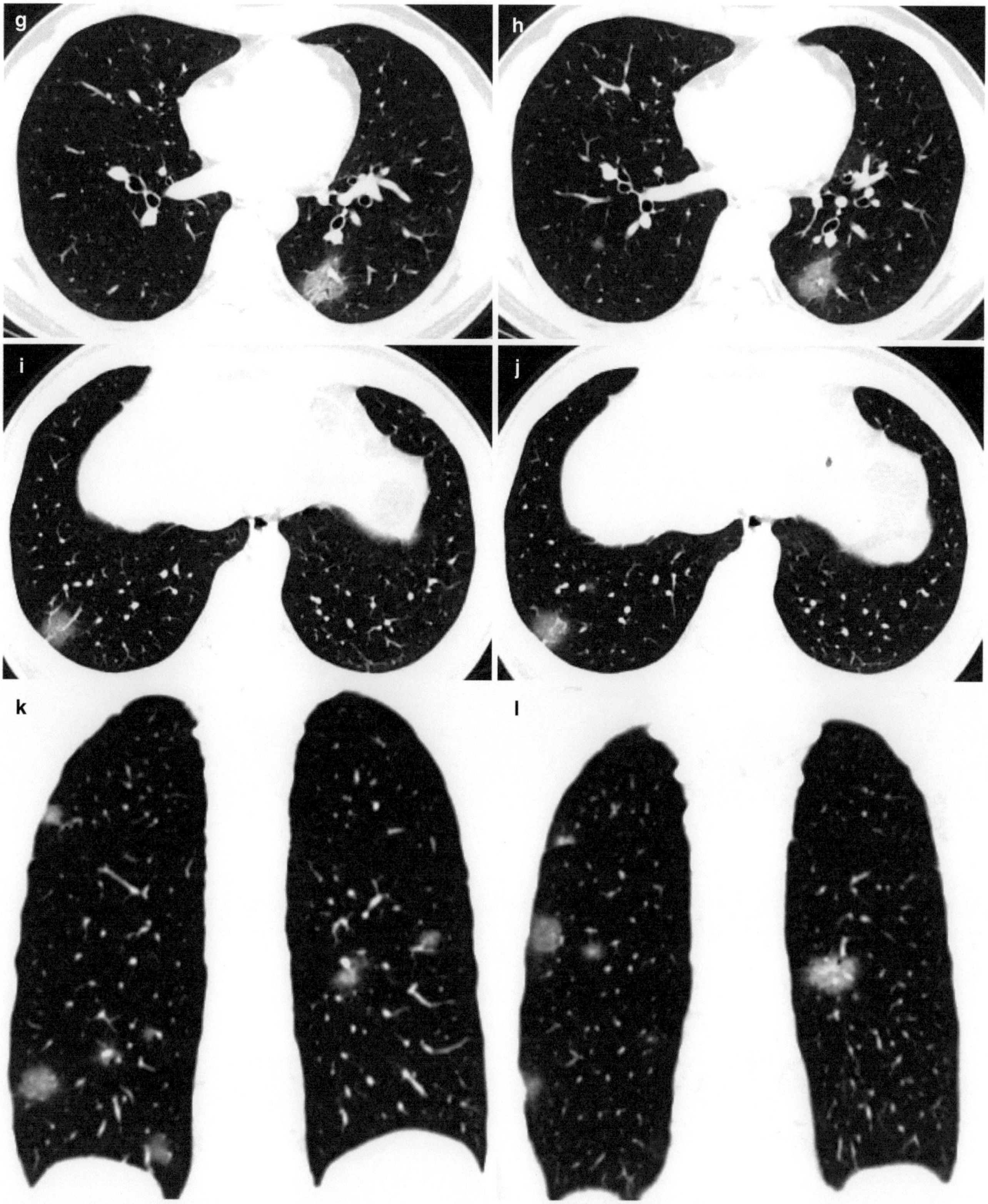

Fig. 3.2 (continued)

Chest CT scan taken 4 days after symptom onset showed multiple patchy ground-glass opacities in both lungs with blurring edge, mainly distributed in the subpleural area of bilateral lower lobes (Fig. 3.2a–l).

3.4 Case 3 (Fig. 3.3a–l)

A 54-year-old female patient presented with fever for 3 days. The body temperature peaked at 38 °C, accompanied by dry cough, and she had the epidemiological history of exposure to

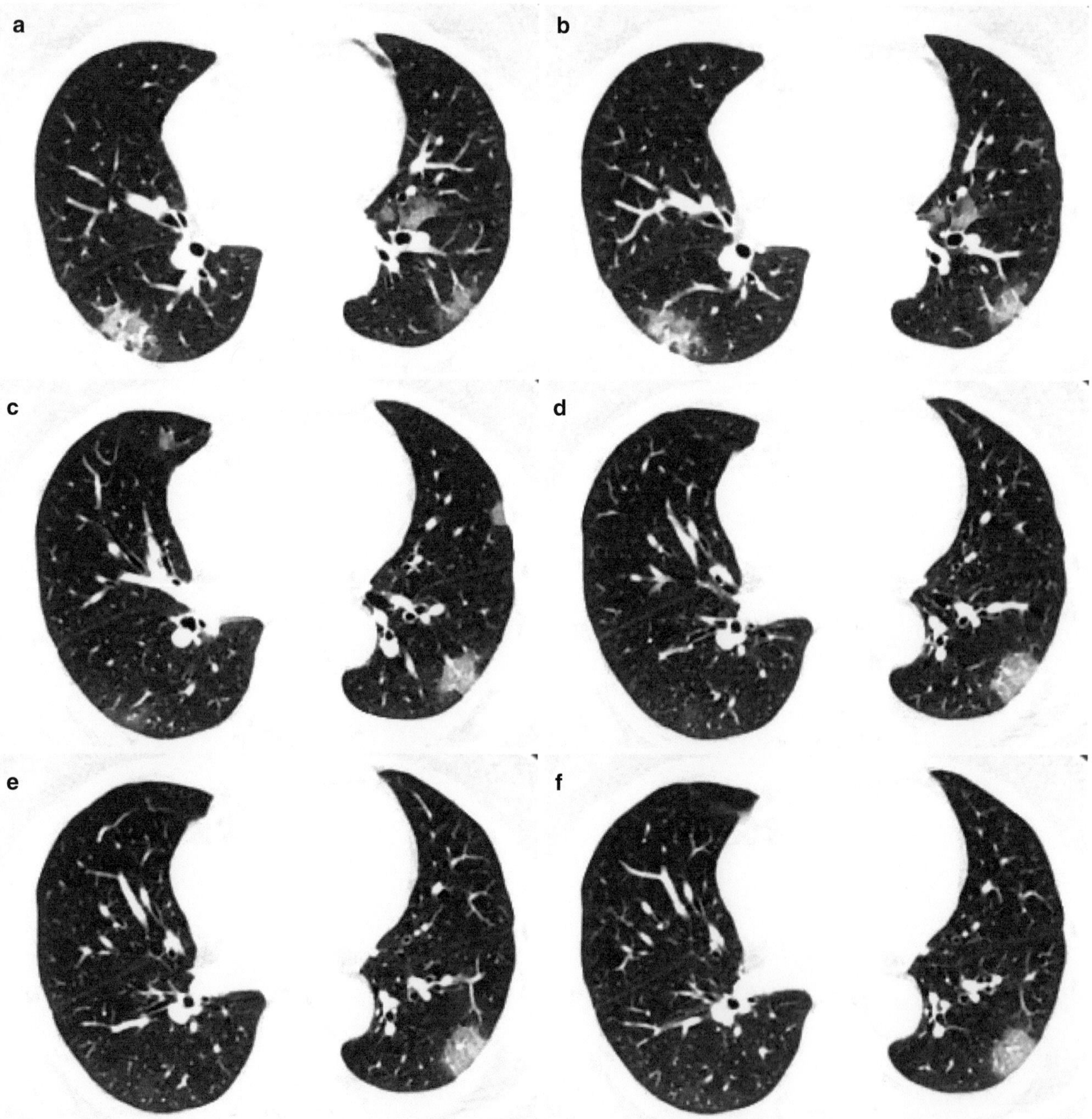

Fig. 3.3 Chest CT examination performed 5 days after symptom onset showed multiple patchy ground-glass opacities in both lungs with blurring edge and subpleural distribution in the bilateral lower lobes. HRCT demonstrated multifocal peripheral ground-glass opacities associated with intralobular septal thickening (**a**–**h**)

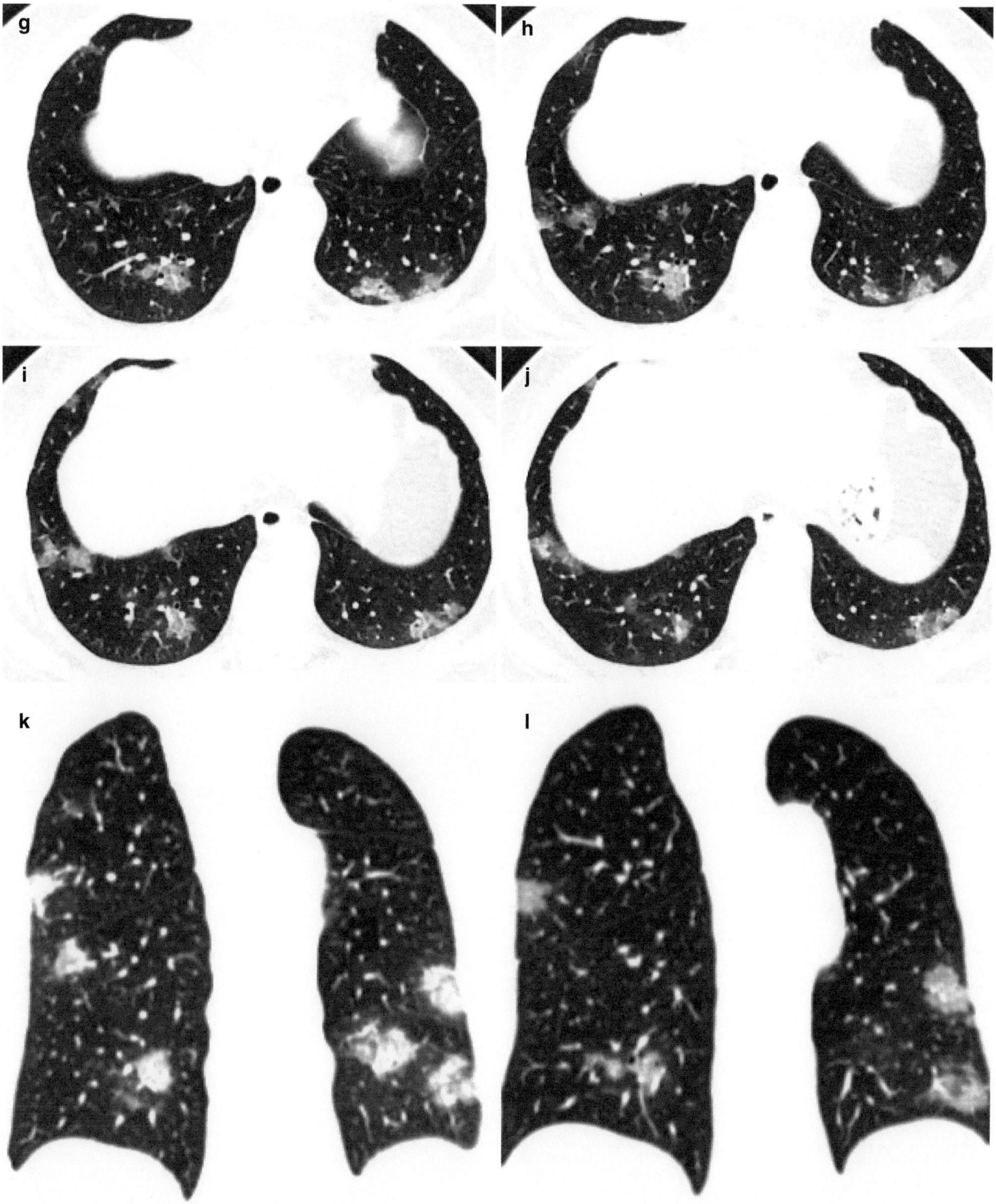

Fig. 3.3 (continued)

patients from epidemic areas. At admission, her body temperature was 37 °C, the pulse rate was 93 beats per minute, the respiratory rate was 18 breaths per minute, and the blood oxygen saturation was 96.7%. Blood routine examination: white-cell count, lymphocyte count, and C-reactive protein were 6.24×10^9/L, 2.18×10^9/L, and 25.68 mg/L, respectively.

Chest CT examination performed 5 days after symptom onset showed multiple patchy ground-glass opacities in both lungs with blurring edge and subpleural distribution in the bilateral lower lobes. High-resolution computed tomography (HRCT) demonstrated multifocal peripheral ground-glass opacities associated with intralobular septal thickening (Fig. 3.3a–h).

3.5 Case 4 (Fig. 3.4a–l)

A 45-year-old male patient presented with dry cough for 3 days without fever and chills, and he had the epidemiological history of exposure to patients from epidemic areas. At admission, the body temperature was 36.8 °C, the pulse rate was 90 beats per minute, the respiratory rate was 18 breaths

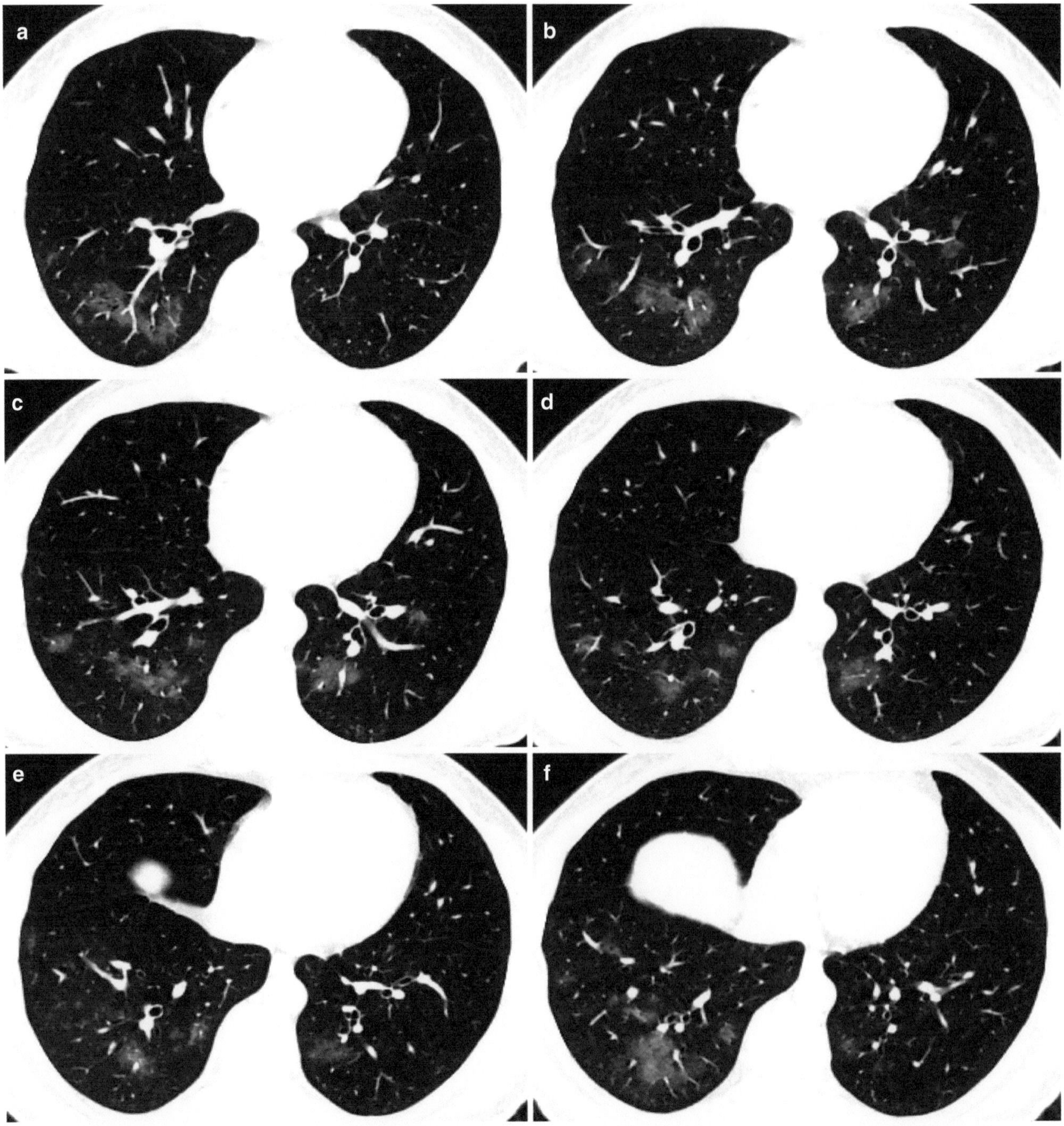

Fig. 3.4 Chest CT examination performed 3 days after symptom onset showed multiple patchy ground-glass opacities in the lower lobe of both lungs with blurring edge, and the lesions were mainly distributed along the bronchovascular bundle (**a**–**l**)

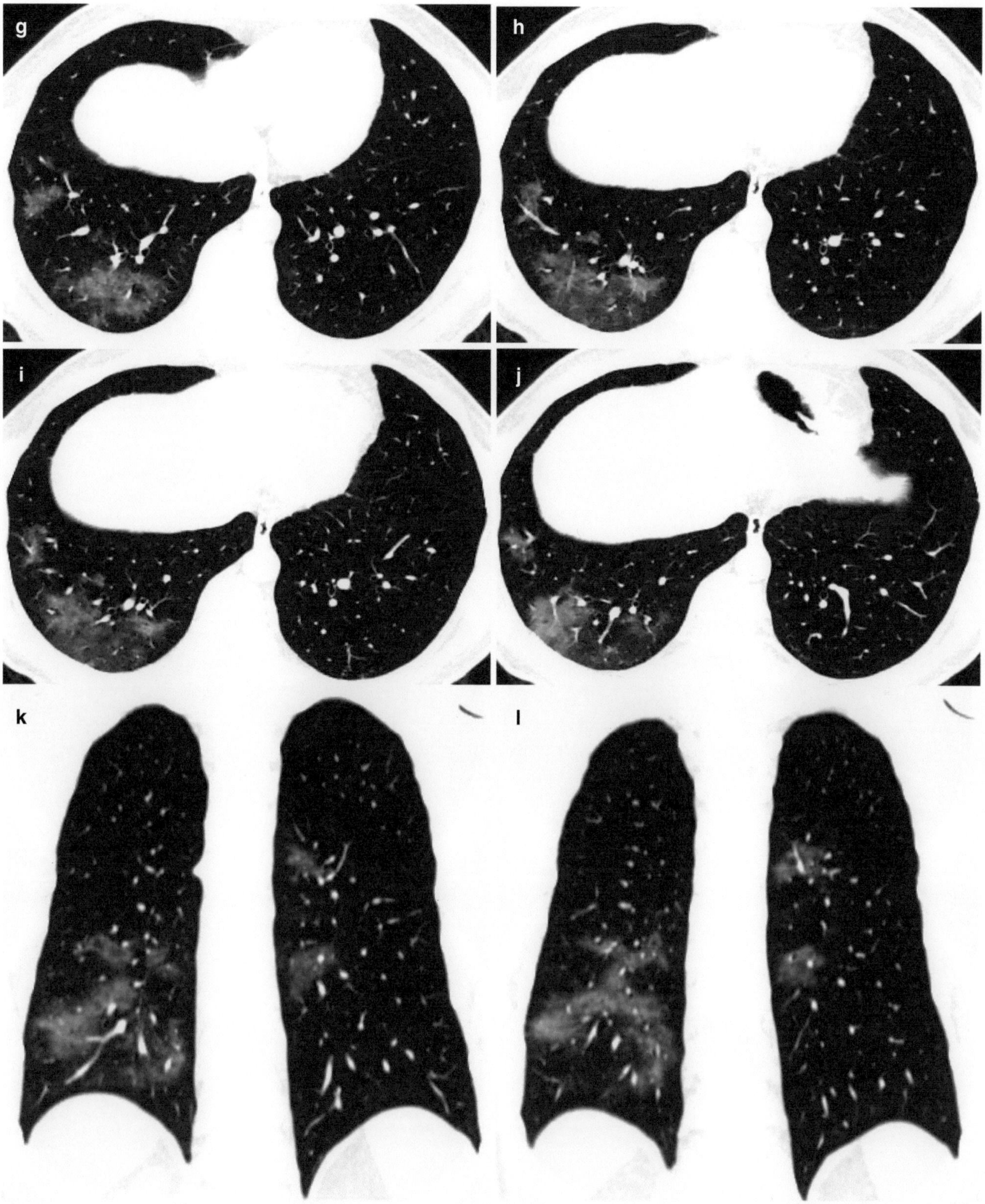

Fig. 3.4 (continued)

per minute, and the blood oxygen saturation was 97.2%. Blood routine examination: white-cell count, lymphocyte count, and C-reactive protein were 9.05×10^9/L, 2.06×10^9/L, and <10 mg/L, respectively.

Chest CT examination performed 3 days after symptom onset showed multiple patchy ground-glass opacities in the lower lobe of both lungs with blurring edge, and the lesions were mainly distributed along the bronchovascular bundle (Fig. 3.4a–l).

3.6 Case 5 (Fig. 3.5a–l)

A 32-year-old male patient presented with fever for 2 days, without chills and shivering. His body temperature peaked at 38.2 °C before admission, accompanied by fatigue and chest tightness, and he had the epidemiological history of exposure to patients from epidemic areas. At admission, the body temperature was 37.8 °C, the pulse rate was 95 beats per minute, the respiratory rate was 20 breaths per minute, and the blood oxygen saturation was 98.5%. Blood routine examination: white-cell count, lymphocyte count, and C-reactive protein were 4.87×10^9/L, 2.11×10^9/L, and <10 mg/L, respectively.

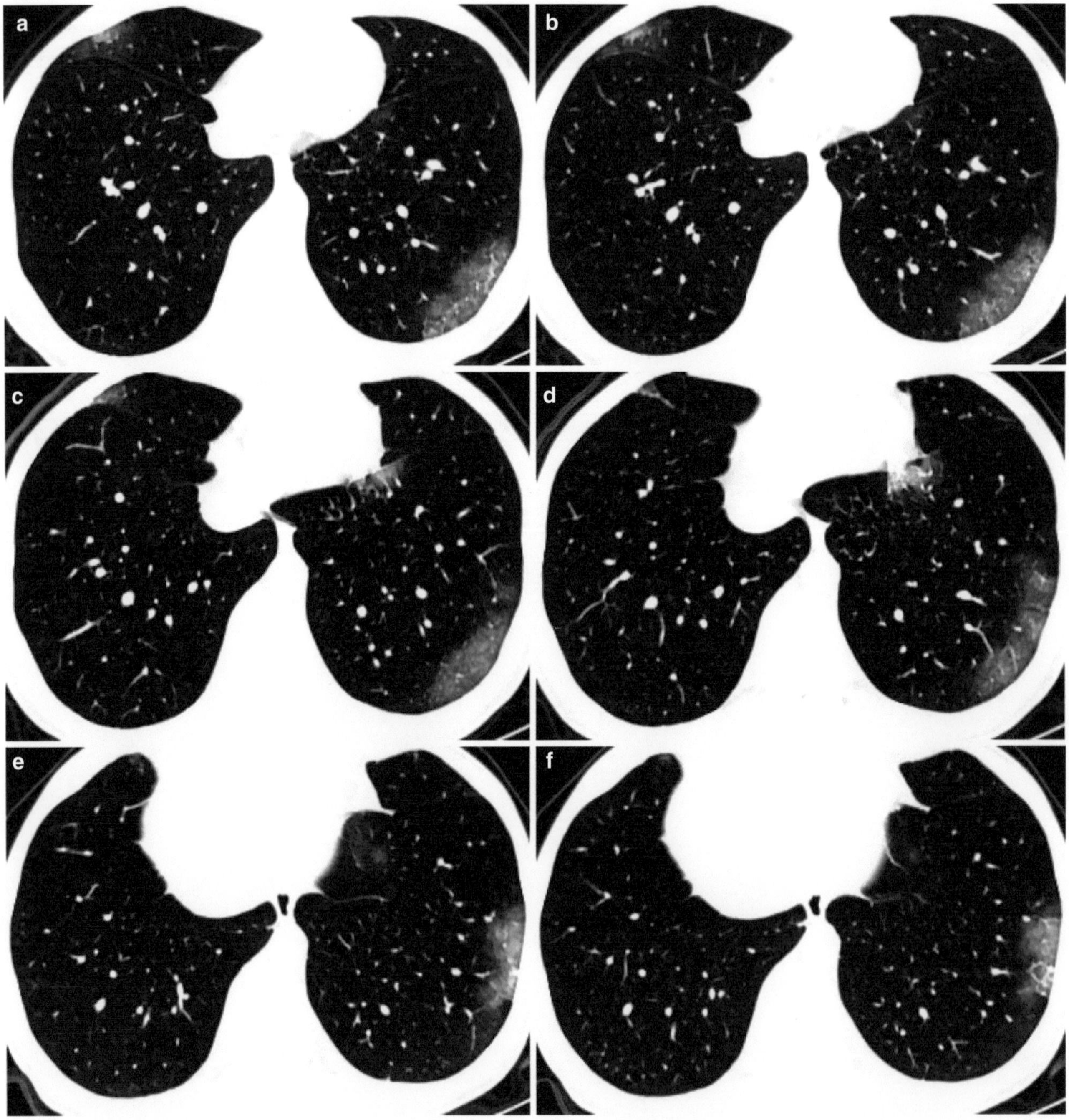

Fig. 3.5 Chest CT scan taken 3 days after symptom onset showed multiple patchy ground-glass opacities with blurring edge located in the subpleural area of the right middle lobe and the left lower lobe, especially in the left lower lobe (**a–l**). Thickened blood vessel shadows were observed in the lesions in the lateral basal segment of the left lower lobe (**e–h**), and subpleural curvilinear line appeared adjacent to the lesion in the posterior basal segment of the left lower lobe (**i**)

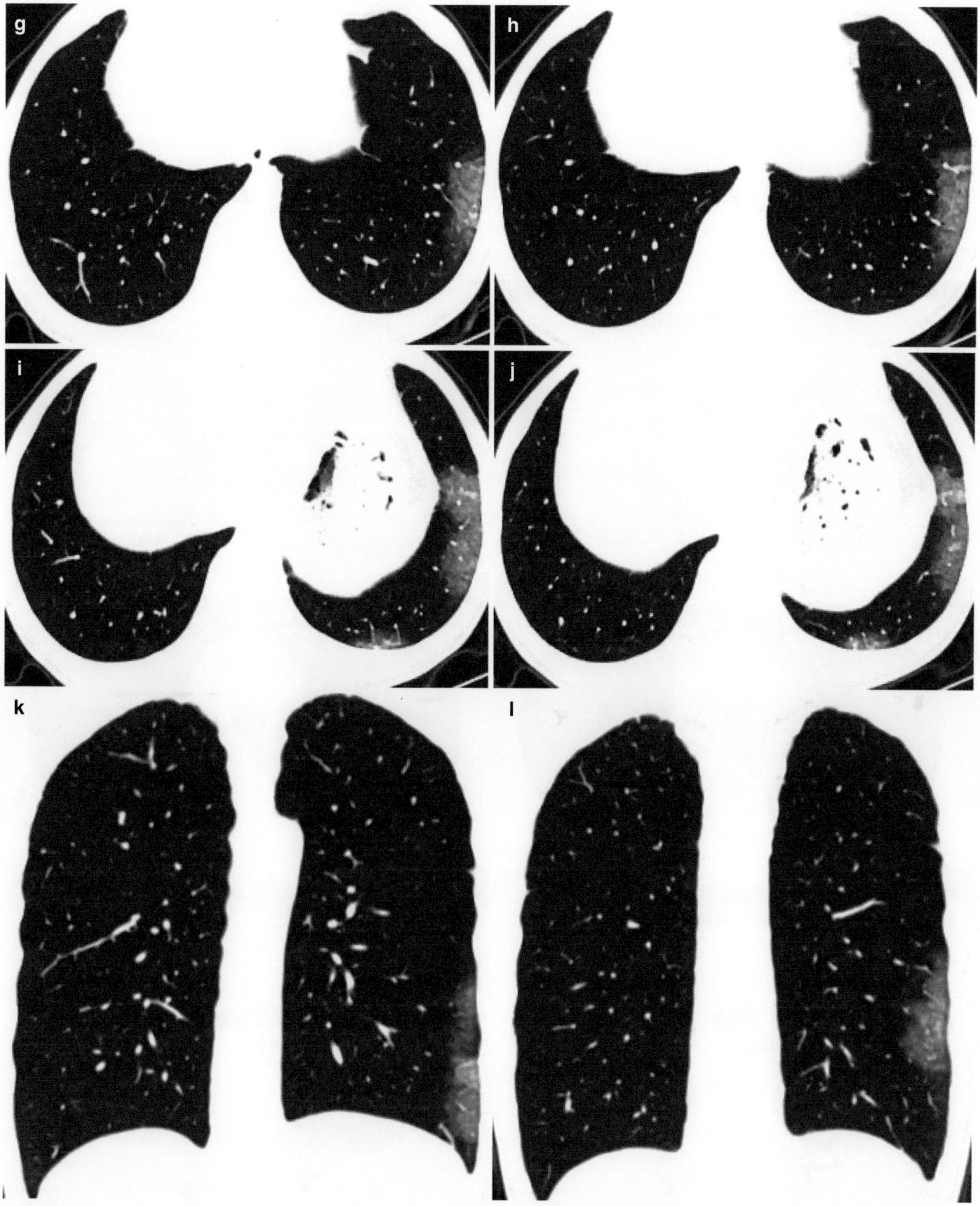

Fig. 3.5 (continued)

Chest CT scan taken 3 days after symptom onset showed multiple patchy ground-glass opacities with blurring edge located in the subpleural area of the right middle lobe and the left lower lobe, especially in the left lower lobe (Fig. 3.5a–l). Thickened blood vessel shadows were observed in the lesions in the lateral basal segment of the left lower lobe (Fig. 3.5e–h), and subpleural curvilinear line appeared adjacent to the lesion in the posterior basal segment of the left lower lobe (Fig. 3.5i).

3.7 Case 6 (Fig. 3.6a–l)

A 40-year-old male patient presented with fever for 3 days, with no chills and shivering, and he had the epidemiological history of exposure to patients from epidemic areas. His body temperature peaked at 38.4 °C before admission. At admission, his body temperature was 37.2 °C, the pulse rate was 94 beats per minute, the respiratory rate was 18 breaths per minute, and the blood oxygen saturation was 97.9%.

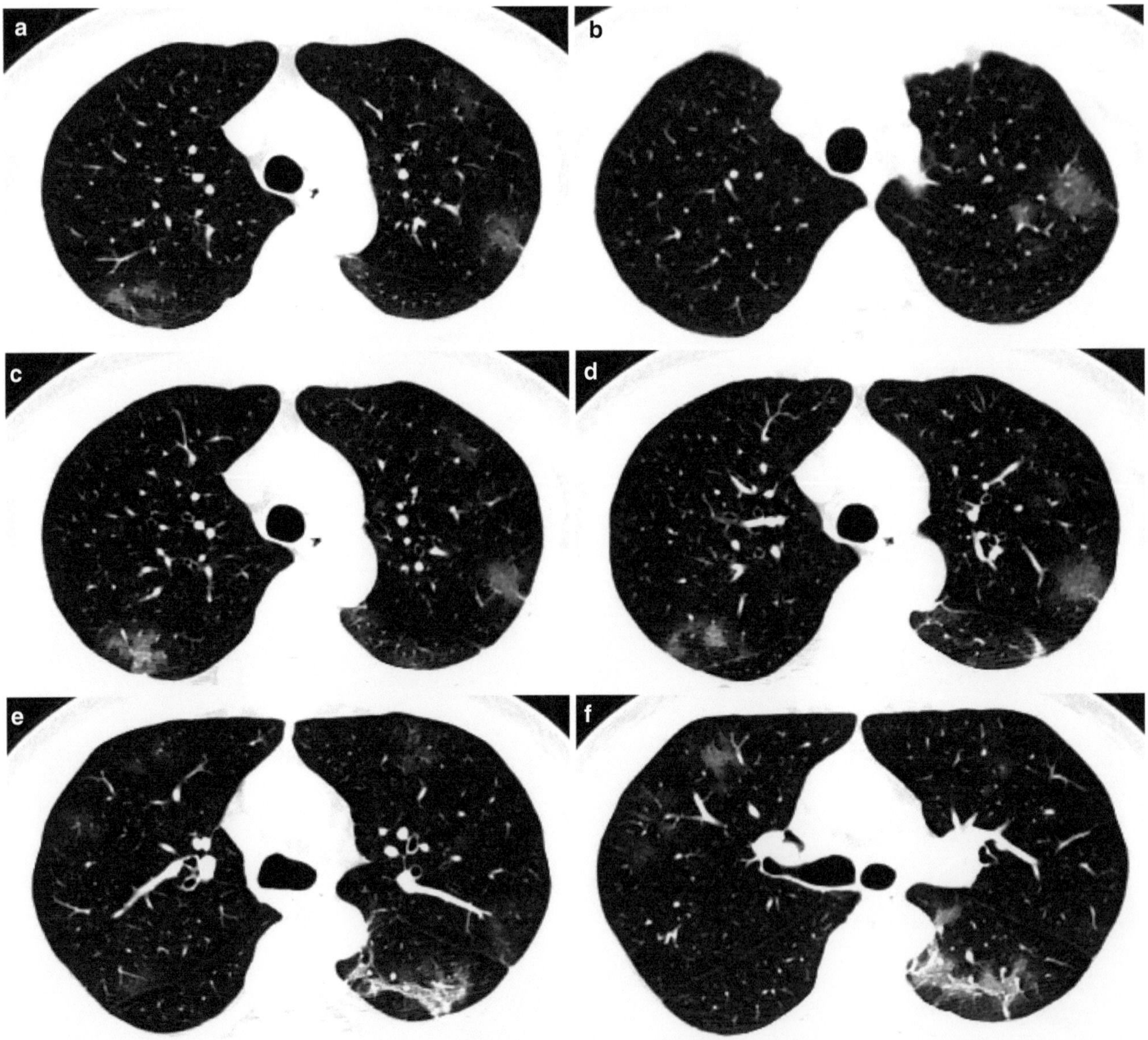

Fig. 3.6 Chest CT scan taken 4 days after symptom onset showed multiple patchy ground-glass opacities in both lungs with blurring edge (**a–l**), and subpleural curvilinear line and *irregular linear opacities* occurred in the bilateral lower lobes (**e–j**)

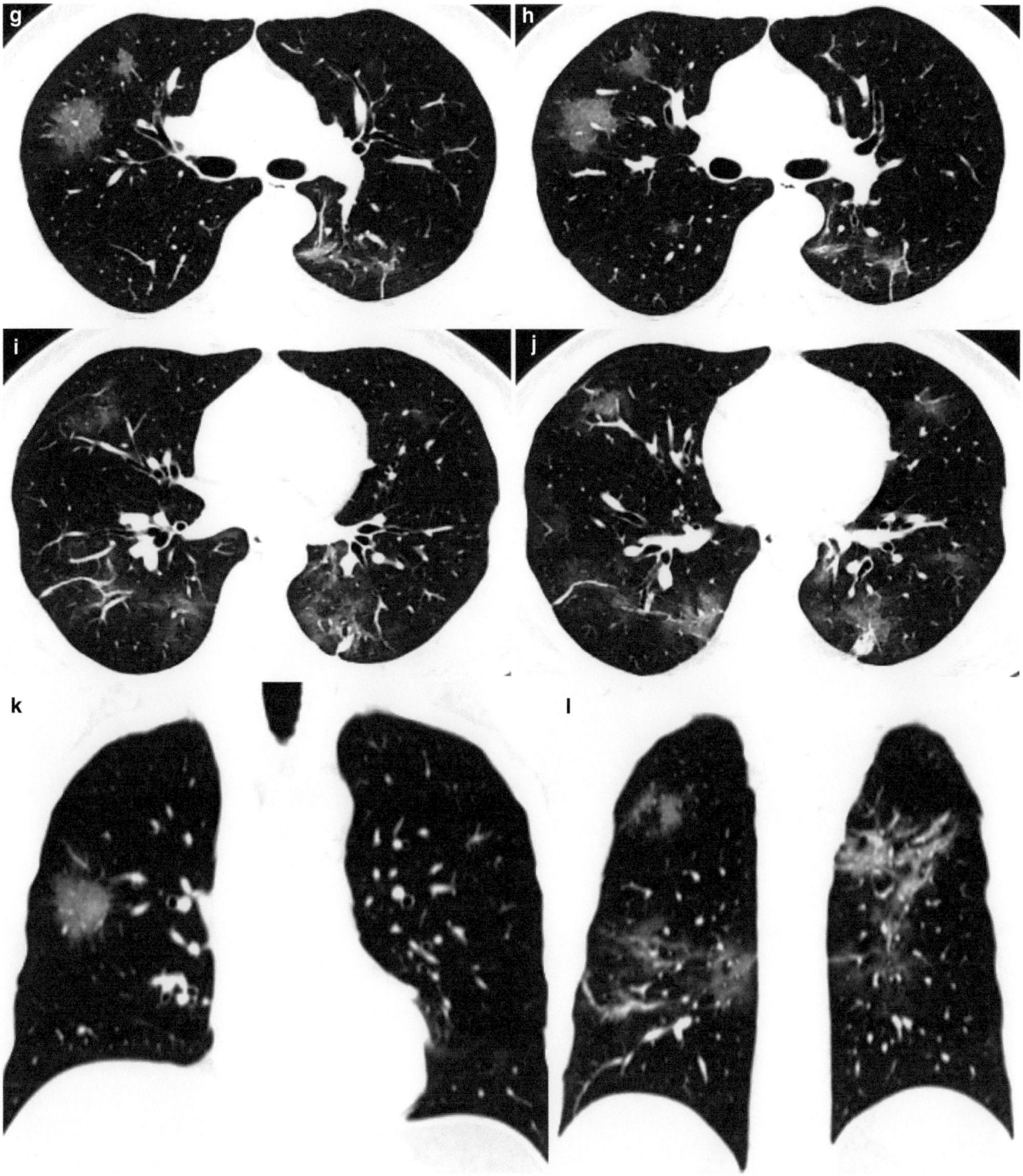

Fig. 3.6 (continued)

Blood routine examination: white-cell count, lymphocyte count, and C-reactive protein were 8.18×10^9/L, 1.24×10^9/L, and 30.84 mg/L, respectively.

Chest CT scan taken 4 days after symptom onset showed multiple patchy ground-glass opacities in both lungs with blurring edge (Fig. 3.6a–l), and subpleural curvilinear line and irregular linear opacities occurred in the bilateral lower lobes (Fig. 3.6e–j).

3.8 Case 7 (Fig. 3.7a–l)

A 26-year-old male patient was admitted to the hospital because of 2 days of fever, accompanied by dry cough, and he had the epidemiological history of exposure to patients from epidemic areas. At admission, his body temperature was 38.5 °C, the pulse rate was 93 beats per minute, the respiratory rate was 18 breaths per minute, and the blood oxygen saturation was 97.6%. Blood routine examination: white-cell count, lymphocyte count, and C-reactive protein were 3.73×10^9/L, 1.04×10^9/L, and 45.40 mg/L, respectively.

Chest CT scan taken 2 days after symptom onset showed multiple patchy ground-glass opacities in both lungs with blur-

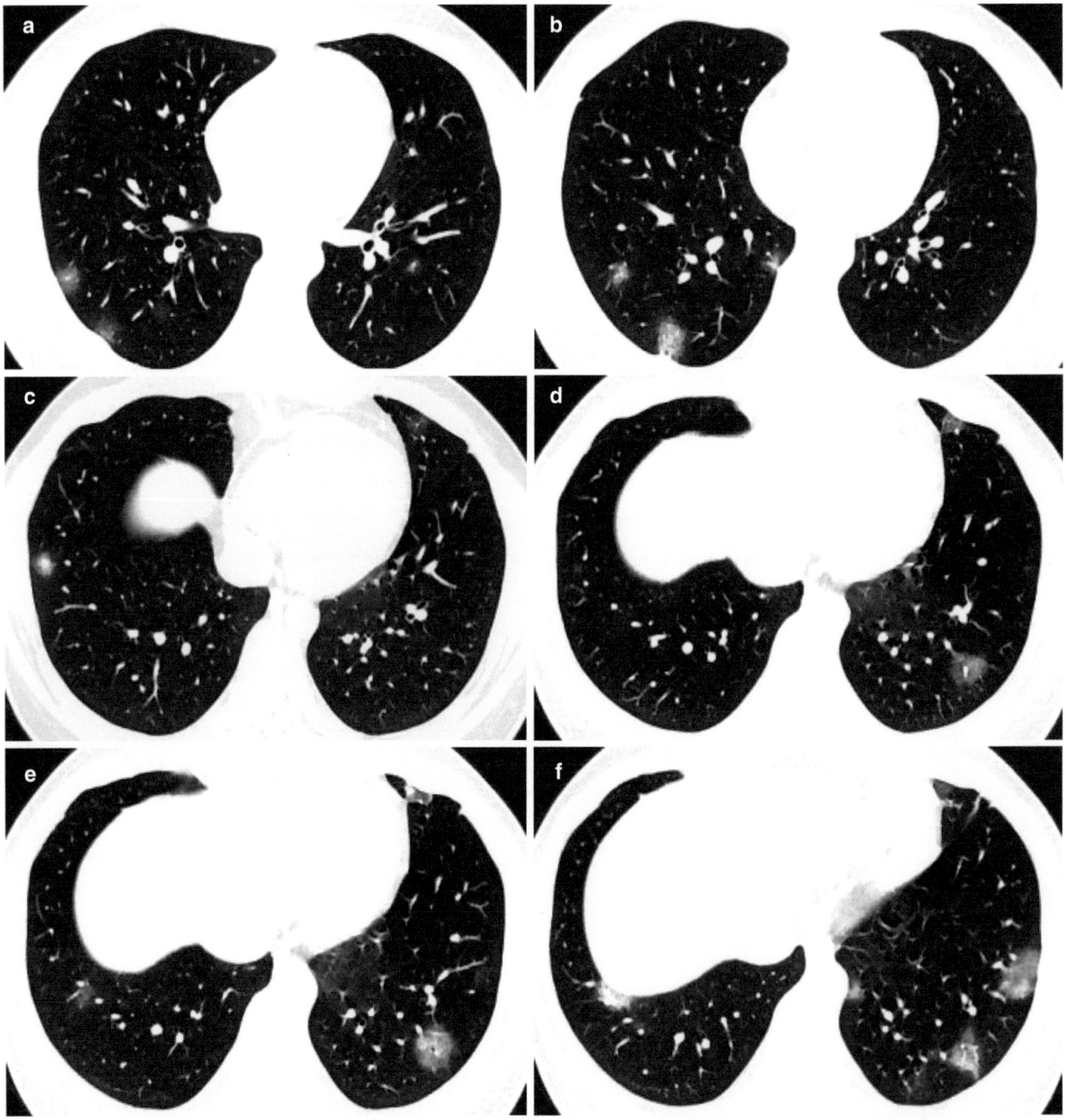

Fig. 3.7 Chest CT scan taken 2 days after symptom onset showed multiple patchy ground-glass opacities in both lungs with blurring edge, and the lesions were mainly distributed in the subpleural area of the lung (**a**–**l**). The central structure of lobules was thickened in the lesions in the bilateral lower lobes, and locally thickened vascular shadows were found (**c**–**j**)

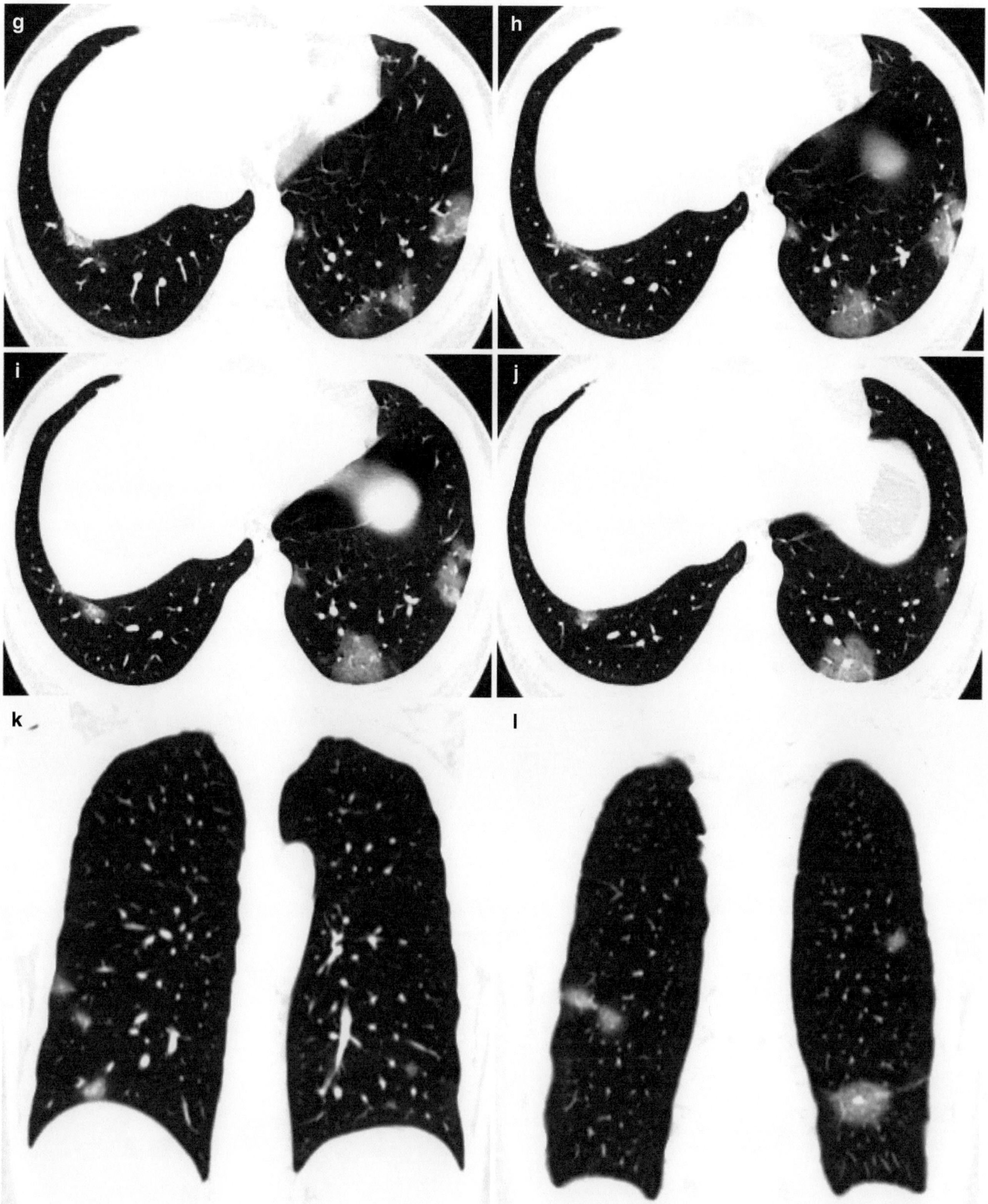

Fig. 3.7 (continued)

ring edge, and the lesions were mainly distributed in the subpleural area of the lung (Fig. 3.7a–l). The central structure of lobules was thickened in the lesions in the bilateral lower lobes, and locally thickened vascular shadows were found (Fig. 3.7c–j).

3.9 Case 8 (Fig. 3.8a–l)

A 54-year-old female patient was admitted to the hospital due to fever and fatigue for 2 days, accompanied by headache and dry cough; the body temperature peaked at 37.7 °C, and she had a history of exposure to patients from epidemic areas. At admission, the body temperature was 37.5 °C, the pulse rate was 56 beats per minute, the respiratory rate was 21 breaths per minute, and the blood oxygen saturation was 99%. Blood routine examination: white-cell count, lymphocyte count, and C-reactive protein were 8.33 × 10^9/L, 2.65 × 10^9/L, and 15.11 mg/L, respectively.

Chest CT examination performed 3 days after symptom onset showed multiple patchy ground-glass opacities in both lungs with blurring edge; the lesions were mainly distributed in the superior segments of the bilateral lower

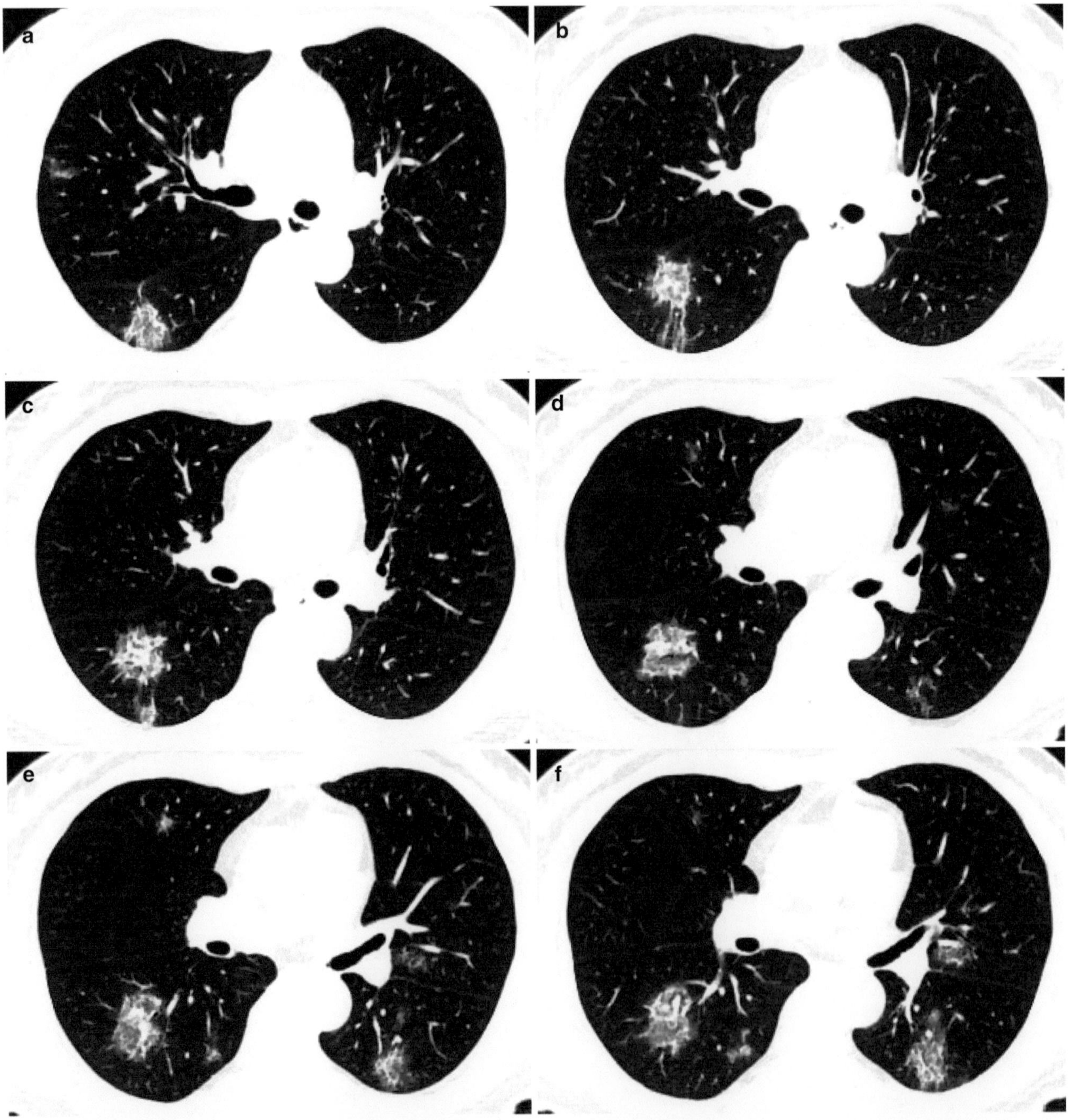

Fig. 3.8 Chest CT examination performed 3 days after symptom onset showed multiple patchy ground-glass opacities in both lungs with blurring edge; the lesions were mainly distributed in the superior segments of the bilateral lower lobe (**a**–**l**). HRCT demonstrated multifocal ground-glass opacities associated with intralobular septal thickening, and a crazy-paving pattern can be seen (**f**–**h**). Besides, reversed halo sign was observed in the lesion in the superior segment of the right lower lobe (**d**–**g**)

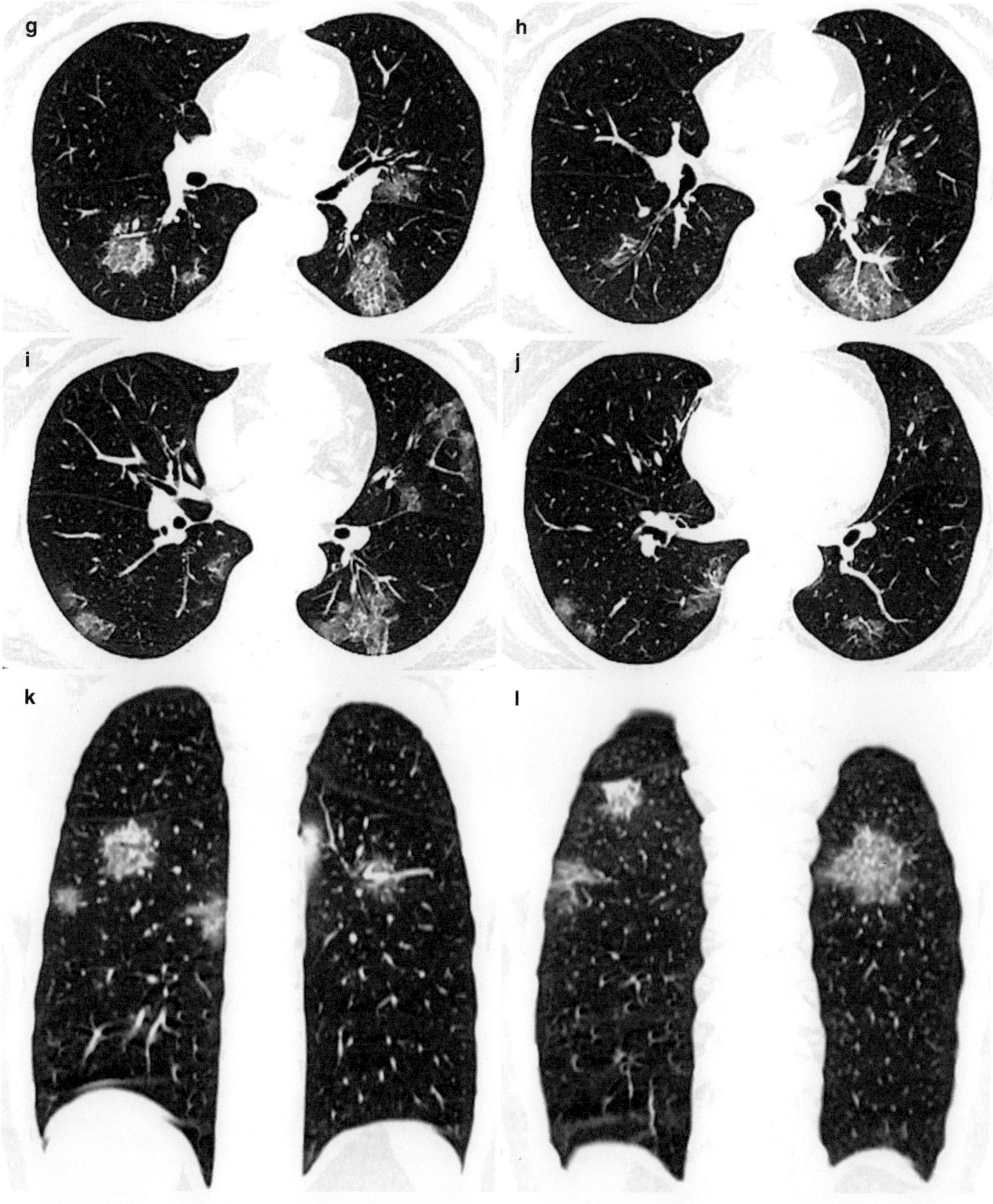

Fig. 3.8 (continued)

lobe (Fig. 3.8a–l). HRCT demonstrated multifocal ground-glass opacities associated with intralobular septal thickening, and a crazy-paving pattern can be seen (Fig. 3.8f–h). Besides, reversed halo sign was observed in the lesion in the superior segment of the right lower lobe (Fig. 3.8d–g).

3.10 Case 9 (Fig. 3.9a–l)

A 30-year-old female patient was admitted to the hospital due to fever for 2 days; the body temperature peaked at 38.7 °C, accompanied by chills and runny nose, with no expectoration; she had the epidemiological history of exposure to patients from epidemic areas. At admission, the body temperature was 38.2 °C, the pulse rate was 110 beats per minute, the respiratory rate was 18 breaths per minute, and the blood oxygen saturation was 97.1%. Blood routine examination: white-cell count, lymphocyte count, and C-reactive protein were 2.70 × 10^9/L, 0.92 × 10^9/L, and <10 mg/L, respectively.

Chest CT examination performed 3 days after symptom onset showed patchy ground-glass opacities and consolidation distributed in the subpleural area of the left

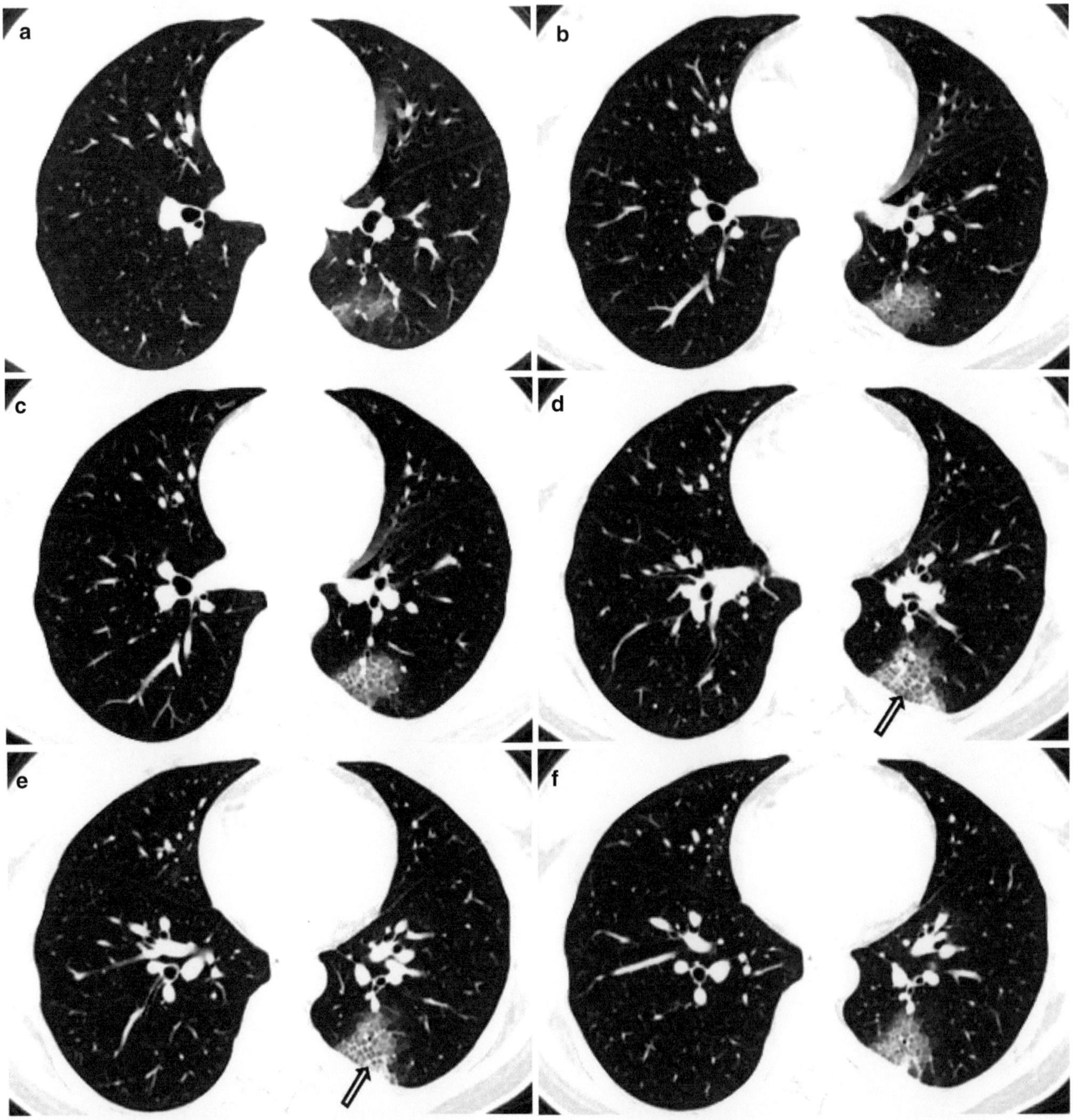

Fig. 3.9 Chest CT examination performed 3 days after symptom onset showed patchy ground-glass opacities and consolidation distributed in the subpleural area of the left lower lobe. HRCT demonstrated focal ground-glass opacities associated with intralobular septal thickening, and a crazy-paving pattern was observed (**d**, **e**, white arrow)

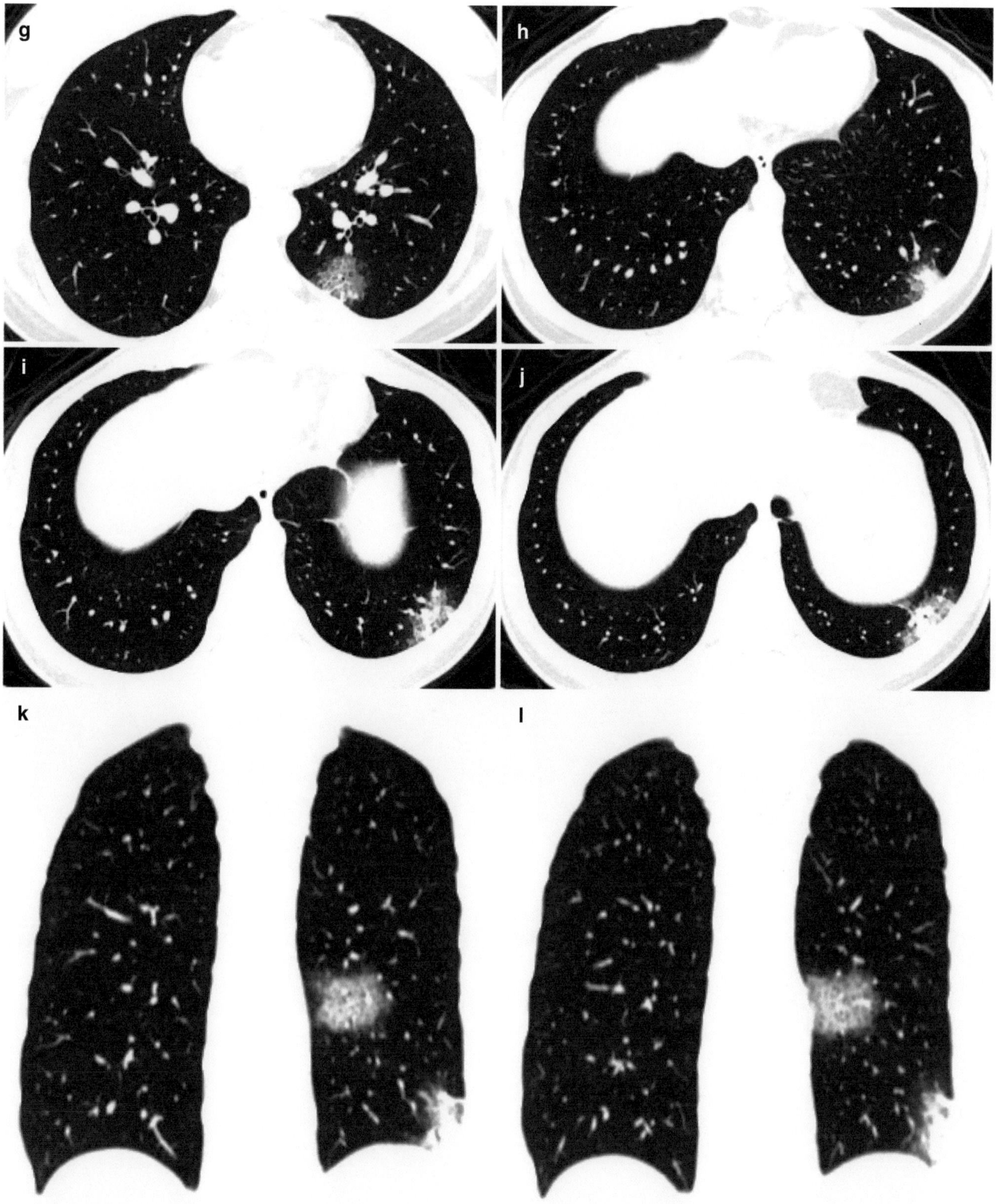

Fig. 3.9 (continued)

lower lobe. HRCT demonstrated focal ground-glass opacities associated with intralobular septal thickening, and a crazy-paving pattern was observed (Fig. 3.9d, e, white arrow).

3.11 Case 10 (Fig. 3.10a–l)

A 65-year-old male patient was admitted to the hospital because of dry cough and chills for 2 days, and he had the epidemiological history of exposure to patients from epidemic areas. At admission, the body temperature was 37.1 °C, the pulse rate was 103 beats per minute, the respiratory rate was 20 breaths per minute, and the blood oxygen saturation was 97.1%. Blood routine examination: white-cell count, lymphocyte count, and C-reactive protein were 4.15 × 10^9/L, 0.76 × 10^9/L, and <10 mg/L, respectively.

Chest CT examination performed 3 days after symptom onset showed multifocal ground-glass opacities mainly distributed in the subpleural area of the bilateral lungs with blurred edge (Fig. 3.10a–l). HRCT demonstrated focal

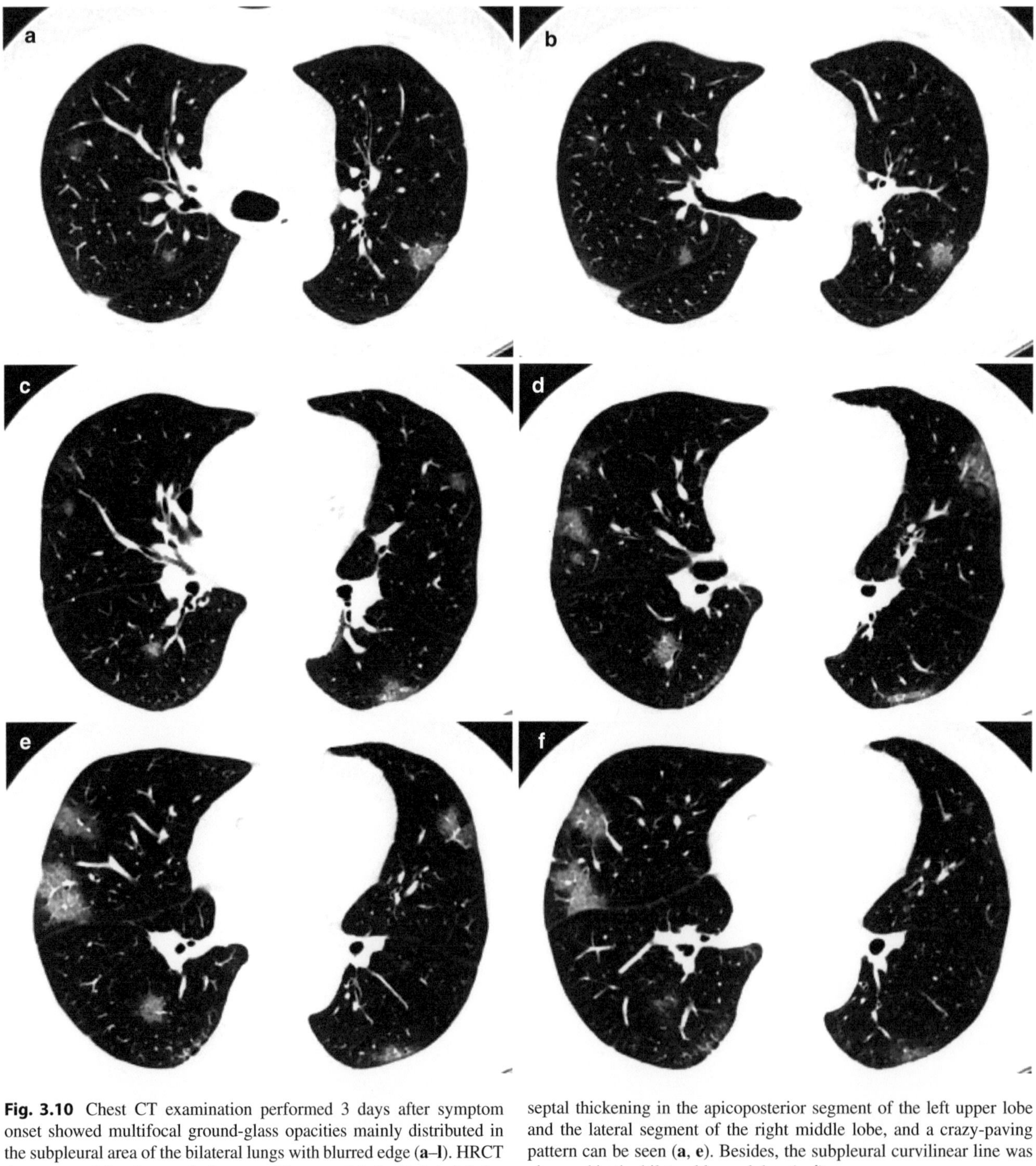

Fig. 3.10 Chest CT examination performed 3 days after symptom onset showed multifocal ground-glass opacities mainly distributed in the subpleural area of the bilateral lungs with blurred edge (**a**–**l**). HRCT demonstrated focal ground-glass opacities associated with intralobular septal thickening in the apicoposterior segment of the left upper lobe and the lateral segment of the right middle lobe, and a crazy-paving pattern can be seen (**a**, **e**). Besides, the subpleural curvilinear line was observed in the bilateral lower lobes (**c**–**j**)

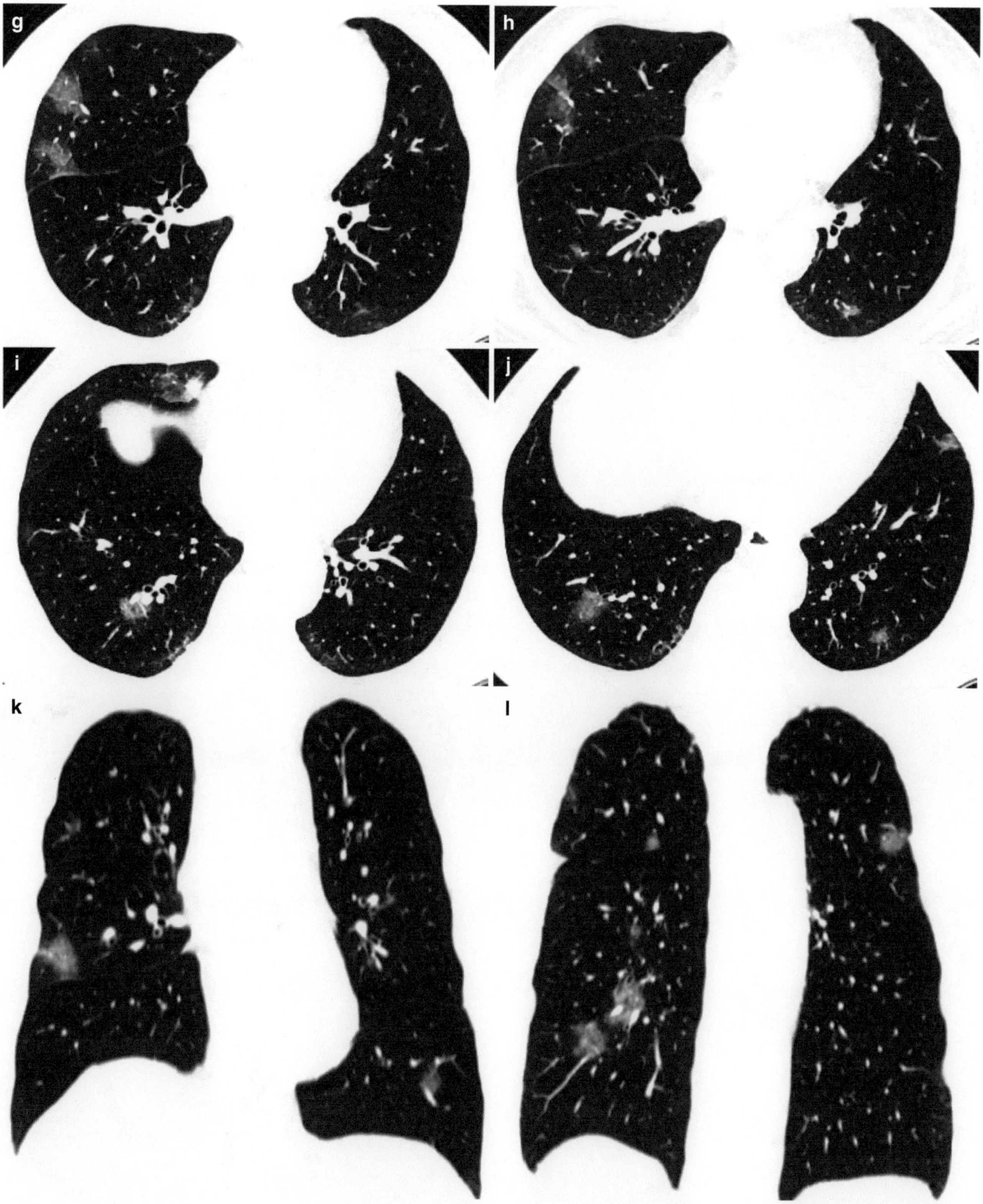

Fig. 3.10 (continued)

ground-glass opacities associated with intralobular septal thickening in the apicoposterior segment of the left upper lobe and the lateral segment of the right middle lobe, and a crazy-paving pattern can be seen (Fig. 3.10a, e). Besides, the subpleural curvilinear line was observed in the bilateral lower lobes (Fig. 3.10c–j).

3.12 Case 11 (Fig. 3.11a–l)

A 47-year-old female patient was admitted to the hospital due to fever for 3 days, accompanied by chills, cough, and expectoration. She had the epidemiological history of exposure to patients from epidemic areas. At admission, the body temperature was 38.5 °C, the pulse rate was 100 beats per minute, the respiratory rate was 20 breaths per minute, and the blood oxygen saturation was 96%. Blood routine examination: white-cell count, lymphocyte count, and C-reactive protein were 4.68×10^9/L, 0.77×10^9/L, and 25.8 mg/L, respectively.

Chest CT examination performed 4 days after symptom onset showed multiple patchy ground-glass opacities mainly distributed in the subpleural area of the bilateral lungs (Fig. 3.11a–l). The subpleural curvilinear line was found in the bilateral lower lobes (Fig. 3.11e–j).

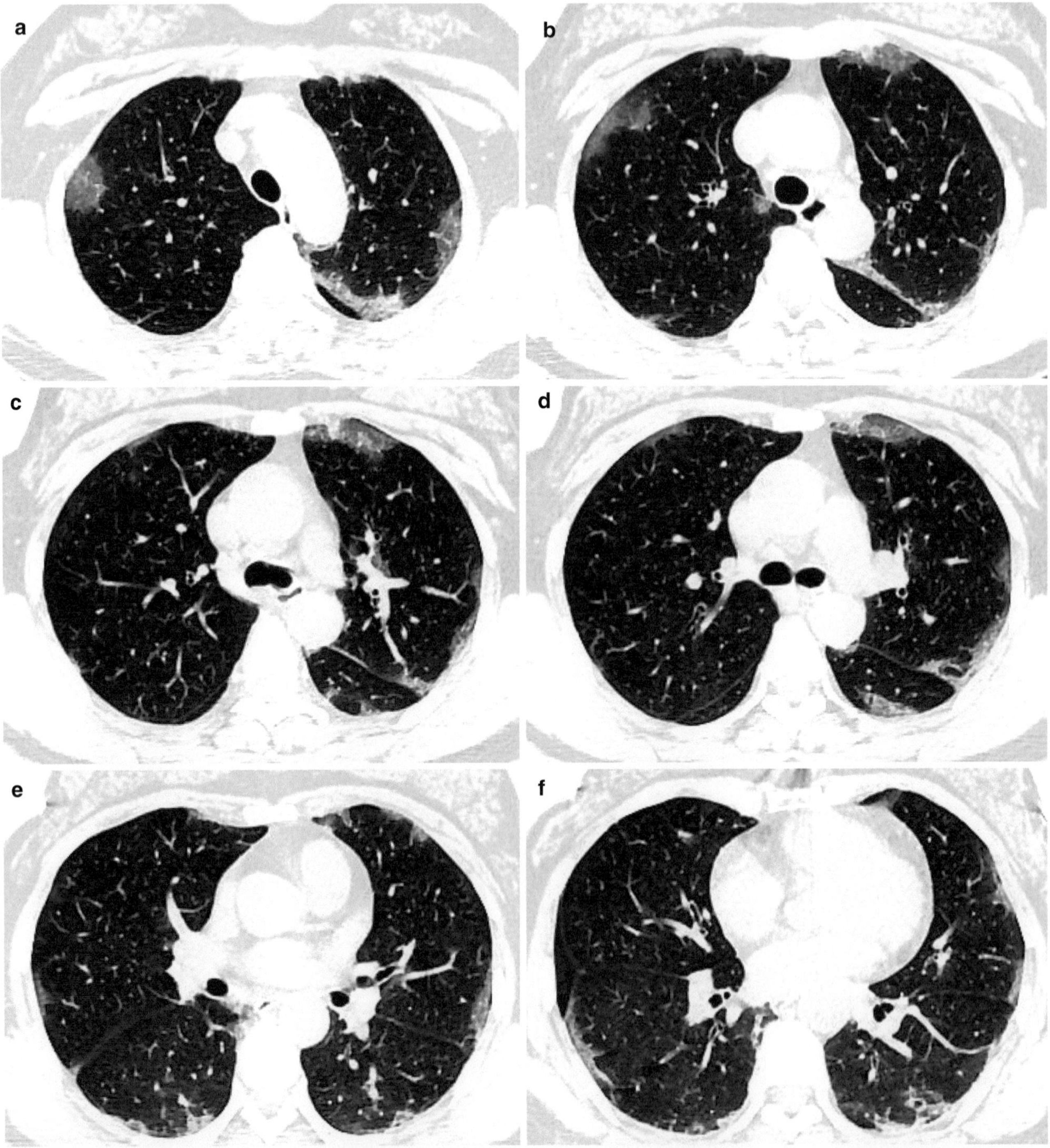

Fig. 3.11 Chest CT examination performed 4 days after symptom onset showed multiple patchy ground-glass opacities mainly distributed in the subpleural area of the bilateral lungs (**a**–**l**). The subpleural curvilinear line was found in the bilateral lower lobes (**e**–**j**)

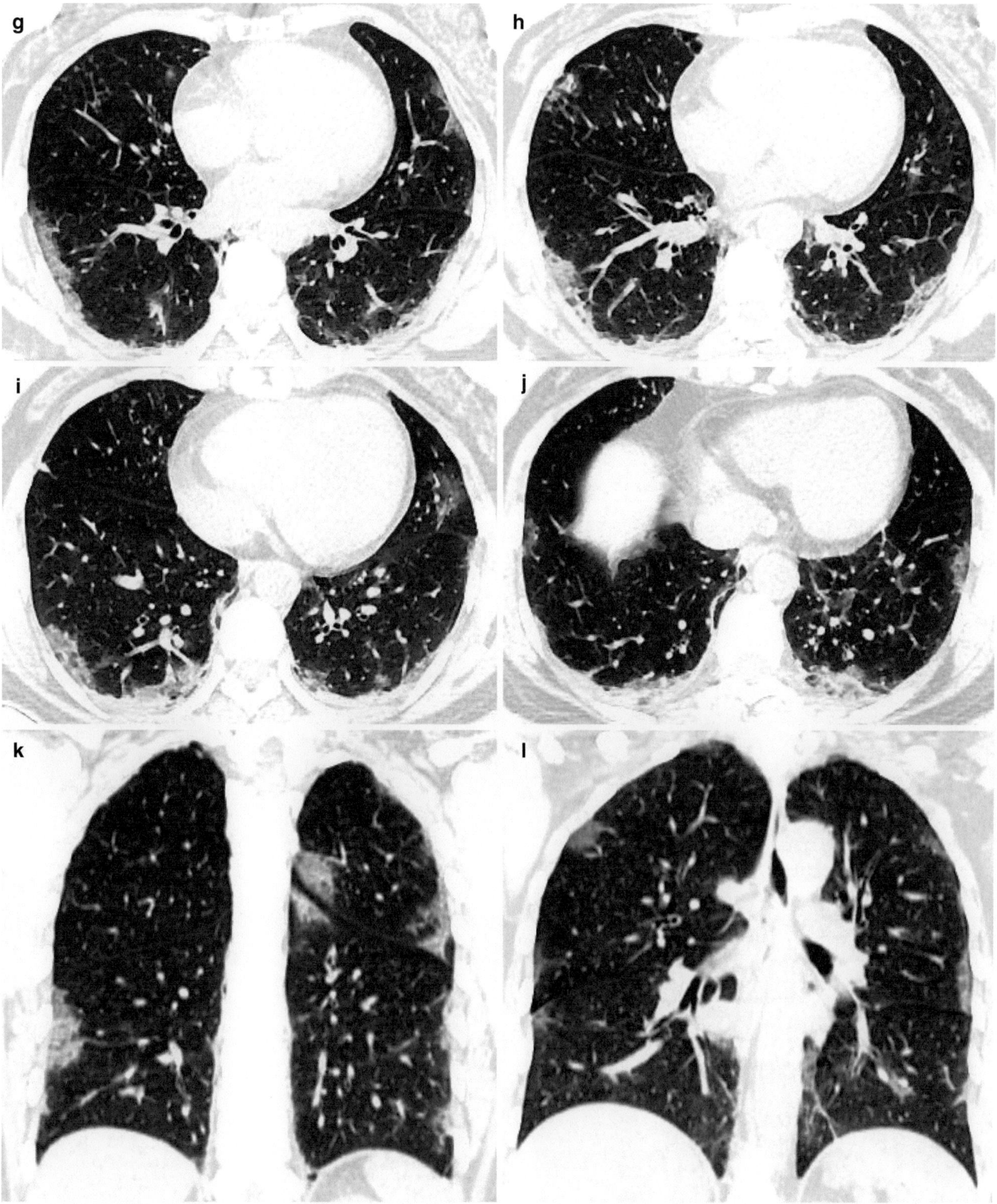

Fig. 3.11 (continued)

3.13 Case 12 (Fig. 3.12a–l)

A 27-year-old male patient was admitted to the hospital due to fever for 4 days; his body temperature peaked at 38.3 °C, accompanied by chills, cough, and expectoration. He had the epidemiological history of exposure to patients from epidemic areas. At admission, the body temperature was 37.8 °C, the pulse rate was 105 beats per minute, the respira-

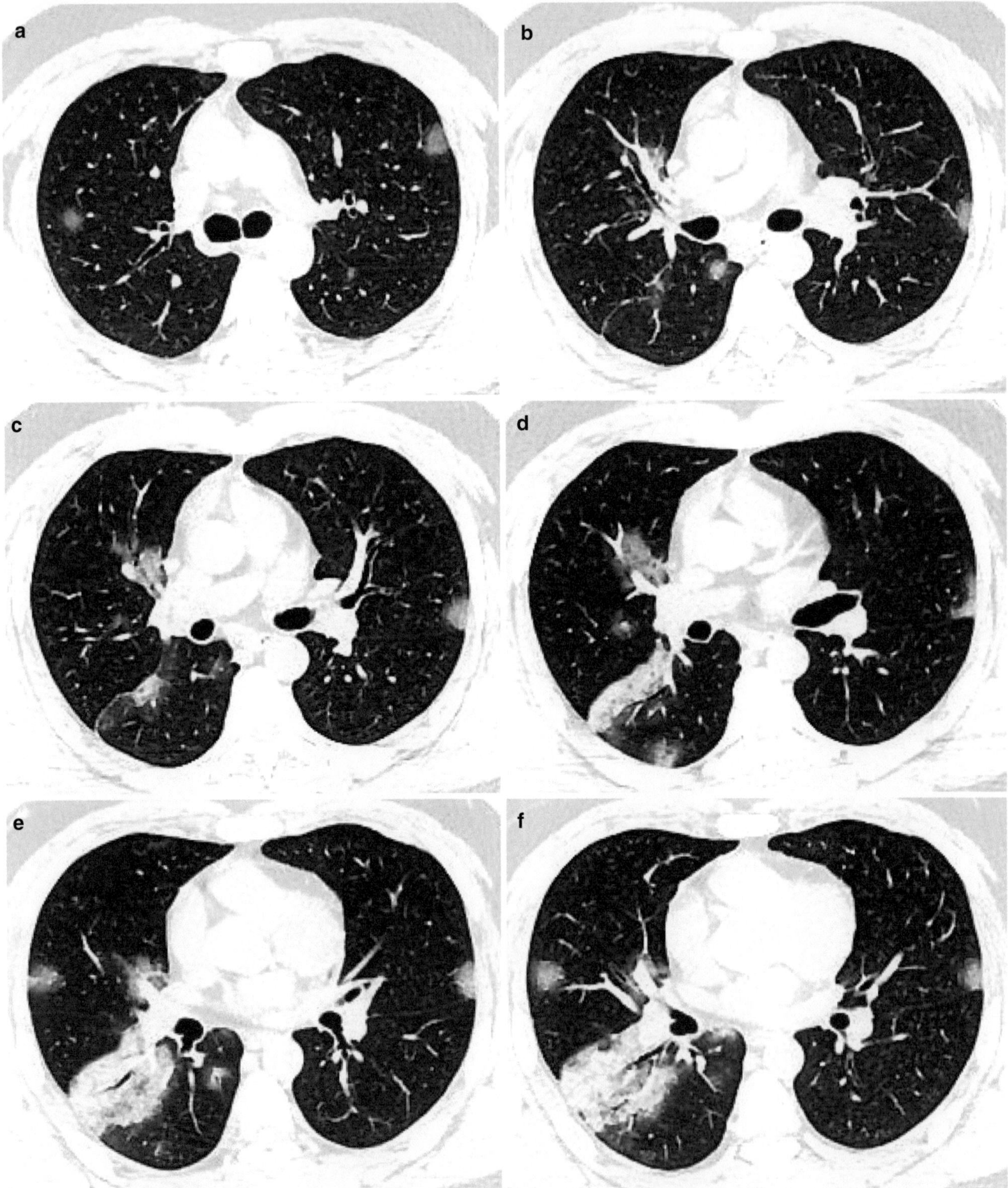

Fig. 3.12 Chest CT examination performed 4 days after symptom onset showed multiple patchy ground-glass opacities mainly distributed in the subpleural area of the bilateral lungs (**a**–**l**). Multifocal lung lesions were predominantly found in the right lower lobe, with presence of consolidation in which the "air bronchogram sign" could be seen (**e**–**h**)

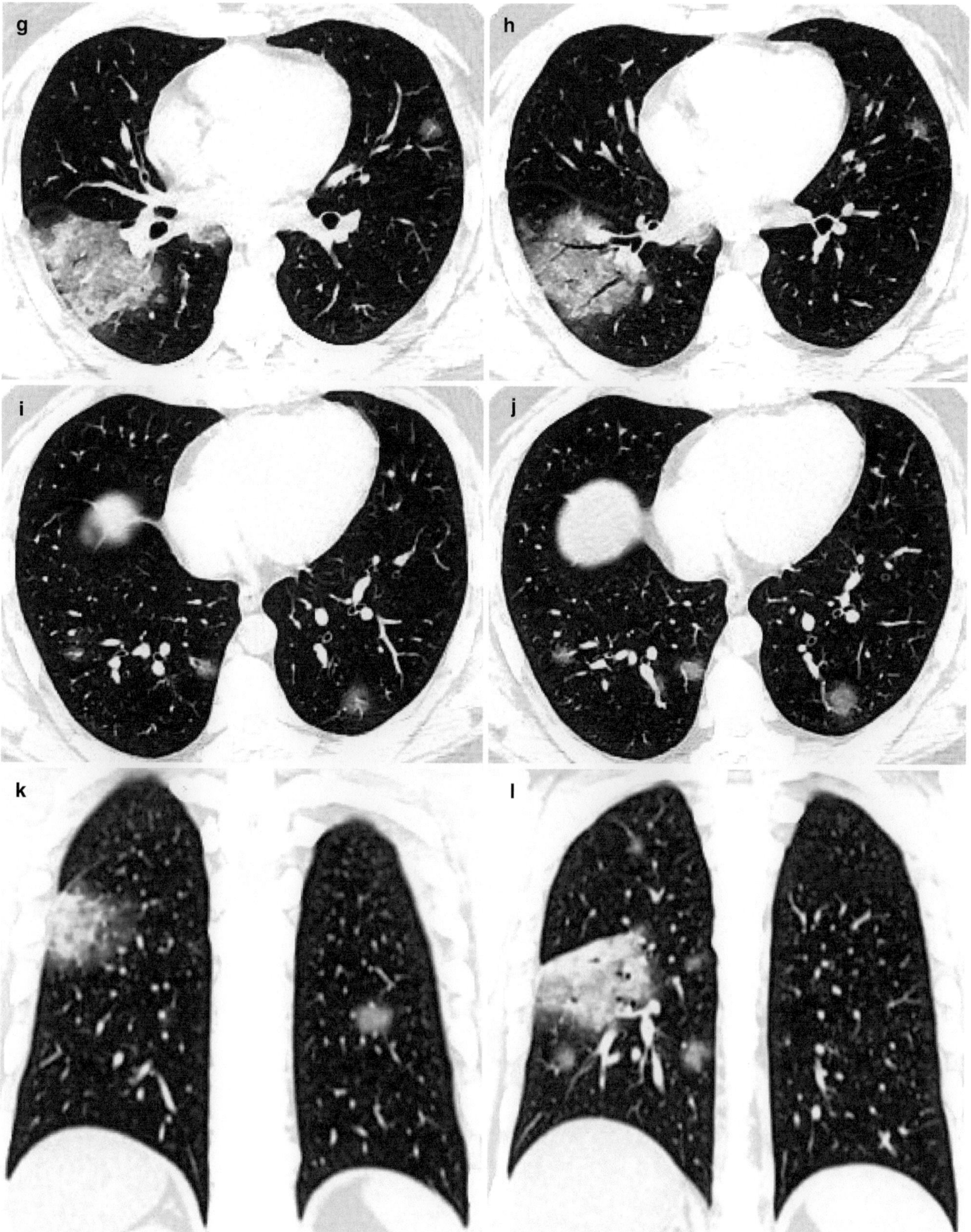

Fig. 3.12 (continued)

tory rate was 20 breaths per minute, and the blood oxygen saturation was 97%. Blood routine examination: white-cell count, lymphocyte count, and C-reactive protein were 3.34 × 10^9/L, 0.89 × 10^9/L, and 12.73 mg/L, respectively.

Chest CT examination performed 4 days after symptom onset showed multiple patchy ground-glass opacities mainly distributed in the subpleural area of the bilateral lungs (Fig. 3.12a–l). Multifocal lung lesions were predominantly found in the right lower lobe, with presence of consolidation in which the "air bronchogram sign" could be seen (Fig. 3.12e–h).

3.14 Case 13 (Fig. 3.13a–l)

A 34-year-old male patient was admitted to the hospital due to fever for 2 days; his body temperature peaked at 38.0 °C, accompanied by chills and cough, with no expectoration. He had the epidemiological history of exposure to patients from epidemic areas. At admission, the body temperature was 37.5 °C, the pulse rate was 82 beats per minute, the respiratory rate was 18 breaths per minute, and the blood oxygen saturation was 96%. Blood routine examination: white-cell

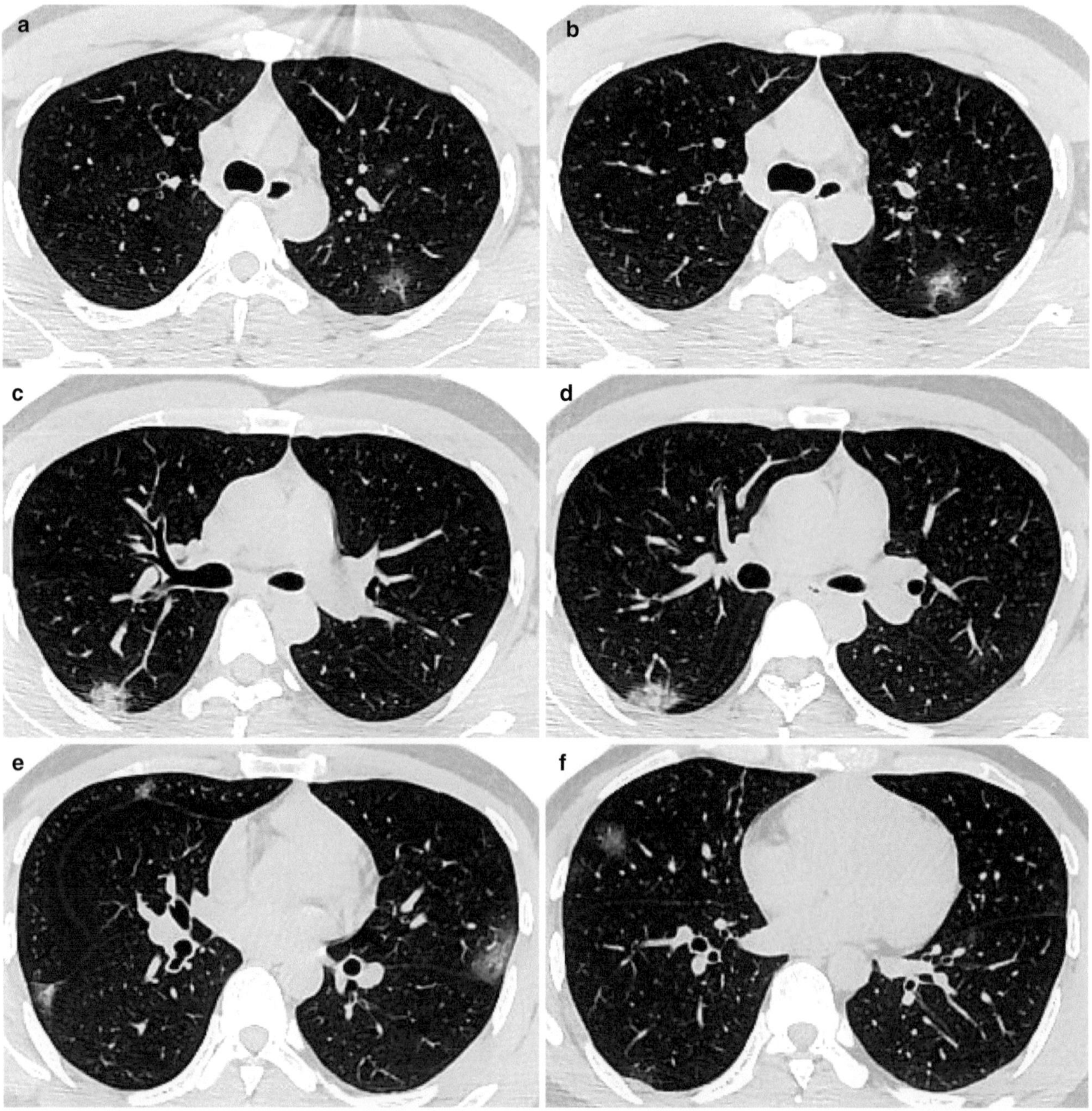

Fig. 3.13 Chest CT examination performed 4 days after symptom onset showed multiple patchy ground-glass opacities in the bilateral lungs with blurred edge and subpleural distribution (**a–l**). A few of lesions manifested as localized consolidation

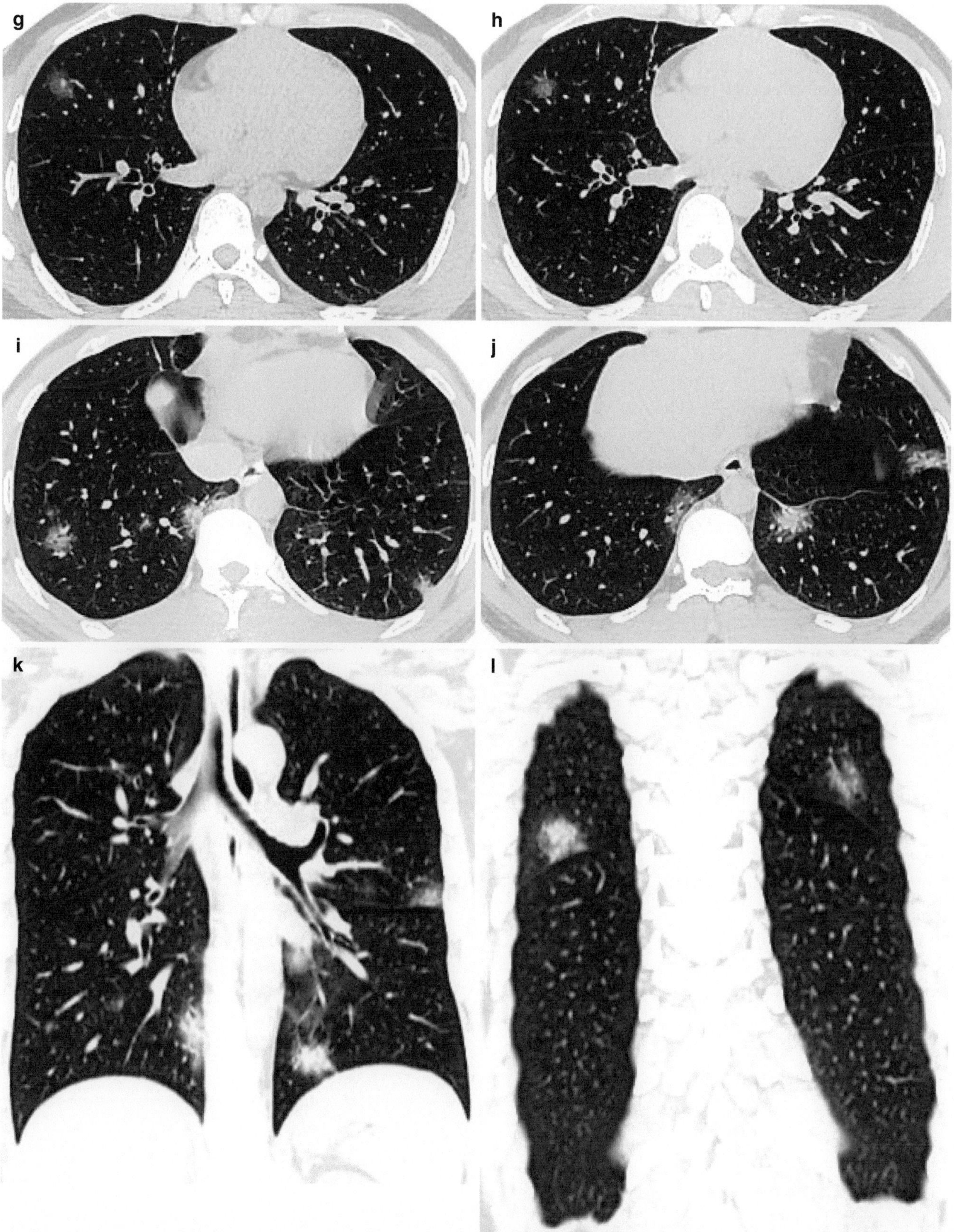

Fig. 3.13 (continued)

count, lymphocyte count, and C-reactive protein were 5.51×10^9/L, 0.99×10^9/L, and <10 mg/L, respectively.

Chest CT examination performed 4 days after symptom onset showed multiple patchy ground-glass opacities in the bilateral lungs with blurred edge and subpleural distribution (Fig. 3.13a–l). A few of lesions manifested as localized consolidation.

References

1. Li Q, Guan X, Wu P, et al. Early transmission dynamics in Wuhan, China, of novel coronavirus-infected pneumonia. N Engl J Med. 2020;382:1199–207.
2. Chen N, Zhou M, Dong X, et al. Epidemiological and clinical characteristics of 99 cases of 2019 novel coronavirus pneumonia in Wuhan, China: a descriptive study. Lancet. 2020;395:507–13.
3. Chung M, Bernheim A, Mei X, et al. CT imaging features of 2019 novel coronavirus (2019-nCoV). Radiology. 2020;295:202–7.
4. Han R, Huang L, Dong J, et al. Early clinical and CT manifestations of coronavirus disease 2019 (COVID-19) pneumonia. Am J Roentgenol. 2020;215:338–43.
5. Paul NS, Roberts H, Butany J, et al. Radiologic pattern of disease in patients with severe acute respiratory syndrome: the Toronto experience. RadioGraphics. 2004;24:553–63.
6. Holshue ML, DeBolt C, Lindquist S, et al. Washington State 2019-nCoV Case Investigation Team. First case of 2019 novel coronavirus in the United States. N Engl J Med. 2020;382:929–36.

CT Features of Intermediate Stage of COVID-19 Pneumonia

4

Lin Lin, Xi Xu, and Weiping Cai

4.1 Introduction

The incubation period of COVID-19 ranges from 1 to 14 days after infection but is typically 3–7 days. Clinically, the majority of patients in the intermediate stage of COVID-19 pneumonia develop deteriorated symptoms with noticeable chest-computed tomography (CT) imaging changes. In contrast, a small proportion of patients only manifest mild or general symptoms, even when chest-CT imaging changes were easily observed. The mismatch between the development of clinical symptoms and function changes of the lung detected by chest CT is probably because of the different immune responses individually. Due to the advantages such as its fastness, high resolution, and direct visualization, chest CT examination plays a critical role for precisely evaluating the patient conditions before initiating proper medical treatment and for predicting the clinical outcome after treatment and thus was regarded as one of the vital references for COVID-19 diagnosis.

There are many publications on the chest CT findings during COVID-19 infection. Jin et al. [1] describe the features of chest CT in different disease courses, and they find large consolidative opacities and air bronchograms on chest CT apart from ground-glass opacity during the progression stage. Song et al. [2] report the increased rate of consolidation on chest CT with disease progression. Pan et al. [3], in a retrospective study involving 63 patients with confirmed COVID-19, demonstrate over 85% of patients having some features on chest CT associated with disease progression including increase in ground-glass opacity, consolidation, and interstitial septal thickening. In another publication, Pan et al. [4] show enlarged lung involvement, increased ground-glasses opacities, and consolidation in the follow-up CT scan of 21 patients with confirmed COVID-19. Moreover, crazy-paving sign was found on chest CT.

Based on our observation, we summarize the chest CT features of intermediate stage of COVID-19 pneumonia. Most of patients enter the rapid disease-progression period within 1 week after disease onset; only a few severe cases progress rapidly within 2 weeks after disease onset. In the early stage, chest CT manifests single or multiple ground-glass opacity combined with thickening of intralobular or interlobular septa in the unilateral or bilateral lung. As the disease progresses, the extent of lung involvement increases, and the most common chest CT findings are ground-glass opacity with consolidation, interstitial septal thickening, and linear opacity. Sometimes, typical crazy-paving sign can be seen. Other than that, some severe cases show bilateral diffuse patchy or massive consolidation with or without air-bronchogram in follow-up chest CT. However, lymphadenopathy and pleural effusions can be found in few cases with confirmed COVID-19. In the following case series, we present different chest CT findings of intermediate stage of COVID-19 pneumonia in detail.

4.2 Case 1 (Fig. 4.1a1–e1, a2–e2)

A 30-year-old female patient with a disease-related exposure history had fever, which occurred 2 days ago, accompanied by chills and runny nose. Admission body temperature was 38.7 °C. White blood cell count, lymphocyte count, and C-reactive protein were 4.31×10^9/L, 1.34×10^9/L, and <10 mg/L, respectively. The patient underwent chest CT scans on day 3 and day 6 after the onset of symptoms and was confirmed by CDC in Guangzhou.

L. Lin (✉) · W. Cai
Guangzhou Eighth People's Hospital, Guangzhou Medical University, Guangzhou, China

X. Xu
The First Affiliated Hospital, Jinan University, Guangzhou, China

J. Liu et al. (eds.), *Atlas of Chest Imaging in COVID-19 Patients*, https://doi.org/10.1007/978-981-16-1082-0_4

Chest CT scans on day 3 (a1–e1) showed patchy ground-glass opacities with thickening of the interlobular and intralobular septa in the right upper lobe and left lower lobe. Chest CT on day 6 (a2–e2) demonstrated enlarged lesions and increased density of the lesions compared with previous images, indicating disease progression. Moreover, the interlobular septal thickening in regions of ground-glass opacification, represented a crazy-paving pattern.

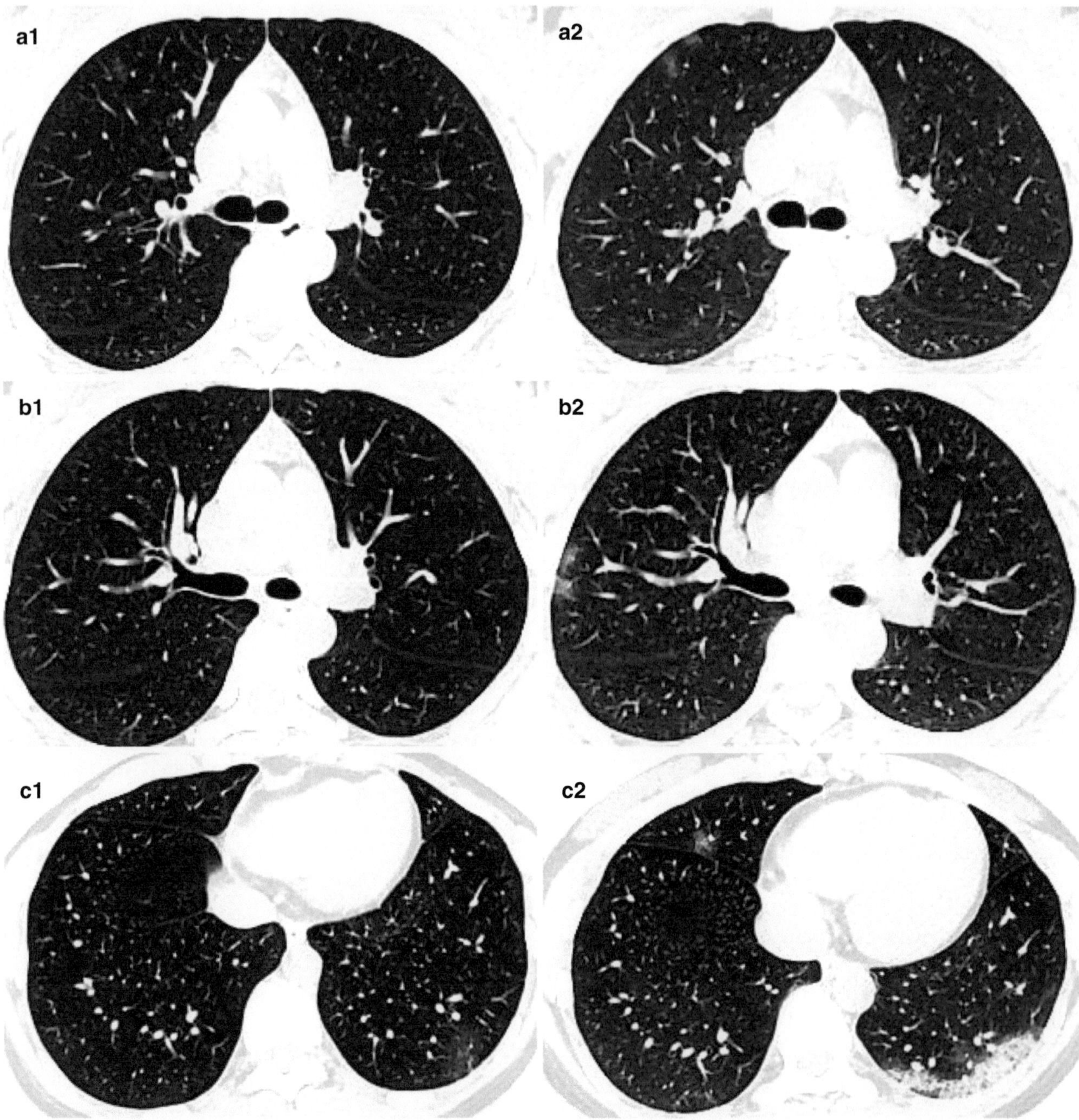

Fig. 4.1 Chest CT scans on day 3 (**a**1–**e**1) showed patchy ground-glass opacities with thickening of the interlobular and intralobular septa in the right upper lobe and left lower lobe. Chest CT on day 6 (**a**2–**e**2) demonstrated enlarged lesions and increased density of the lesions compared with previous images, indicating disease progression. Moreover, the interlobular septal thickening in regions of ground-glass opacification, represented a crazy-paving pattern

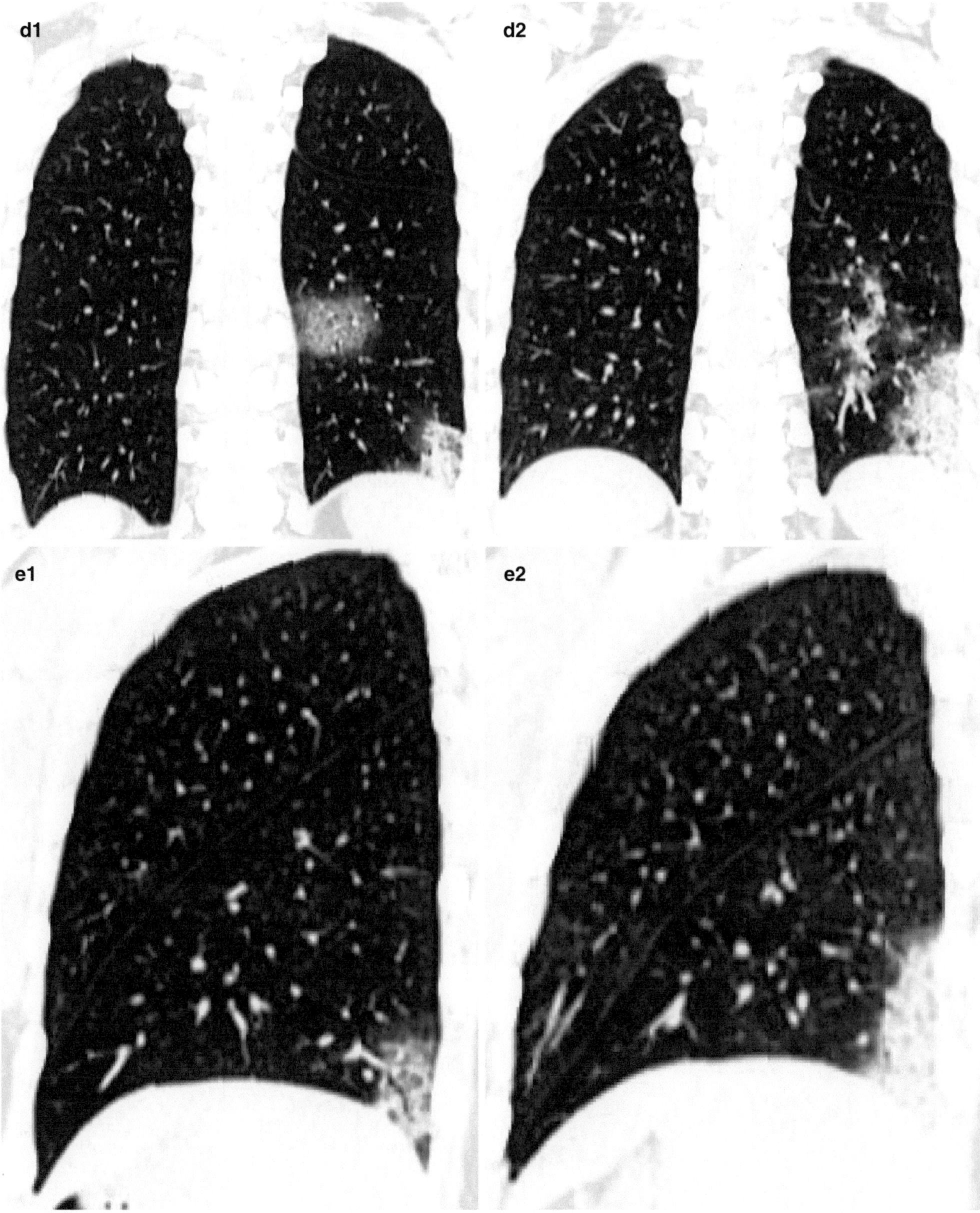

Fig. 4.1 (continued)

4.3 Case 2 (Fig. 4.2a1–e1, a2–e2)

A 65-year-old female patient with a disease-related exposure history presented with pharyngalgia for 1 day. Admission body temperature was 36.7 °C. White blood cell count, lymphocyte count, and C-reactive protein were 4.61 × 10^9/L, 0.95 × 10^9/L, and <10 mg/L, respectively. The patient underwent chest CT scans on day 3 and day 6 after the onset of symptoms and was confirmed by CDC in Guangzhou.

Chest CT on day 3 (a1–e1) showed patchy ground-glass opacities with thickened interlobular septa and intralobular septa and focal consolidation in the bilateral lung. Chest CT on day 6 (a2–e2) demonstrated an enlargement of lesions and increased consolidation. Most of lesions were located in the peripheral field of the lung.

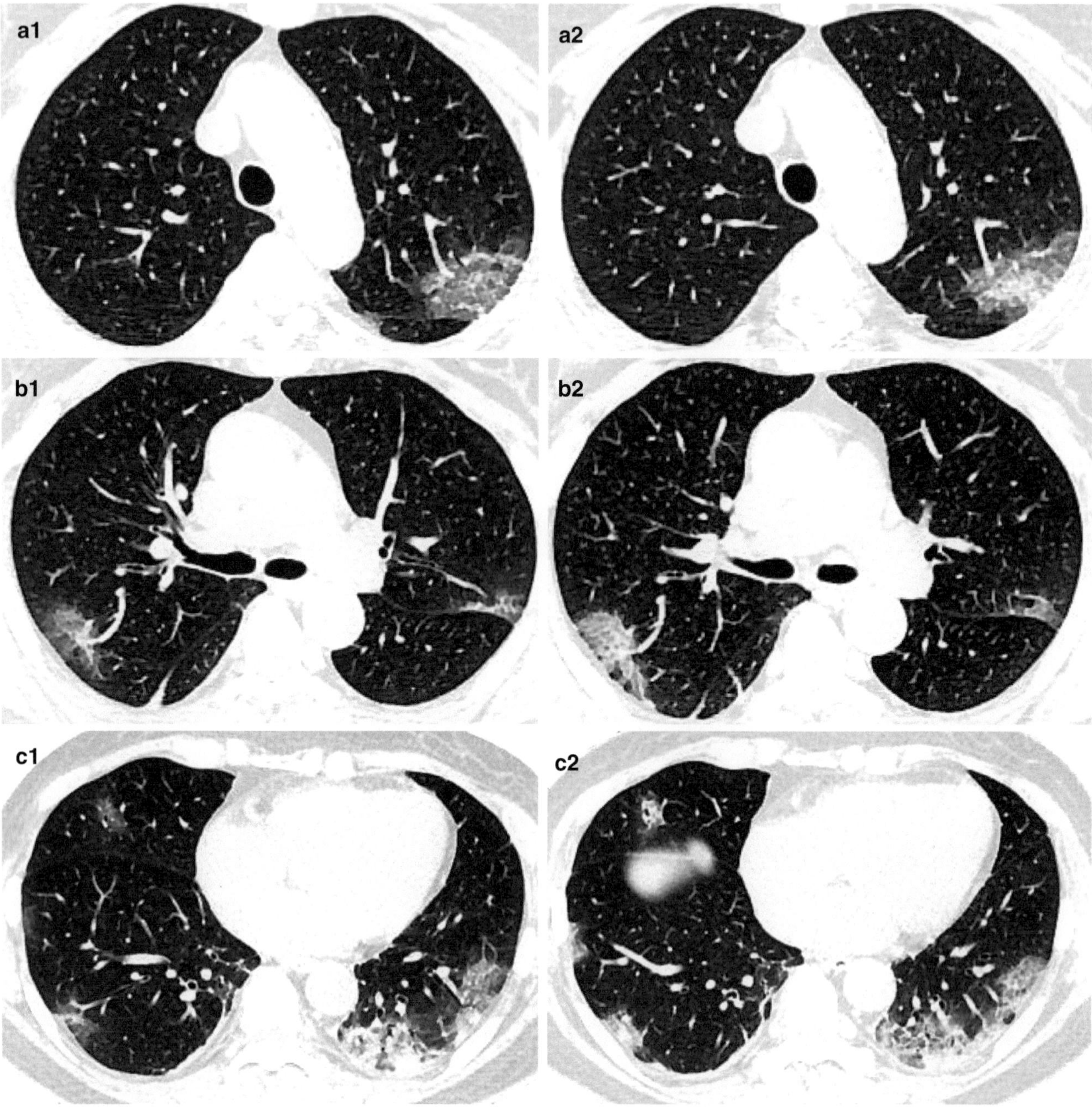

Fig. 4.2 Chest CT on day 3 (**a**1–**e**1) showed patchy ground-glass opacities with thickened interlobular septa and intralobular septa and focal consolidation in the bilateral lung. Chest CT on day 6 (**a**2–**e**2) demonstrated an enlargement of lesions and increased consolidation. Most of lesions were located in the peripheral field of the lung

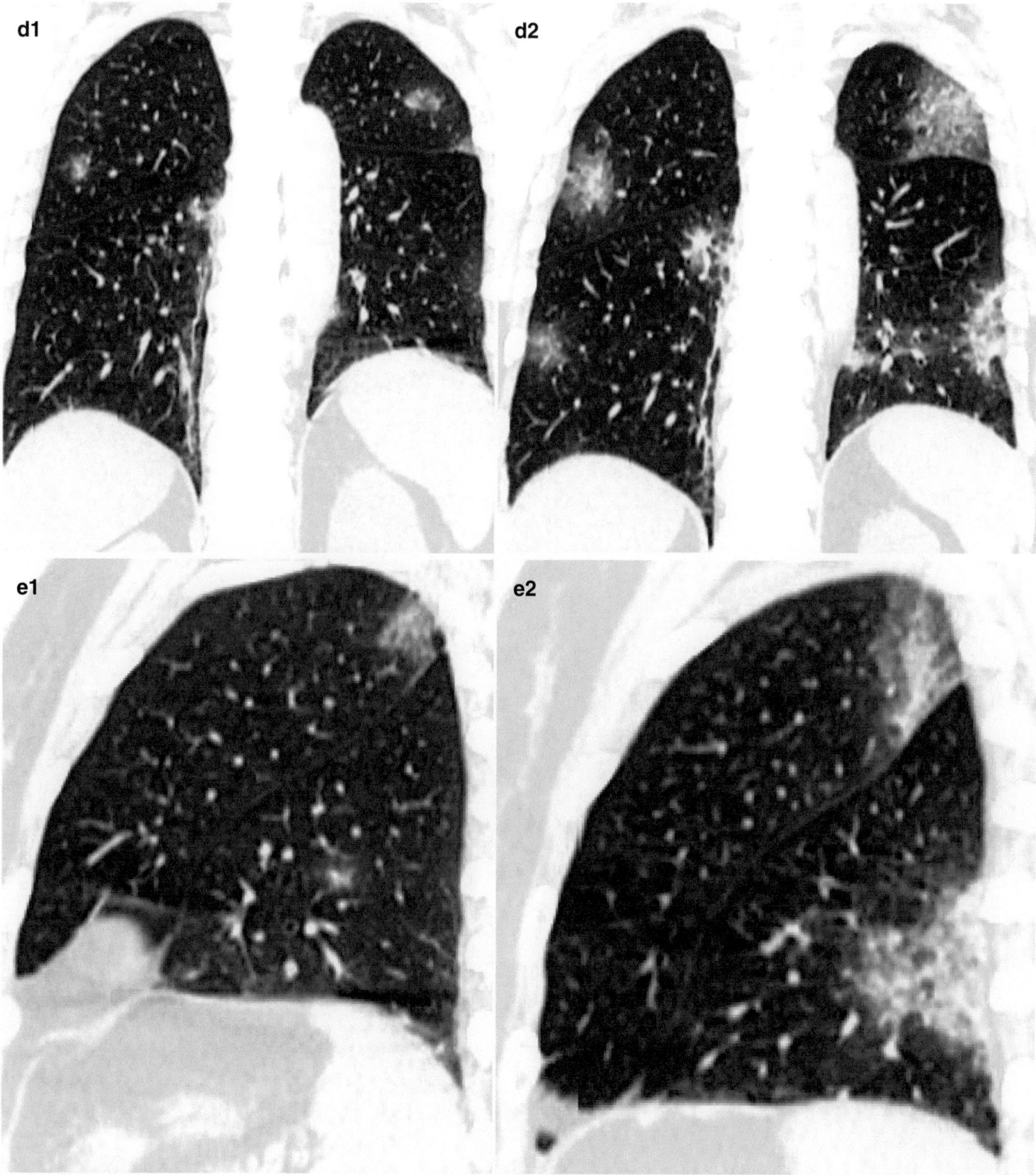

Fig. 4.2 (continued)

4.4 Case 3 (Fig. 4.3a1–e1, a2–e2)

A 63-year-old male patient presented with shortness of breath for 10 days. Fever occurred 3 days ago, and admission body temperature was 37.8 °C. White blood cell count, lymphocyte count, and C-reactive protein were 6.70×10^9/L, 1.34×10^9/L, and 39.68 mg/L, respectively. The patient underwent chest CT scans on day 13 and day 17 after the onset of symptoms and was confirmed by CDC in Guangzhou.

Chest CT on day 13 (a1–e1) showed diffuse ground-glass opacities with thickened interlobular septa and intralobular septa, manifested as typical crazy-paving sign. Chest CT on day 17 (a2–e2) demonstrated a significantly increase of consolidation.

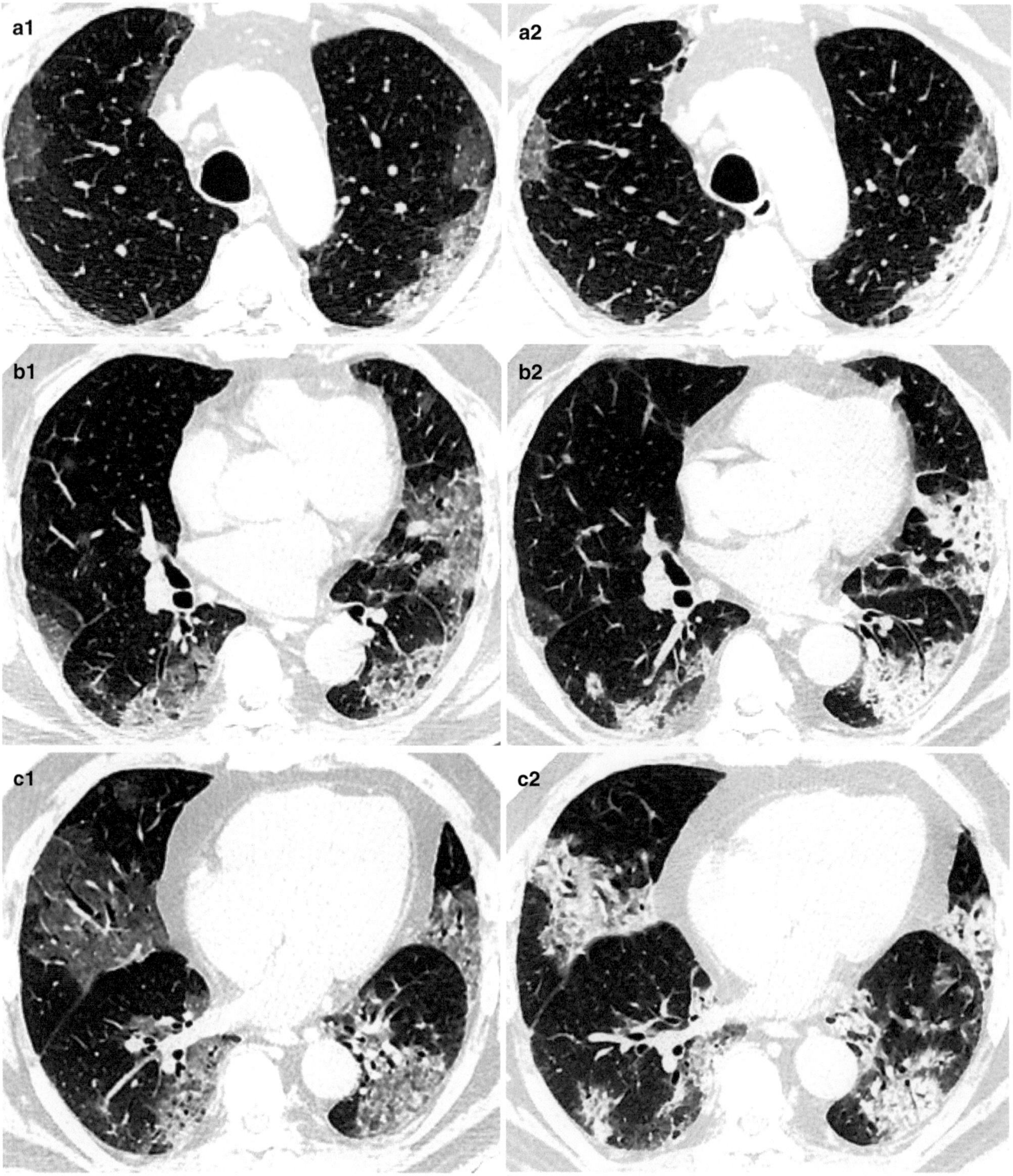

Fig. 4.3 Chest CT on day 13 (**a**1–**e**1) showed diffuse ground-glass opacities with thickened interlobular septa and intralobular septa, manifested as typical crazy-paving sign. Chest CT on day 17 (**a2**–**e2**) demonstrated a significantly increase of consolidation

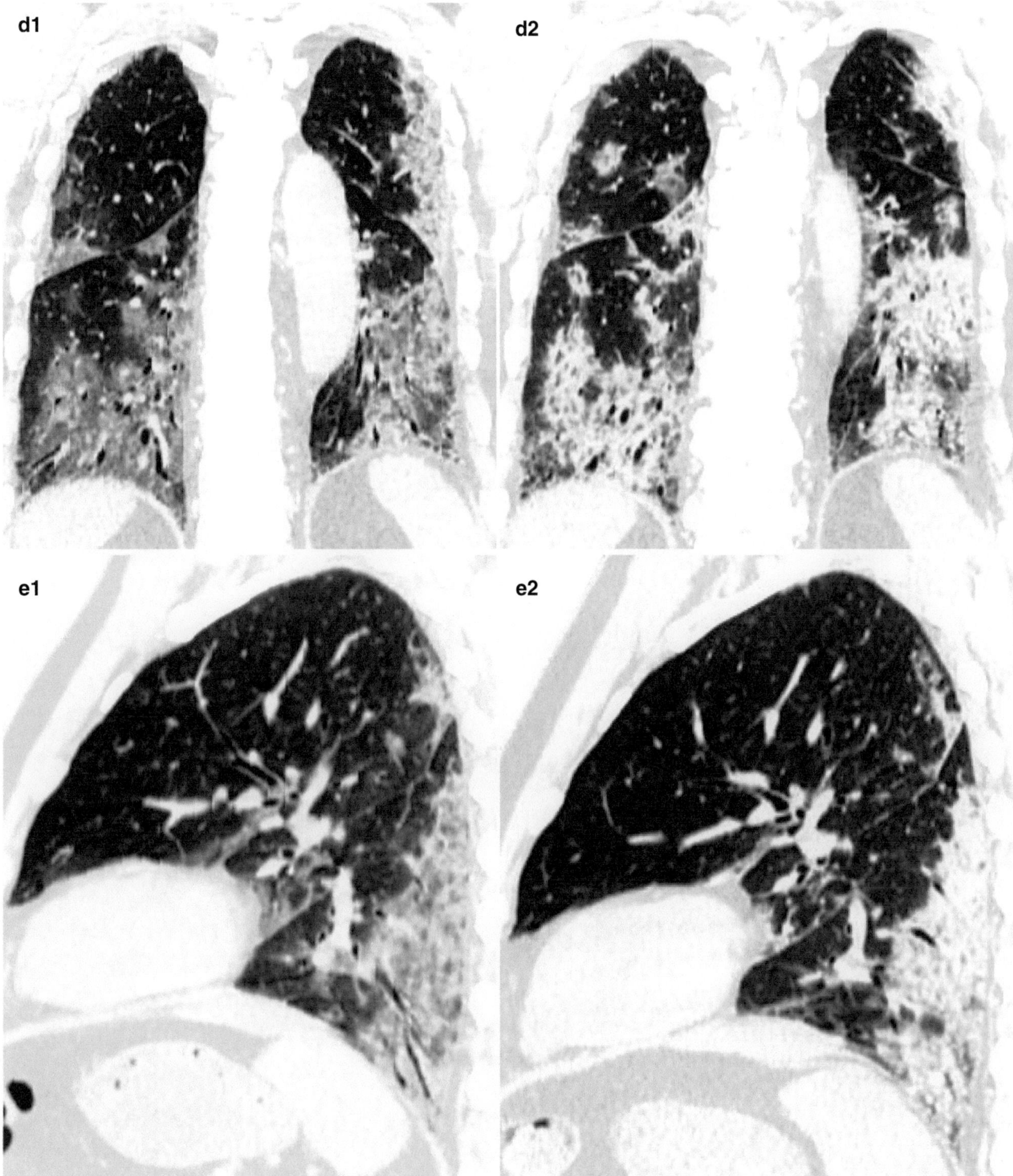

Fig. 4.3 (continued)

4.5 Case 4 (Fig. 4.4a1–e1, a2–e2)

A 37-year-old male patient with a disease-related exposure history had fever, which occurred 4 days ago, and admission body temperature was 39.2 °C. White blood cell count, lymphocyte count, and C-reactive protein were 5.50×10^9/L, 1.95×10^9/L, and 34.59 mg/L, respectively. The patient underwent chest CT scans on day 6 and day 10 after the onset of symptoms and was confirmed by CDC in Guangzhou.

Chest CT on day 6 (a1–e1) showed multifocal ground-glass opacities with interlobular and intralobular septal thickening and linear opacities in the bilateral lung, mainly in the peripheral field of the lung. Typical crazy-paving sign (black arrow) and subpleural linear opacity can be seen (white arrow). Chest CT on day 10 (a2–e2) demonstrated the enlargement of lesions.

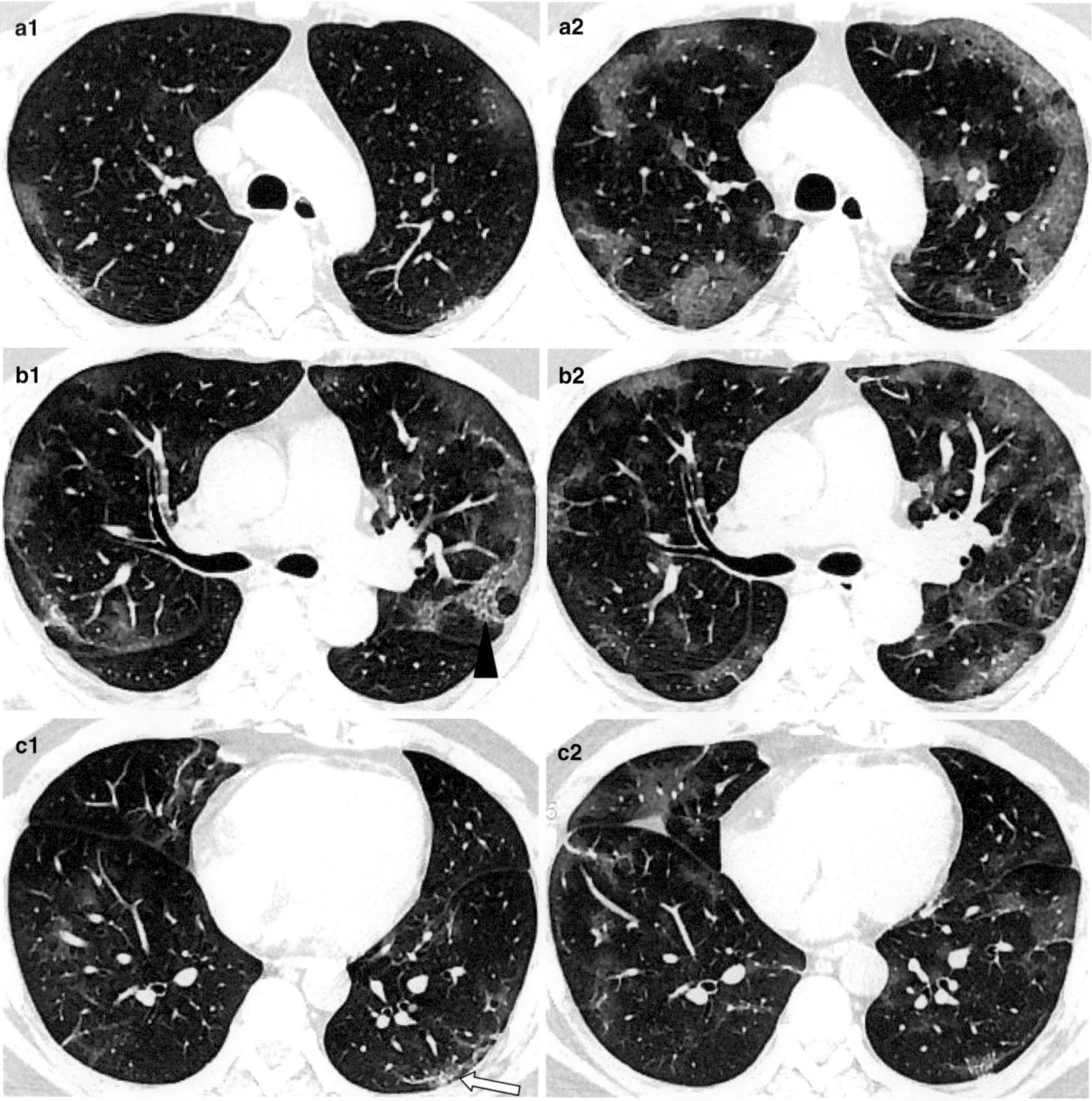

Fig. 4.4 Chest CT on day 6 (**a**1–**e**1) showed multifocal ground-glass opacities with interlobular and intralobular septal thickening and linear opacities in the bilateral lung, mainly in the peripheral field of the lung. Typical crazy-paving sign (black arrow) and subpleural linear opacity can be seen (white arrow). Chest CT on day 10 (**a**2–**e**2) demonstrated the enlargement of lesions

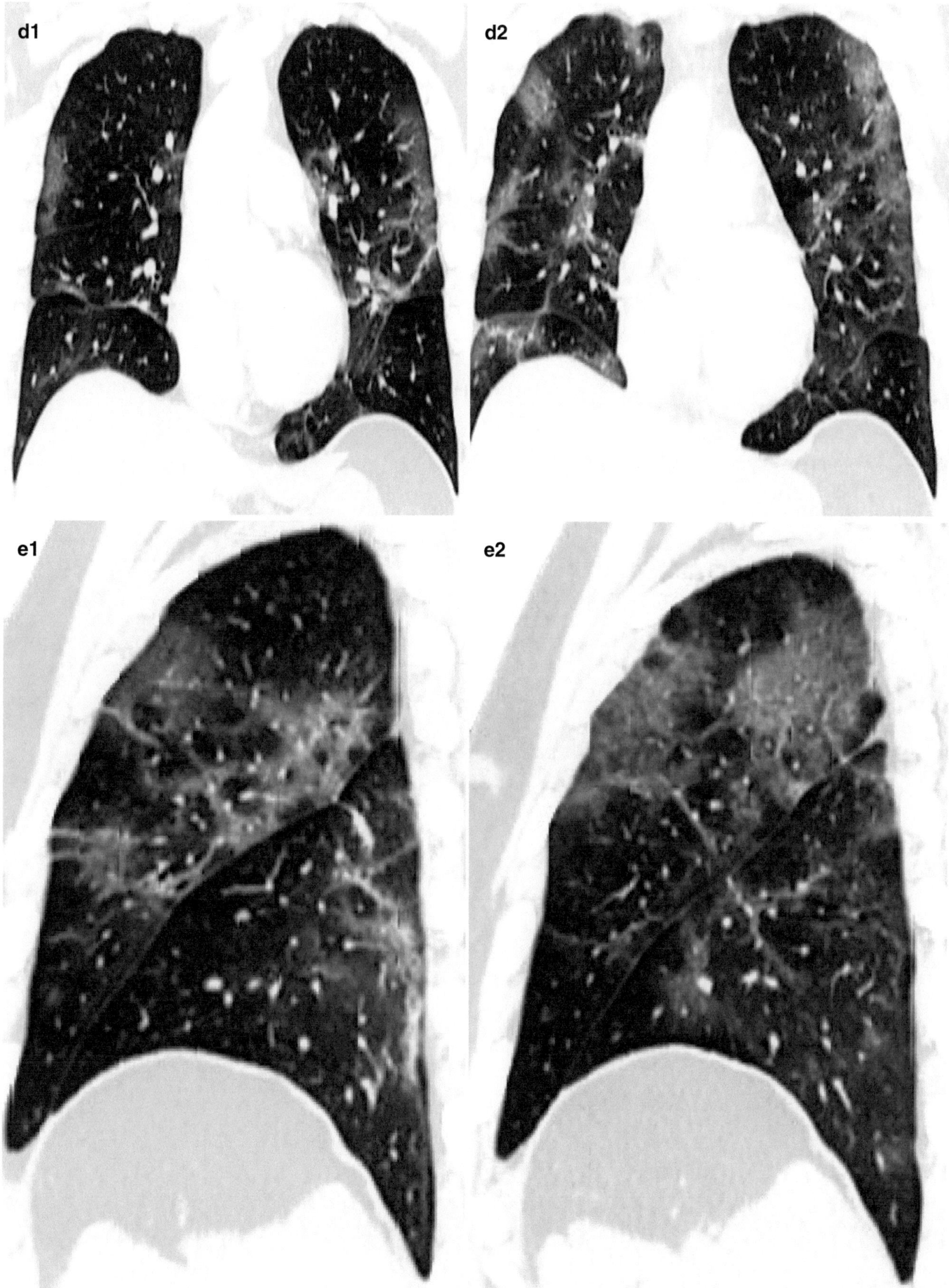

Fig. 4.4 (continued)

4.6 Case 5 (Fig. 4.5a1–e1, a2–e2)

A 33-year-old male patient with a disease-related exposure history presented with runny nose for 3 days. Fever occurred 1 day ago, accompanied by cough. Admission body temperature was 38.1 °C. White blood cell count, lymphocyte count, and C-reactive protein were 5.46×10^9/L, 1.10×10^9/L, and 16.77 mg/L, respectively. The patient underwent chest CT scans on day 5 and day 9 after the onset of symptoms and was confirmed by CDC in Guangzhou.

Chest CT on day 5 (a1–e1) showed nodular and patchy ground-glass opacities in the bilateral lung, mainly in the right lower lobe. Chest CT on day 9 (a2–e2) demonstrated rapid progression of lesions with patchy consolidation and linear opacities.

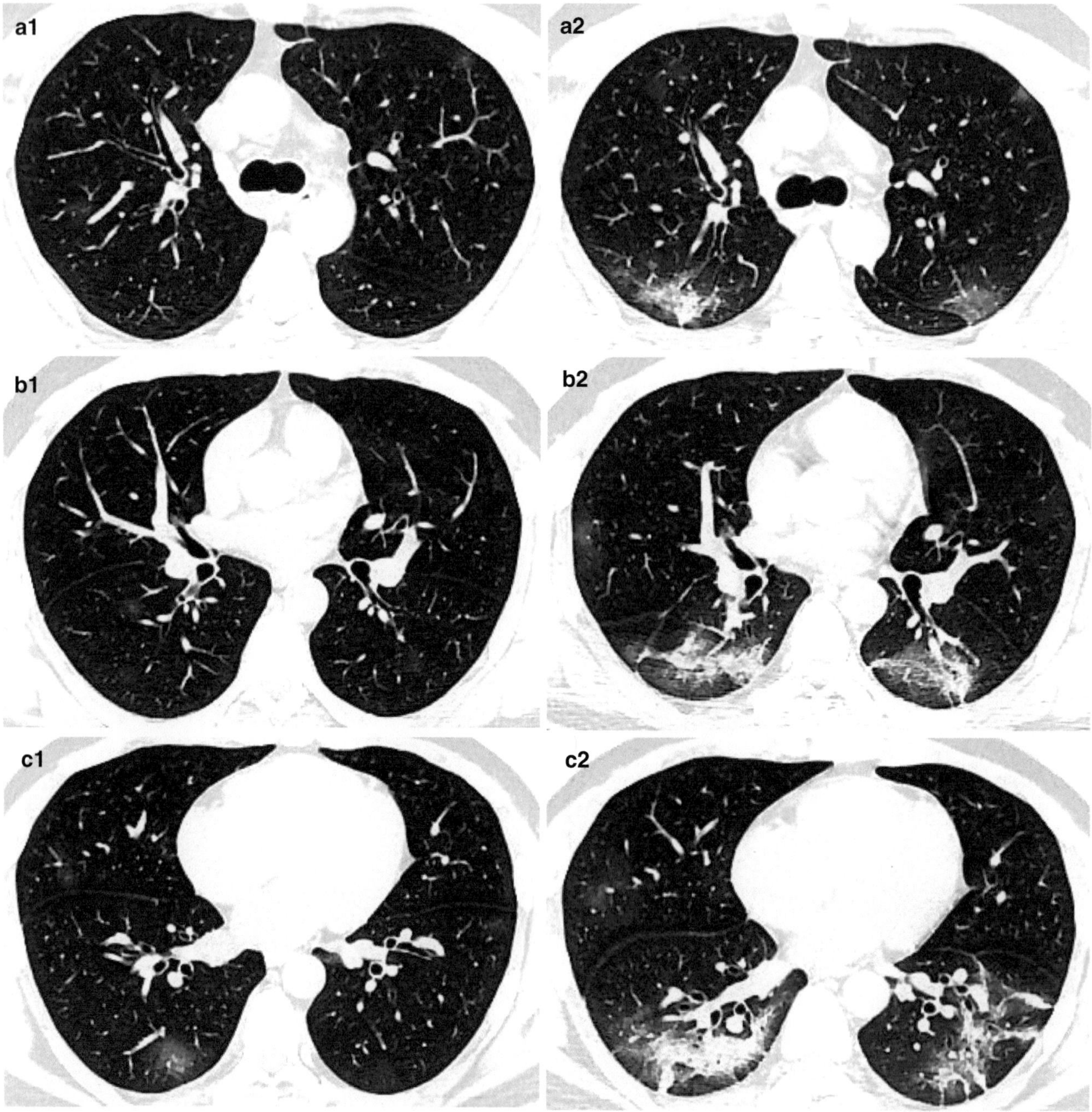

Fig. 4.5 Chest CT on day 5 (**a**1–**e**1) showed nodular and patchy ground-glass opacities in the bilateral lung, mainly in the right lower lobe. Chest CT on day 9 (**a**2–**e**2) demonstrated rapid progression of lesions with patchy consolidation and linear opacities

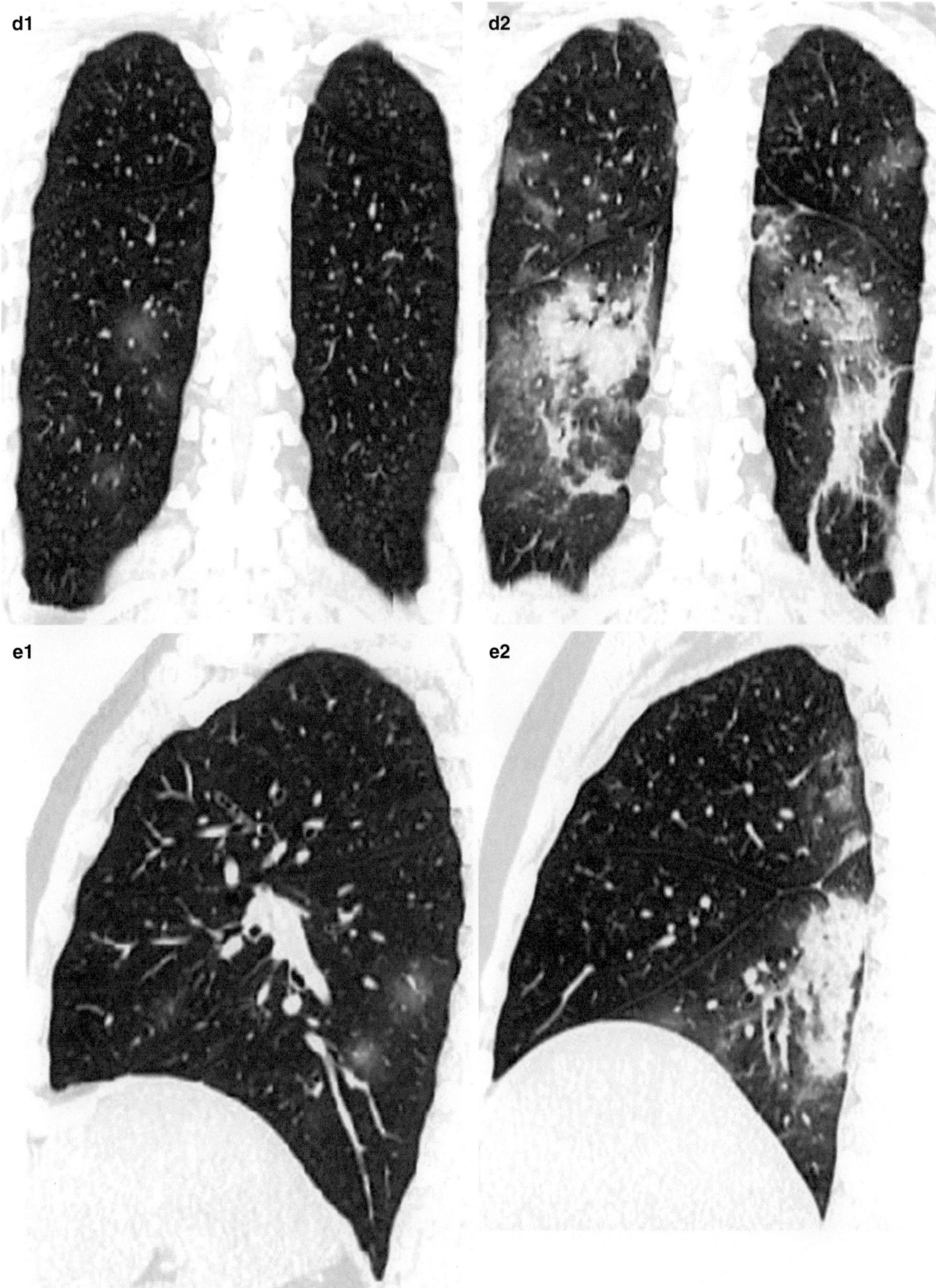

Fig. 4.5 (continued)

4.7 Case 6 (Fig. 4.6a1–e1, a2–e2)

A 29-year-old male patient with a disease-related exposure history presented with cough for 3 days. Admission body temperature was 37.8 °C. White blood cell count, lymphocyte count, and C-reactive protein were 7.93×10^9/L, 1.33×10^9/L, and 21.54 mg/L, respectively. The patient underwent chest CT scans on day 5 and day 9 after the onset of symptoms and was confirmed by CDC in Guangzhou.

Chest CT on day 5 (a1–e1) showed nodular and patchy ground-glass opacities in the bilateral lung. Chest CT on day 9 (a2–e2) demonstrated rapid progression of lesions with patchy consolidation and thickened intralobular septa.

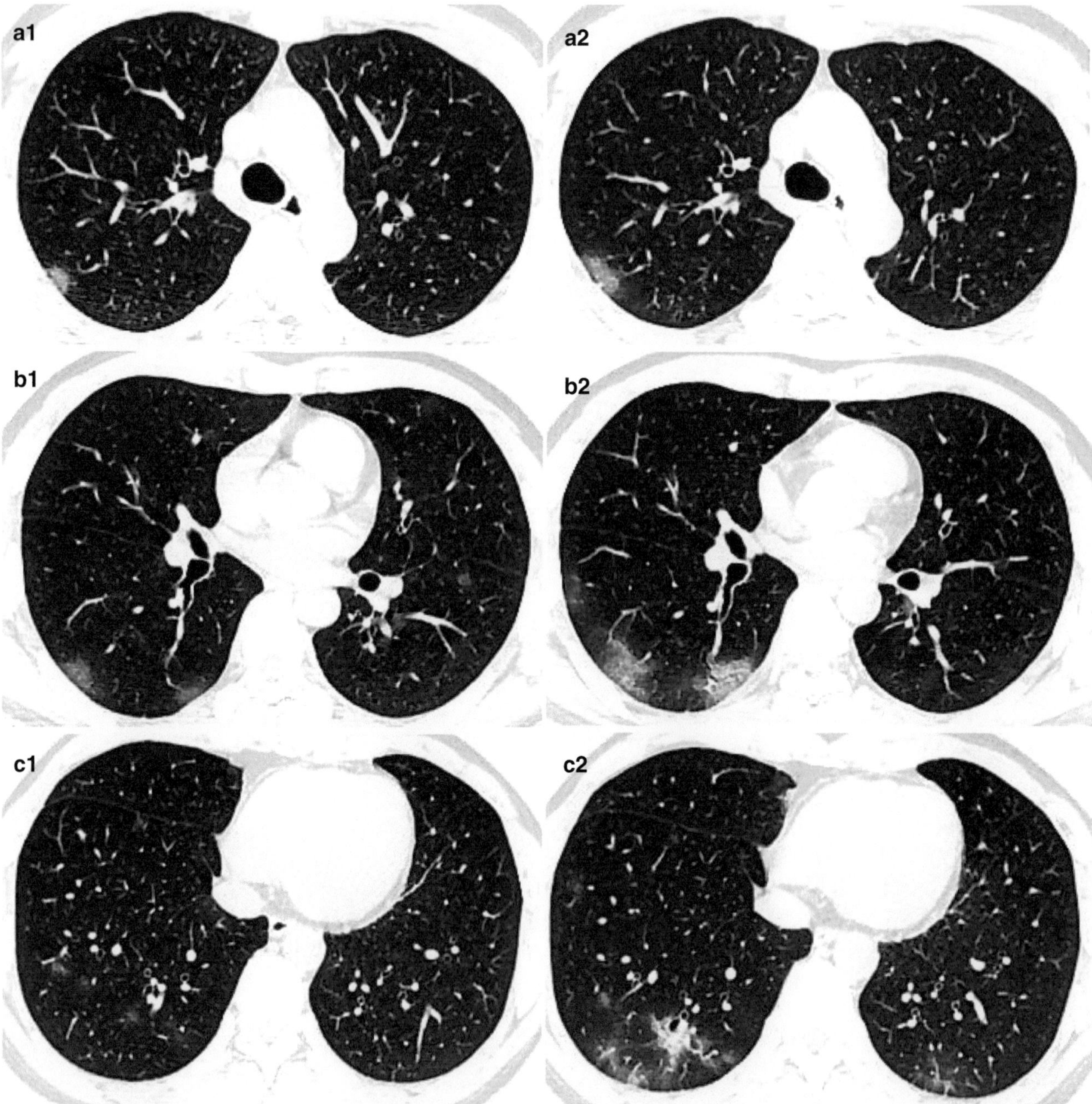

Fig. 4.6 Chest CT on day 5 (**a**1–**e**1) showed nodular and patchy ground-glass opacities in the bilateral lung. Chest CT on day 9 (**a**2–**e**2) demonstrated rapid progression of lesions with patchy consolidation and thickened intralobular septa

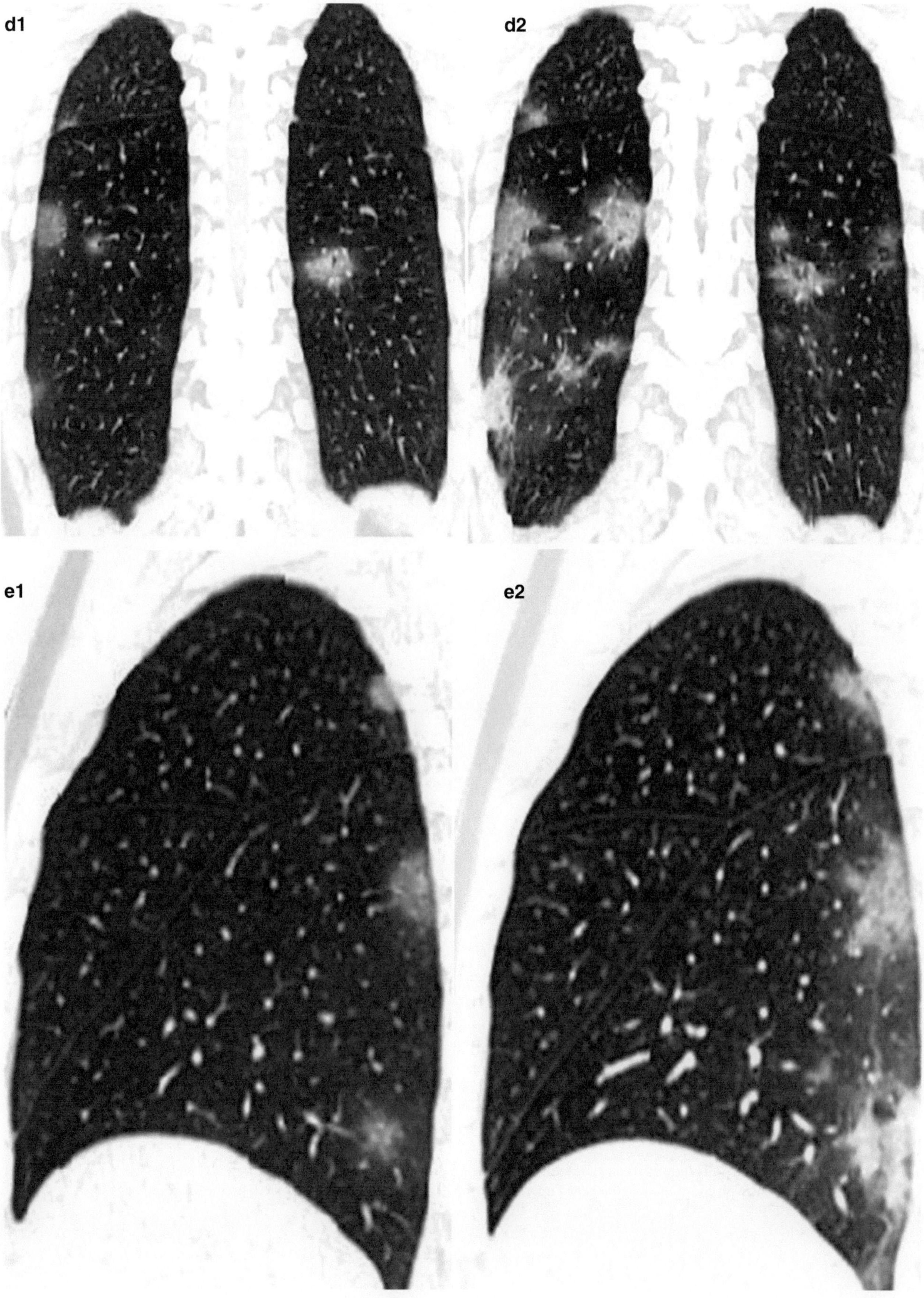

Fig. 4.6 (continued)

4.8 Case 7 (Fig. 4.7a1–e1, a2–e2)

A 30-year-old male patient with a disease-related exposure history had fever, which occurred 4 days ago, accompanied by cough, chills, myalgia, and headache. Admission body temperature was 39.1 °C. White blood cell count, lymphocyte count, and C-reactive protein were 5.25×10^9/L, 2.64×10^9/L, and <10 mg/L, respectively. The patient underwent chest CT scans on day 7 and day 11 after the onset of symptoms and was confirmed by CDC in Guangzhou.

Chest CT on day 7 (a1–e1) showed patchy consolidation in the lower lobe of the bilateral lung. Chest CT on day 11 (a2–e2) demonstrated rapid progression of lesions with consolidation, thickened interlobular septa, and subpleural linear opacity in the bilateral lung.

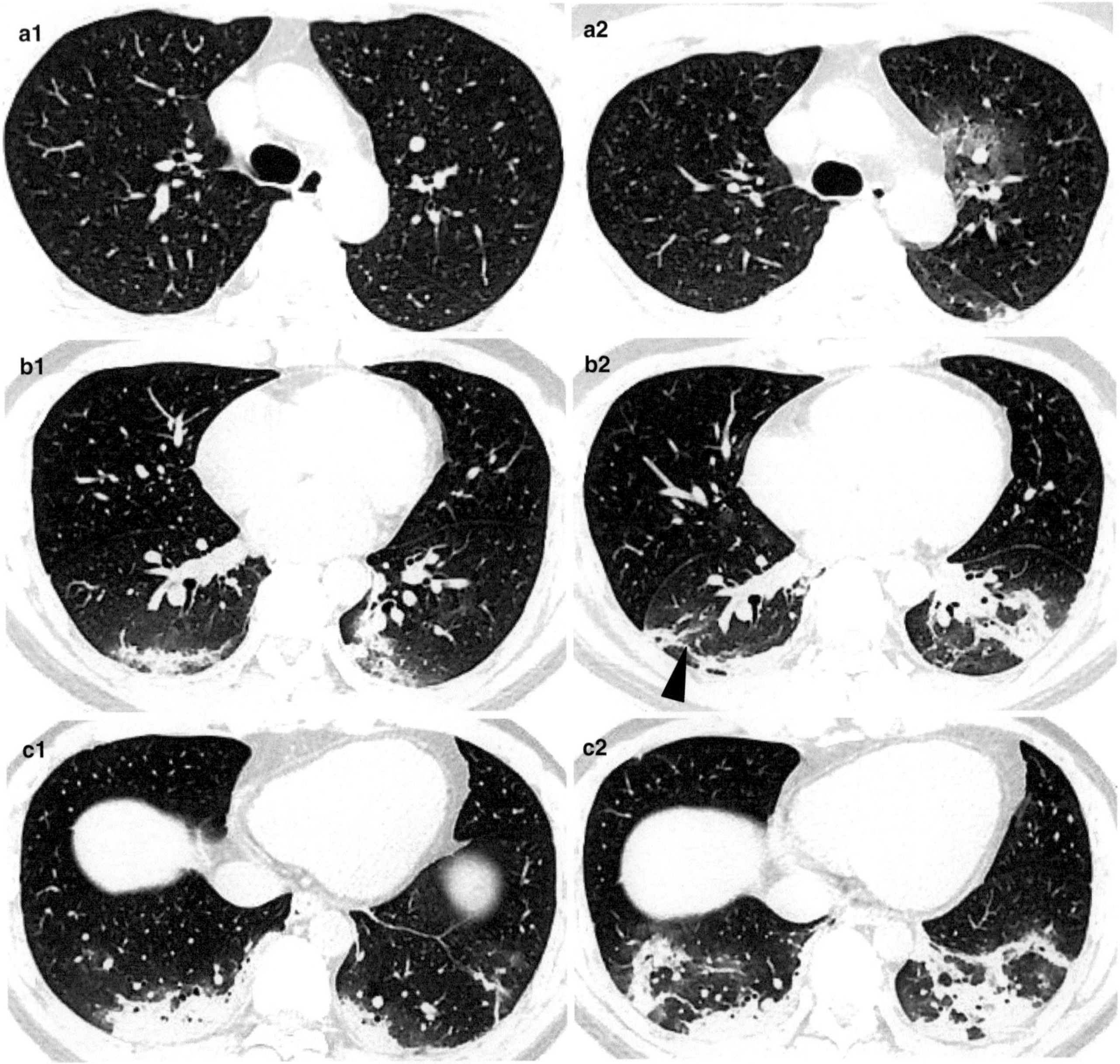

Fig. 4.7 Chest CT on day 7 (**a**1–**e**1) showed patchy consolidation in the lower lobe of the bilateral lung. Chest CT on day 11 (**a**2–**e**2) demonstrated rapid progression of lesions with consolidation, thickened interlobular septa, and subpleural linear opacity in the bilateral lung

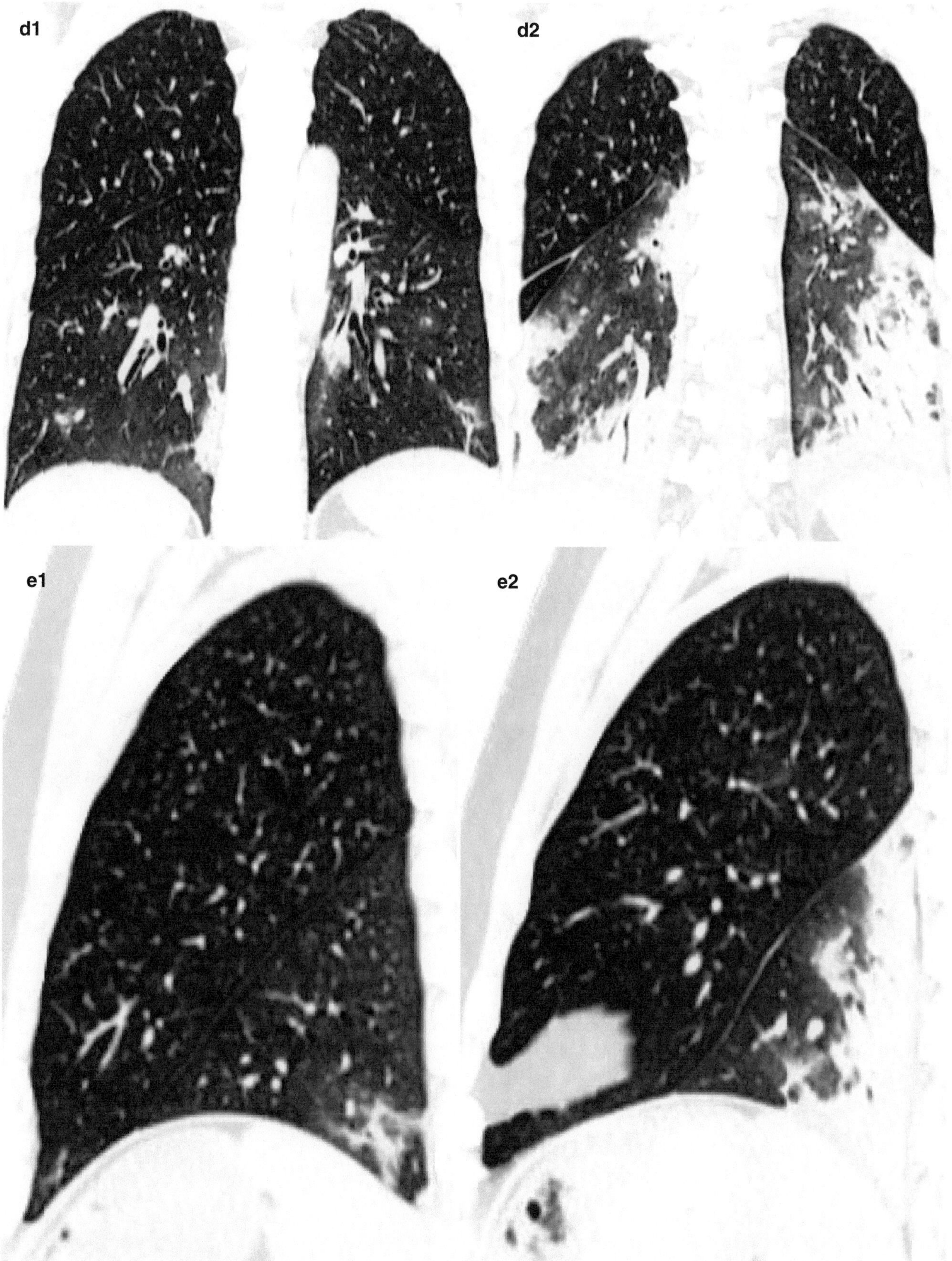

Fig. 4.7 (continued)

4.9 Case 8 (Fig. 4.8a1–e1, a2–e2)

A 50-year-old female patient with a disease-related exposure history presented with cough for 3 days. Fever occurred 1 day ago, and admission body temperature was 38.0 °C. White blood cell count, lymphocyte count, and C-reactive protein were 4.35×10^9/L, 1.44×10^9/L, and 12.16 mg/L, respectively. The patient underwent chest CT scans on day 5 and day 9 after the onset of symptoms and was confirmed by CDC in Guangzhou.

Chest CT on day 5 (a1–e1) showed nodular ground-glass opacities with reversed halo sign in the right lung (white arrow). Chest CT on day 9 (a2–e2) demonstrated the shrink of reversed halo sign, replaced by the enlargement of lesions with consolidation and linear opacities in the bilateral lung.

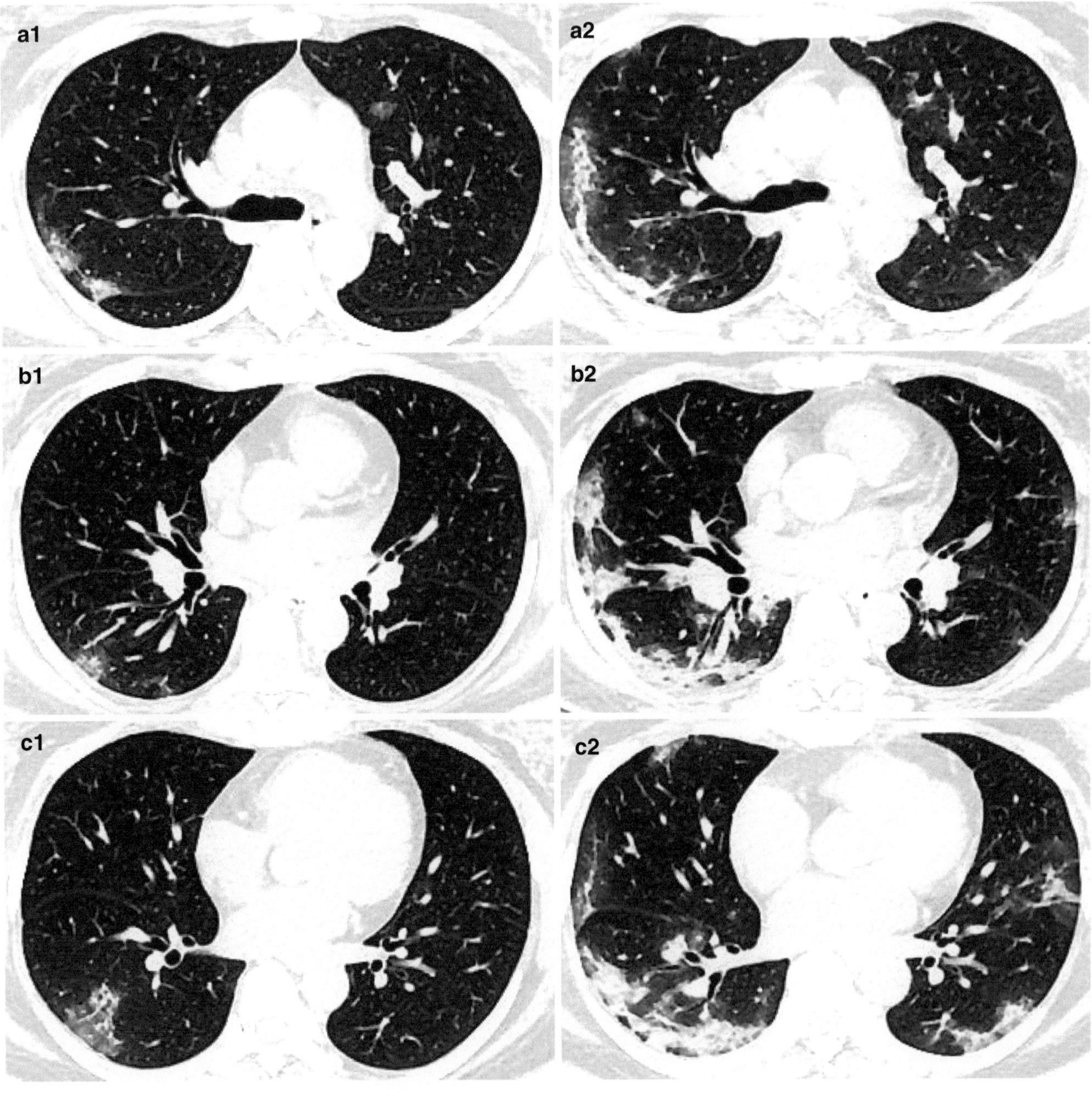

Fig. 4.8 Chest CT on day 5 (**a**1–**e**1) showed nodular ground-glass opacities with reversed halo sign in the right lung (white arrow). Chest CT on day 9 (**a**2–**e**2) demonstrated the shrink of reversed halo sign, replaced by the enlargement of lesions with consolidation and linear opacities in the bilateral lung

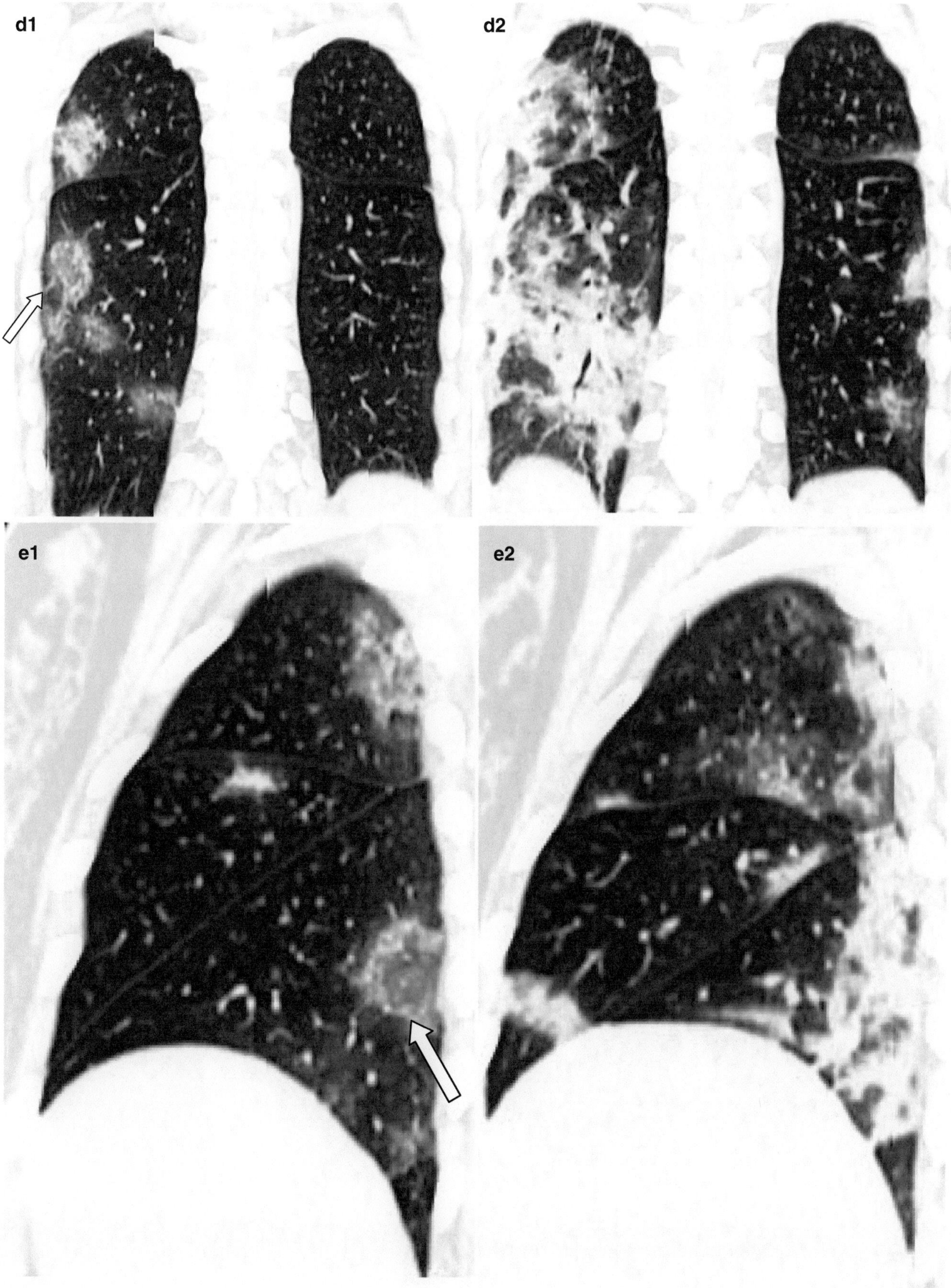

Fig. 4.8 (continued)

4.10 **Case 9** (Fig. 4.9a1–e1, a2–e2)

A 39-year-old female patient with a disease-related exposure history had fever, which occurred 1 day ago, and admission body temperature was 36.7 °C. White blood cell count, lymphocyte count, and C-reactive protein were 4.83×10^9/L, 1.11×10^9/L, and <10 mg/L, respectively. The patient underwent chest CT scans on day 9 and day 12 after the onset of symptoms and was confirmed by CDC in Guangzhou.

Chest CT on day 9 (a1–e1) showed patchy ground-glass opacities in the right lower lobe. Chest CT on day 12 (a2–e2) demonstrated the enlargement of lesions with intralobular and interlobular septal thickening.

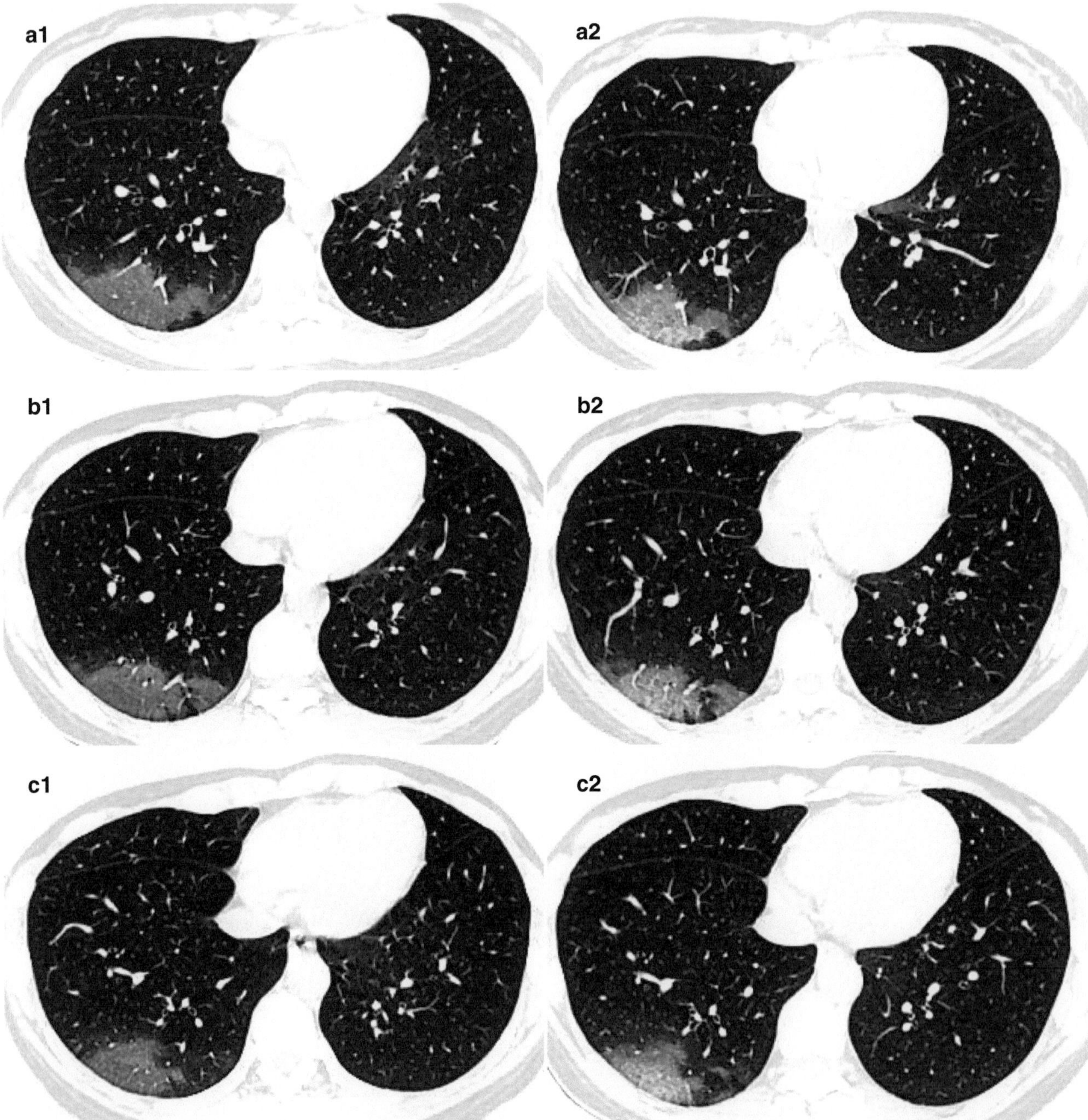

Fig. 4.9 Chest CT on day 9 (**a**1–**e**1) showed patchy ground-glass opacities in the right lower lobe. Chest CT on day 12 (**a**2–**e**2) demonstrated the enlargement of lesions with intralobular and interlobular septal thickening

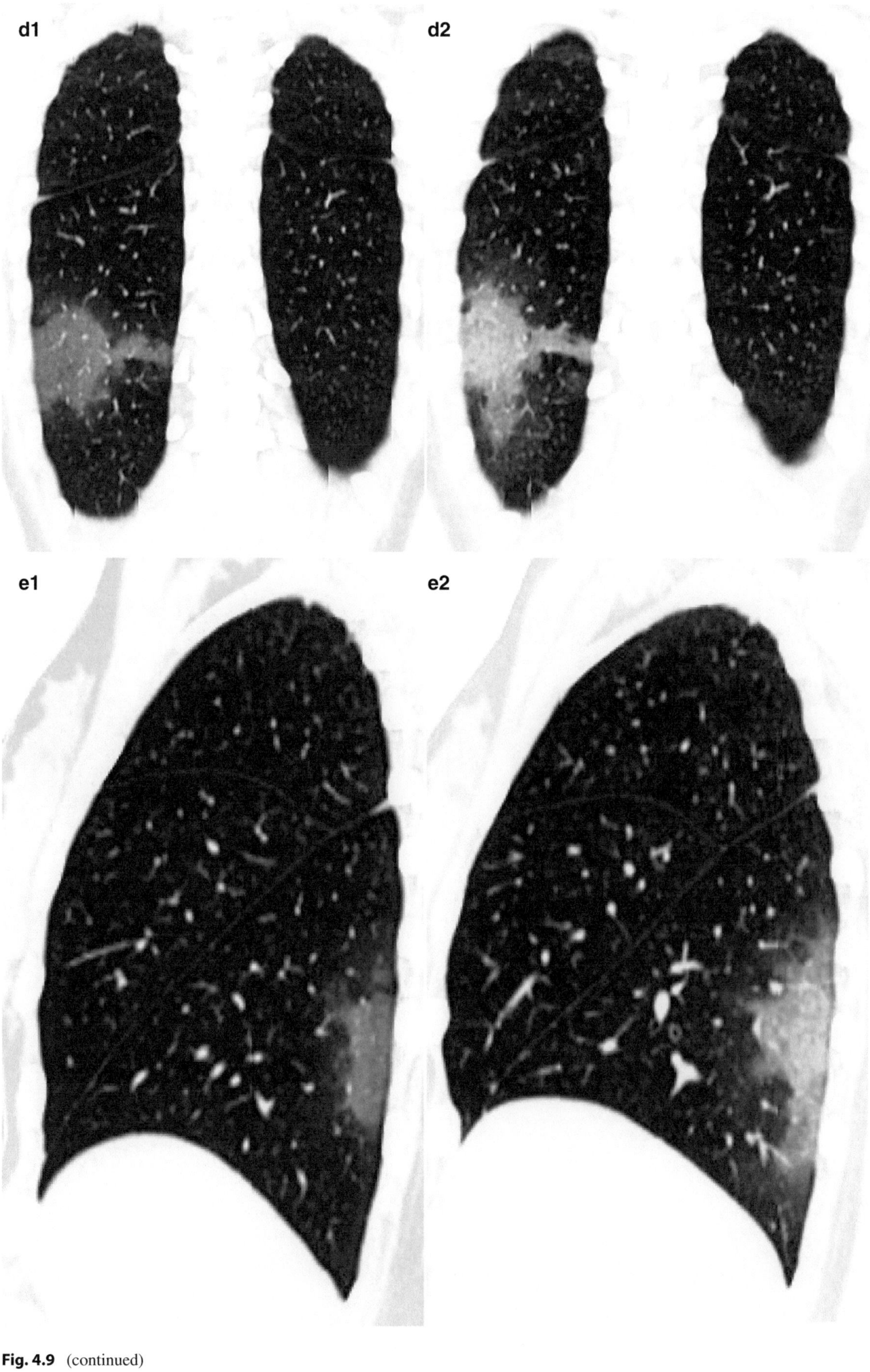

Fig. 4.9 (continued)

4.11 Case 10 (Fig. 4.10a1–e1, a2–e2)

A 70-year-old male patient with a disease-related exposure history had fever, which occurred 8 days ago, accompanied by cough, chills, myalgia, and fatigue. Admission body temperature was 37.8 °C. White blood cell count, lymphocyte count, and C-reactive protein were 7.05 × 10^9/L, 0.56 × 10^9/L, and 92.82 mg/L, respectively. The patient underwent chest CT scans on day 11 and day 15 after the onset of symptoms and was confirmed by CDC in Guangzhou.

Chest CT on day 11 (a1–e1) showed diffuse patchy ground-glass opacities with thickened intralobular and interlobular septa in the bilateral lung. Chest CT on day 15 (a2–e2) demonstrated the enlargement of lesions with typical crazy-paving sign and lobular consolidation.

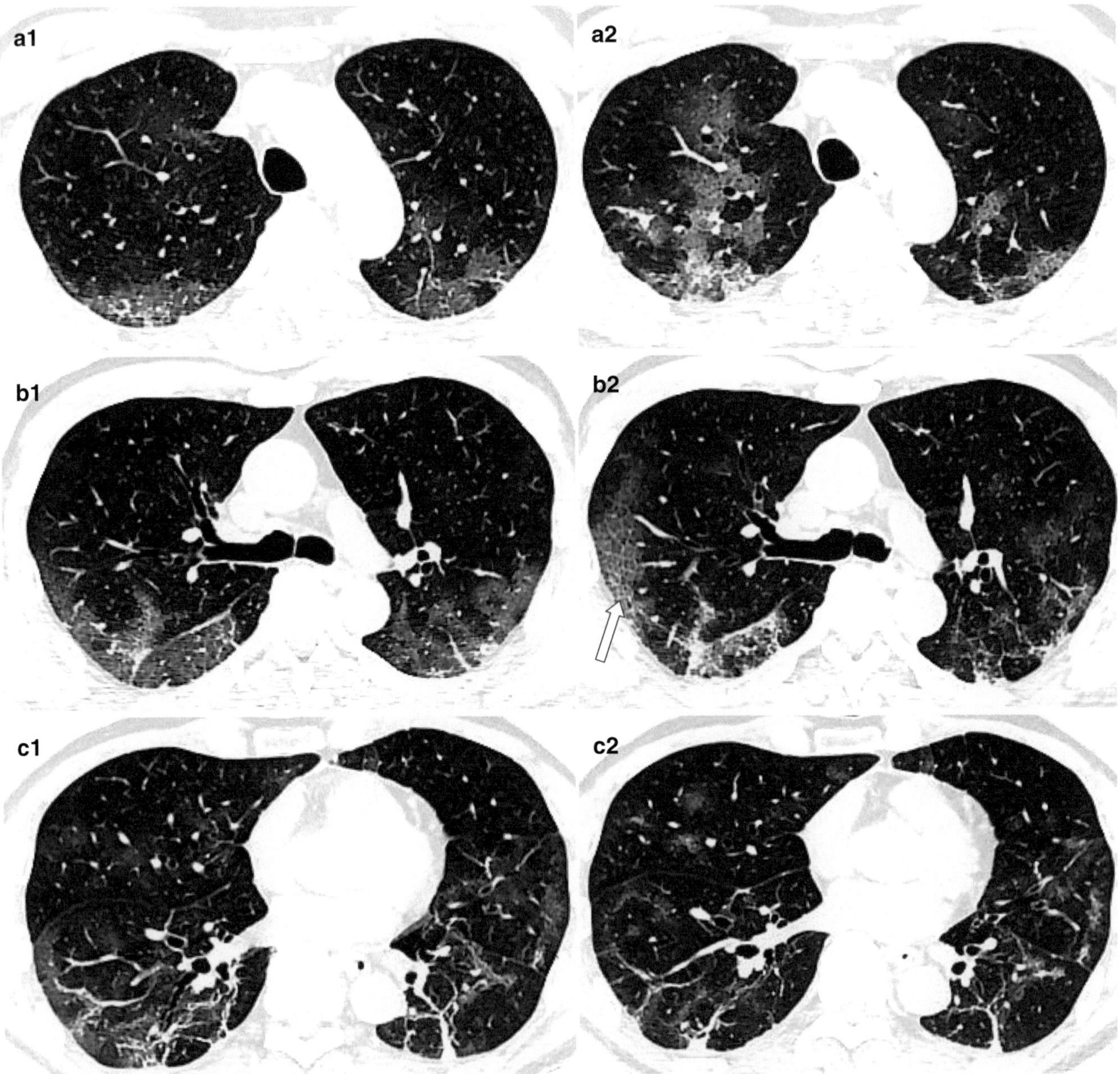

Fig. 4.10 Chest CT on day 11 (**a**1–**e**1) showed diffuse patchy ground-glass opacities with thickened intralobular and interlobular septa in the bilateral lung. Chest CT on day 15 (**a**2–**e**2) demonstrated the enlargement of lesions with typical crazy-paving sign and lobular consolidation

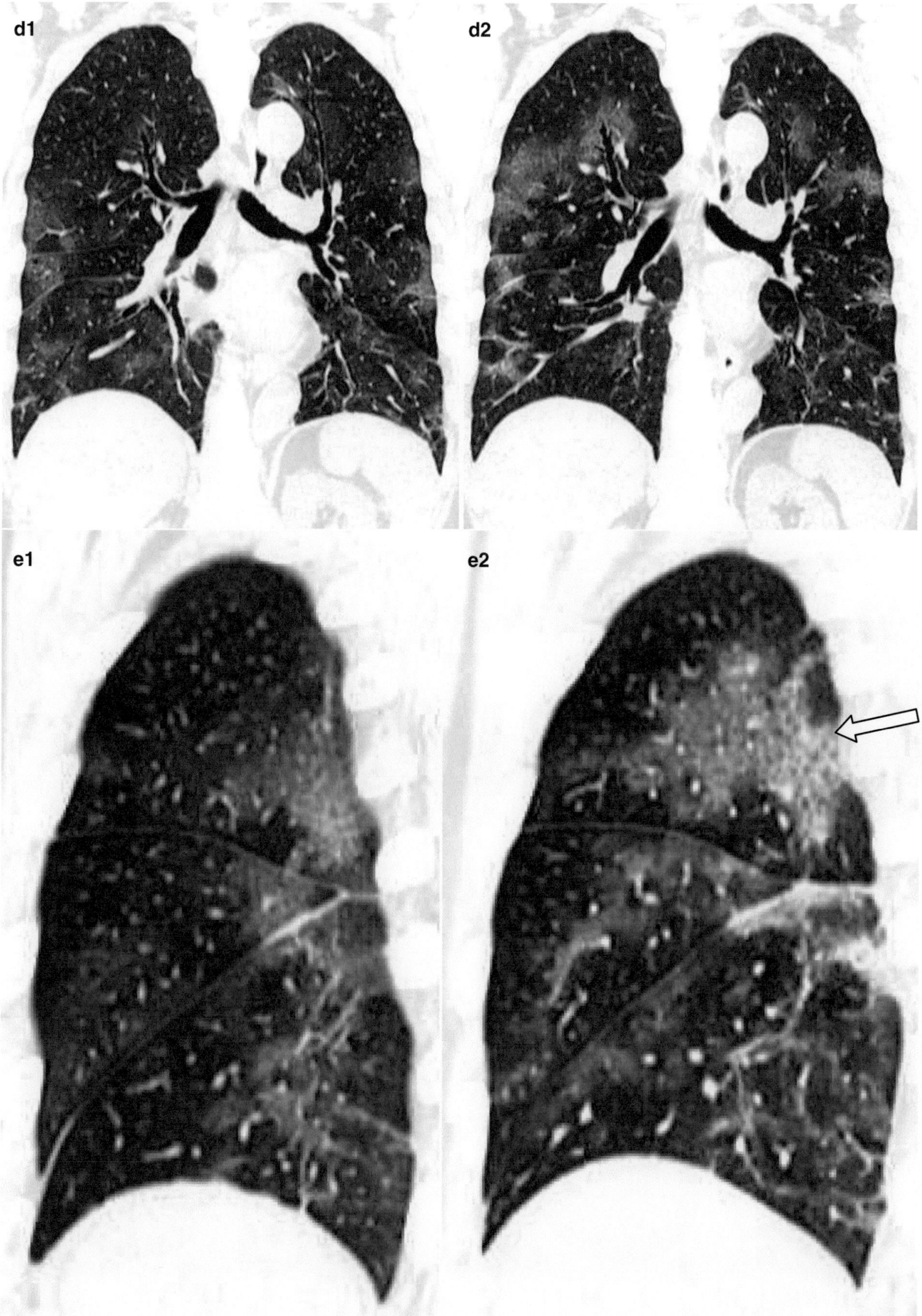

Fig. 4.10 (continued)

4.12 Case 11 (Fig. 4.11a1–e1, a2–e2)

A 64-year-old female patient with a disease-related exposure history presented with fever for 8 days. Admission body temperature was 38.2 °C. White blood cell count, lymphocyte count, and C-reactive protein were 3.48×10^9/L, 1.56×10^9/L, and 25.68 mg/L, respectively. The patient underwent chest CT scans on day 10 and day 13 after the onset of symptoms and was confirmed by CDC in Guangzhou.

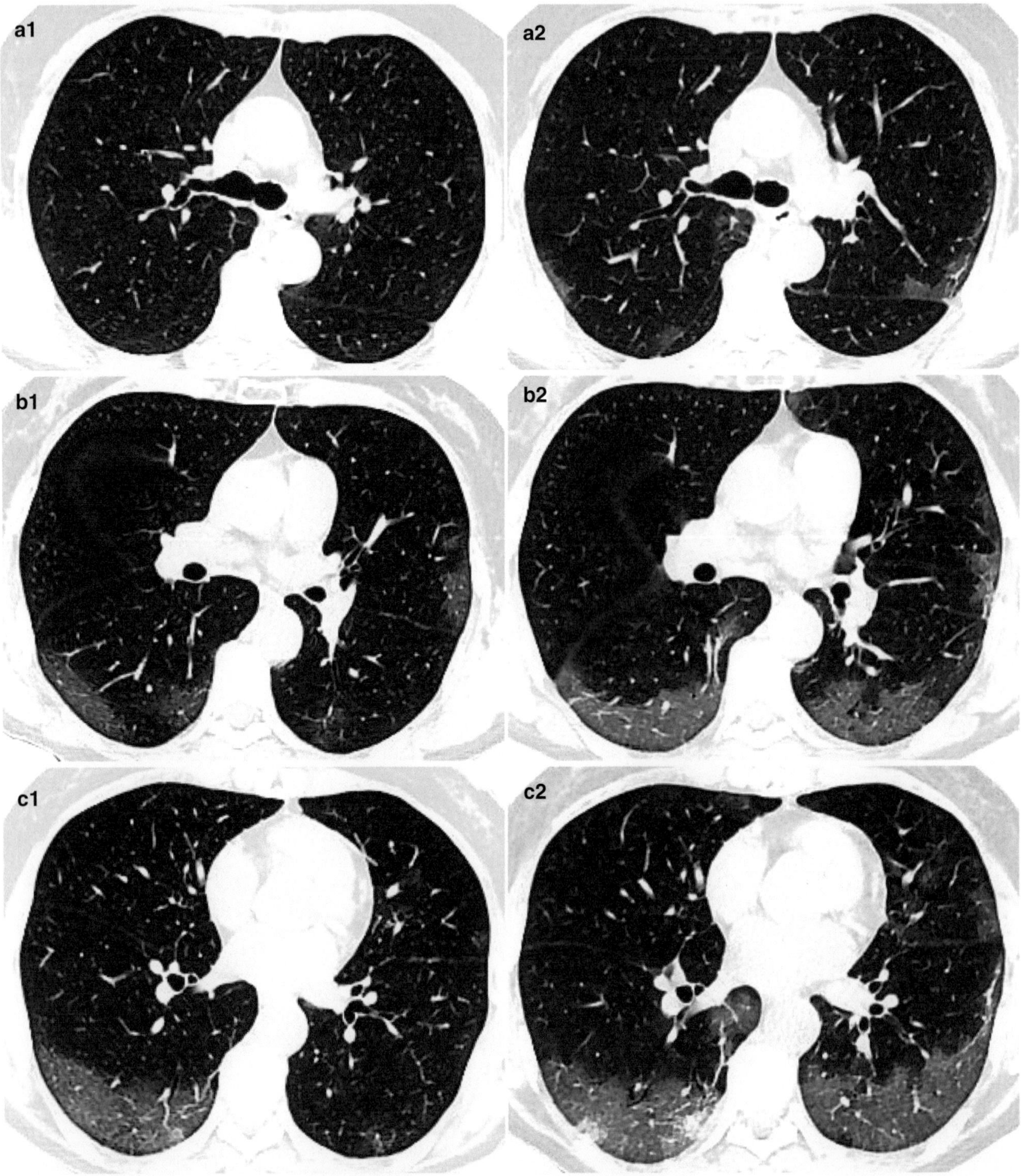

Fig. 4.11 Chest CT on day 10 (**a**1–**e**1) showed multifocal patchy ground-glass opacities in the bilateral lung. Chest CT on day 13 (**a**2–**e**2) demonstrated the enlargement of lesions with lobular consolidation and linear opacities

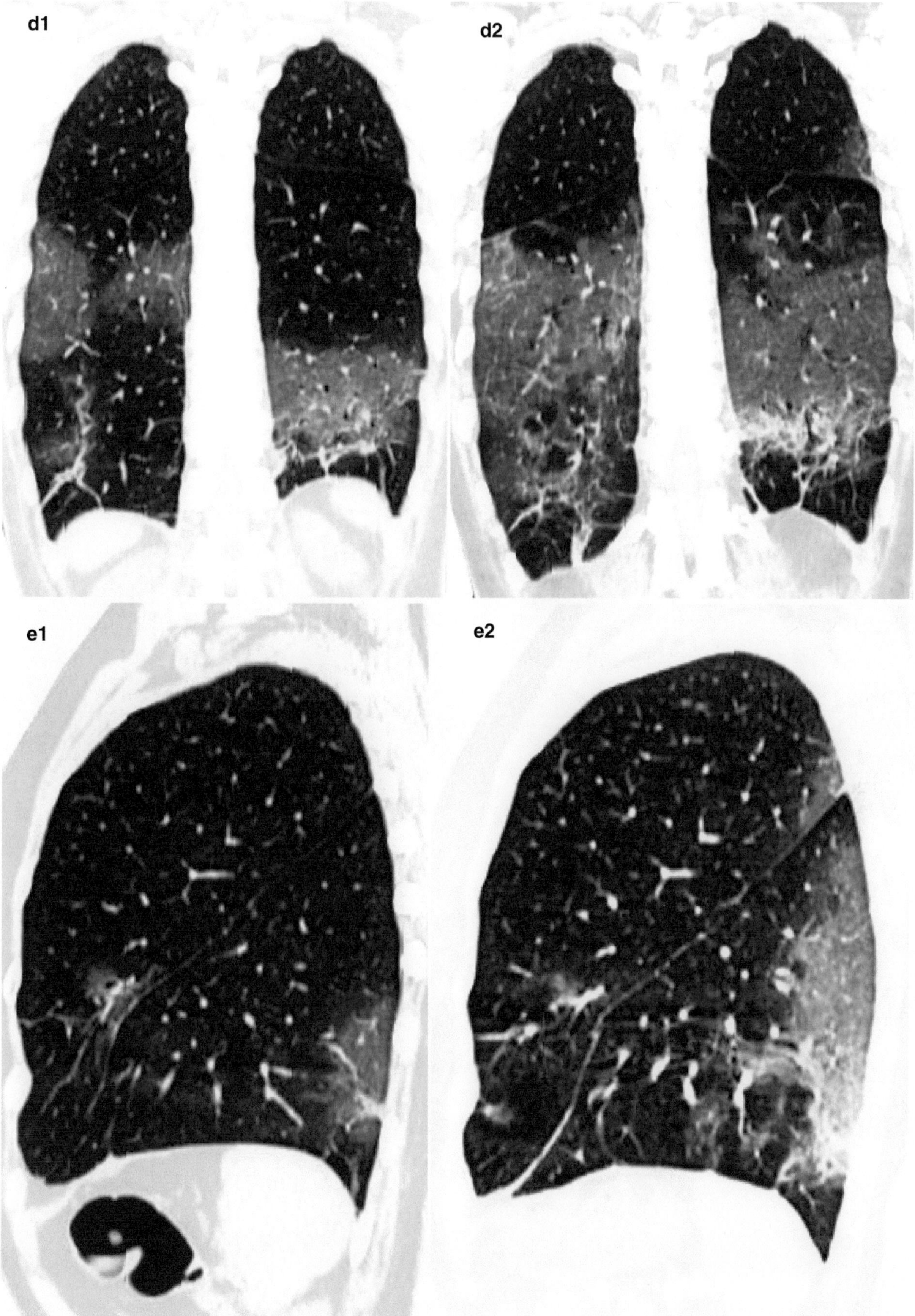

Fig. 4.11 (continued)

Chest CT on day 10 (a1–e1) showed multifocal patchy ground-glass opacities in the bilateral lung. Chest CT on day 13 (a2–e2) demonstrated the enlargement of lesions with lobular consolidation and linear opacities.

4.13 Case 12 (Fig. 4.12a1–e1, a2–e2)

A 58-year-old male patient with a disease-related exposure history presented with cough for 7 days. Fever occurred 1 day ago, and admission body temperature was 38.5 °C. White

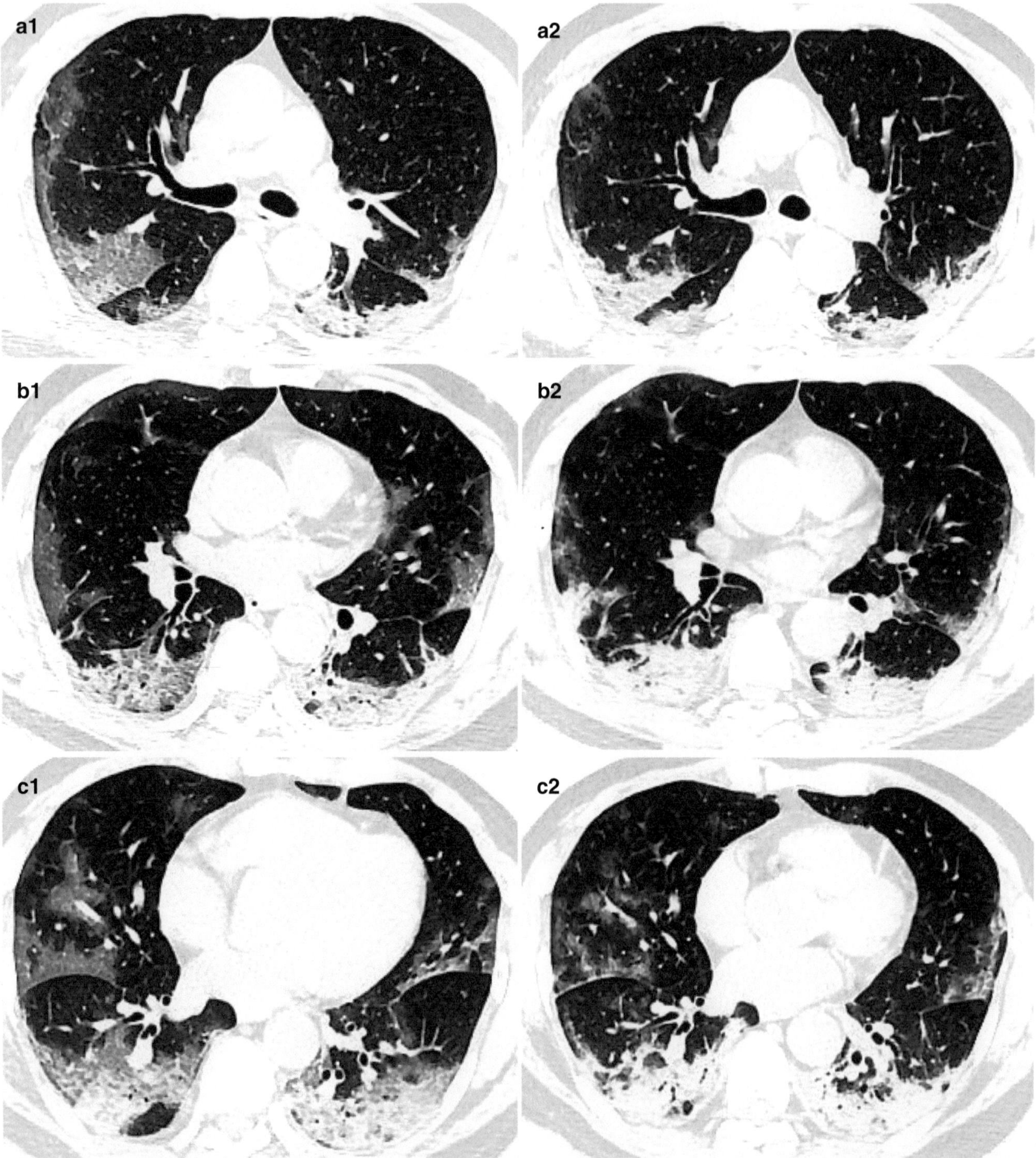

Fig. 4.12 Chest CT on day 10 (**a**1–**e**1) showed multifocal patchy ground-glass opacities with thickened interlobular septa and lobular consolidation in the bilateral lung. Chest CT on day 15 (**a**2–**e**2) demonstrated the enlargement of lesions with patchy consolidation

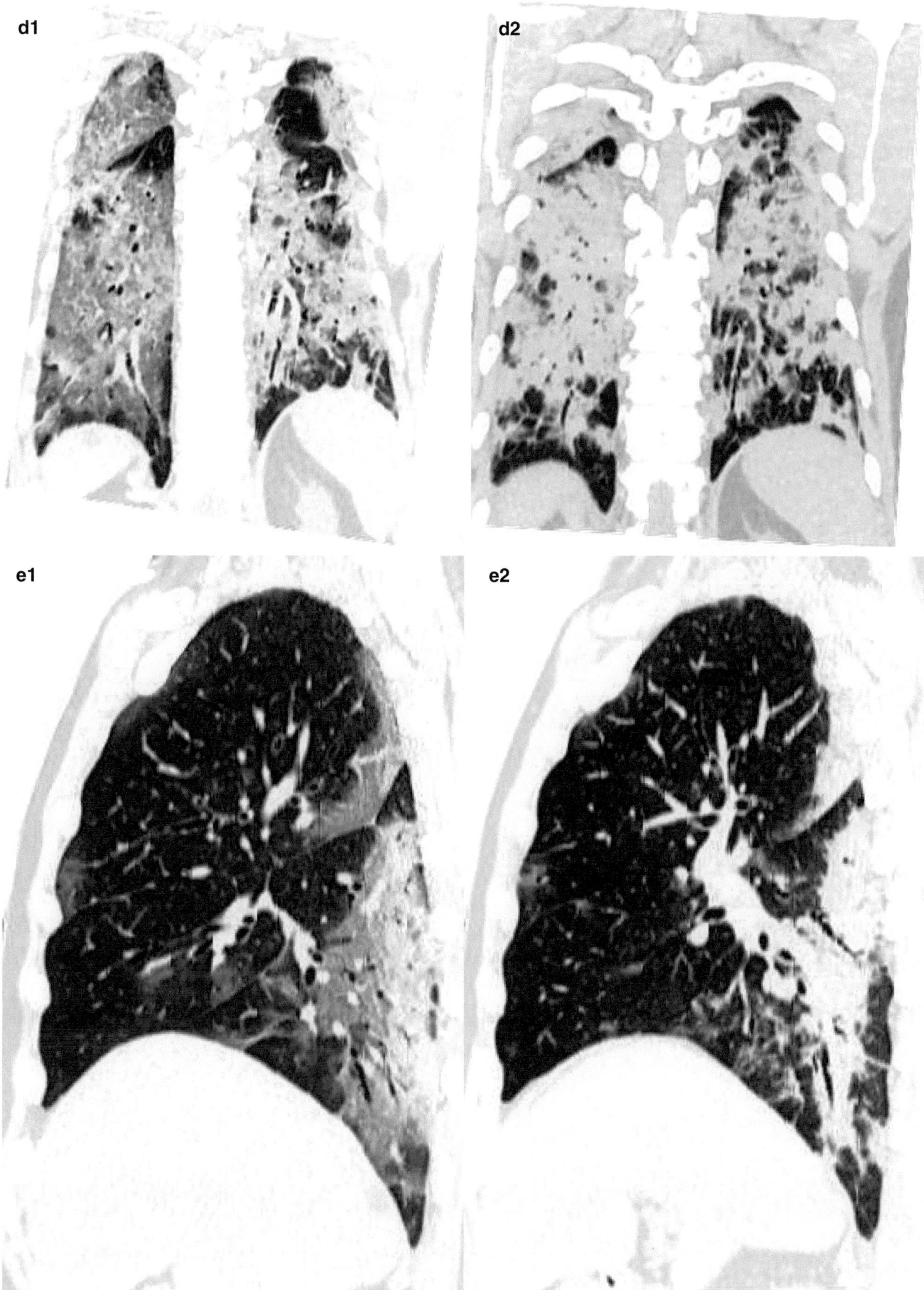

Fig. 4.12 (continued)

blood cell count, lymphocyte count, and C-reactive protein were 2.61 × 10^9/L, 0.53 × 10^9/L, and 74.43 mg/L, respectively. The patient underwent chest CT scans on day 10 and day 15 after the onset of symptoms and was confirmed by CDC in Guangzhou.

Chest CT on day 10 (a1–e1) showed multifocal patchy ground-glass opacities with thickened interlobular septa and lobular consolidation in the bilateral lung. Chest CT on day 15 (a2–e2) demonstrated the enlargement of lesions with patchy consolidation.

References

1. Jin YH, Cai L, Cheng ZS, et al. A rapid advice guideline for the diagnosis and treatment of 2019 novel coronavirus (2019-nCoV) infected pneumonia (standard version). Mil Med Res. 2020;7(1):4. https://doi.org/10.1186/s40779-020-0233-6.
2. Song F, Shi N, Shan F, et al. Emerging coronavirus 2019-nCoV pneumonia. Radiology. 2020;295(1):210–7. https://doi.org/10.1148/radiol.2020200274. Epub 2020 Feb 6
3. Pan Y, Guan H, Zhou S, et al. Initial CT findings and temporal changes in patients with the novel coronavirus pneumonia (2019-nCoV): a study of 63 patients in Wuhan, China. Eur Radiol. 2020;30(6):3306–9. https://doi.org/10.1007/s00330-020-06731-x. Epub 2020 Feb 13
4. Pan F, Ye T, Sun P, et al. Time course of lung changes on chest CT during recovery from 2019 novel coronavirus (COVID-19) pneumonia. Radiology. 2020;295(3):715–21. https://doi.org/10.1148/radiol.2020200370. Epub 2020 Feb 13

CT Features of Late Stage of COVID-19 Pneumonia

5

Yanhong Yang, Peixu Wang, and Fengjuan Chen

5.1 Introduction

In the late stage of COVID-19 pneumonia, the patients' clinical symptoms improved as the lung lesions gradually disappeared. After approximately 14 days, the absorption of lung lesions on chest computed tomography (CT) was reported in 75% of the patients, and the imaging features included decreased number of involved lobes, reduction of crazy-paving pattern, and consolidative opacities [1].

According to the database collected from the patients admitted to Guangzhou Eighth People's Hospital, we found that the absorption time of the lesions on chest-CT imaging was later than that of the improvement of clinical symptoms or negative conversion of viral RNA and the imaging features associated with clinical improvement usually occur after 2 weeks of onset [2–4]. Chest-CT findings in late stage usually showed a reduction in the size and density of lung lesions. Most of the lung lesions can be gradually absorbed and can disappear.

Chest-CT imaging showed that inflammation absorption was one of the indicators to evaluate whether patients can be discharged from the hospital. The image recommendations for patients meeting discharge standards are the following:

(1) The scope of the lesions in the lung is significantly reduced (the volume of the lesion is reduced by 50% and the density is reduced by 50%); most of it is absorbed or completely dissipated.

(2) Only a few linear opacities remain in the lungs.

(3) No new lesions are detected in the lungs.

5.2 Case 1 (Fig. 5.1a1–e1, a2–e2)

A 58-year-old woman was admitted to the hospital with repeated cough and expectoration for 12 days and fever for 9 days, accompanied by chest tightness and shortness of breath. She had no exposure to an infected patient or epidemic area. The body temperature at admission was 38.4 °C. White blood cell count, neutrophil count, lymphocyte count, and C-reactive protein were 7.56 × 10^9/L, 5.98 × 10^9/L, 1.21 × 10^9/L, and 95.96 mg/L, respectively. The patient was laboratory confirmed by novel coronavirus nucleic acid throat swab test in Guangzhou CDC. Chest CT examination was performed 12 days and 22 days after the onset of symptoms.

On day 12 after the onset of symptoms, chest CT images (Fig. 5.1a1–e1) showed that patchy ground-glass opacities with thickening of the interlobular septa were found in the bilateral lung, representing a crazy-paving pattern (Fig. 5.1a1, white arrow), with focal consolidation. After oxygen therapy, anti-infection and anti-asthmatic therapy, phlegm elimination, treatment with traditional Chinese medicine, and other treatment, the body temperature returned to normal for 1 week, the symptoms of the patient were improved significantly, and the real-time fluorescence polymerase chain reaction of the patient's pharyngeal swab was negative for two consecutive times of COVID-19 nucleic acid. On day 22 after the onset of symptoms, chest CT images (Fig. 5.1a2–e2) showed most of the lesions in the bilateral lung decreased and disappeared, compared with previous images, but a few linear opacities remained, compared with previous images (Fig. 5.1e2).

5.3 Case 2 (Fig. 5.2a1–e1, a2–e2)

A 36-year-old male with fever for 9 days, accompanied by aggravated rash, dry cough, and limb joint muscle soreness for 1 day, was admitted, and he was exposed to confirmed cases with novel coronavirus pneumonia. The body temperature at admission was 39.1 °C. White blood cell count, neutrophil count, lymphocyte count, and C-reactive protein were 3.74 × 10^9/L, 1.59 × 10^9/L, 1.64 × 10^9/L, and <10 mg/L, respectively. The patient was laboratory confirmed by novel coronavirus nucleic acid throat swab test in

Y. Yang (✉) · P. Wang · F. Chen
Guangzhou Eighth People's Hospital, Guangzhou Medical University, Guangzhou, China

J. Liu et al. (eds.), *Atlas of Chest Imaging in COVID-19 Patients*, https://doi.org/10.1007/978-981-16-1082-0_5

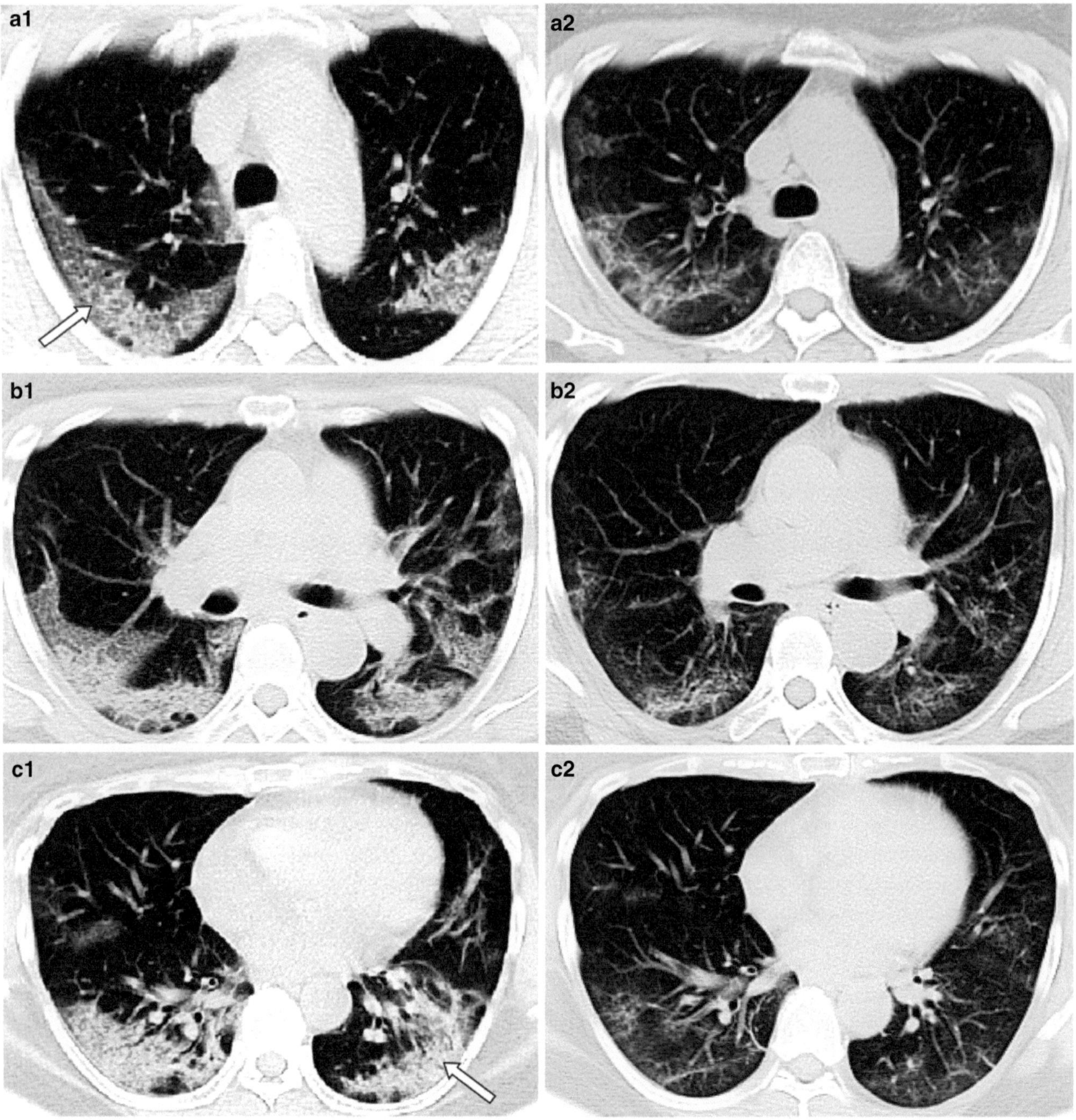

Fig. 5.1 On day 12 after the onset of symptoms, chest CT images (**a**1–**e**1) showed that patchy ground-glass opacities with thickening of the interlobular septa were found in the bilateral lung, representing a crazy-paving pattern (**a**1 white arrow), with focal consolidation. After oxygen therapy, anti-infection and anti-asthmatic therapy, phlegm elimination, treatment with traditional Chinese medicine, and other treatments, the body temperature returned to normal for 1 week, the symptoms of the patient were improved significantly, and the real-time fluorescence polymerase chain reaction of the patient's pharyngeal swab was negative for two consecutive times of COVID-19 nucleic acid. On day 22 after the onset of symptoms, chest CT images (**a**2–**e**2) showed most of the lesions in the bilateral lung decreased and disappeared, compared with previous images, but a few linear opacities remained, compared with previous images (**e**2)

Guangzhou CDC. Chest CT examination was performed 10 days and 21 days after the onset of symptoms (Fig. 5.2a1–e1, a2–e2).

On day 10 after the onset of symptoms, chest CT images (Fig. 5.2a1–e1) showed that patchy ground-glass opacities were found in the bilateral lung. After antiviral, anti-infection, and anti-asthmatic therapy, phlegm elimination, and treatment with traditional Chinese medicine, the body temperature returned to normal for 10 days, the clinical symptoms of the patient were improved significantly, and

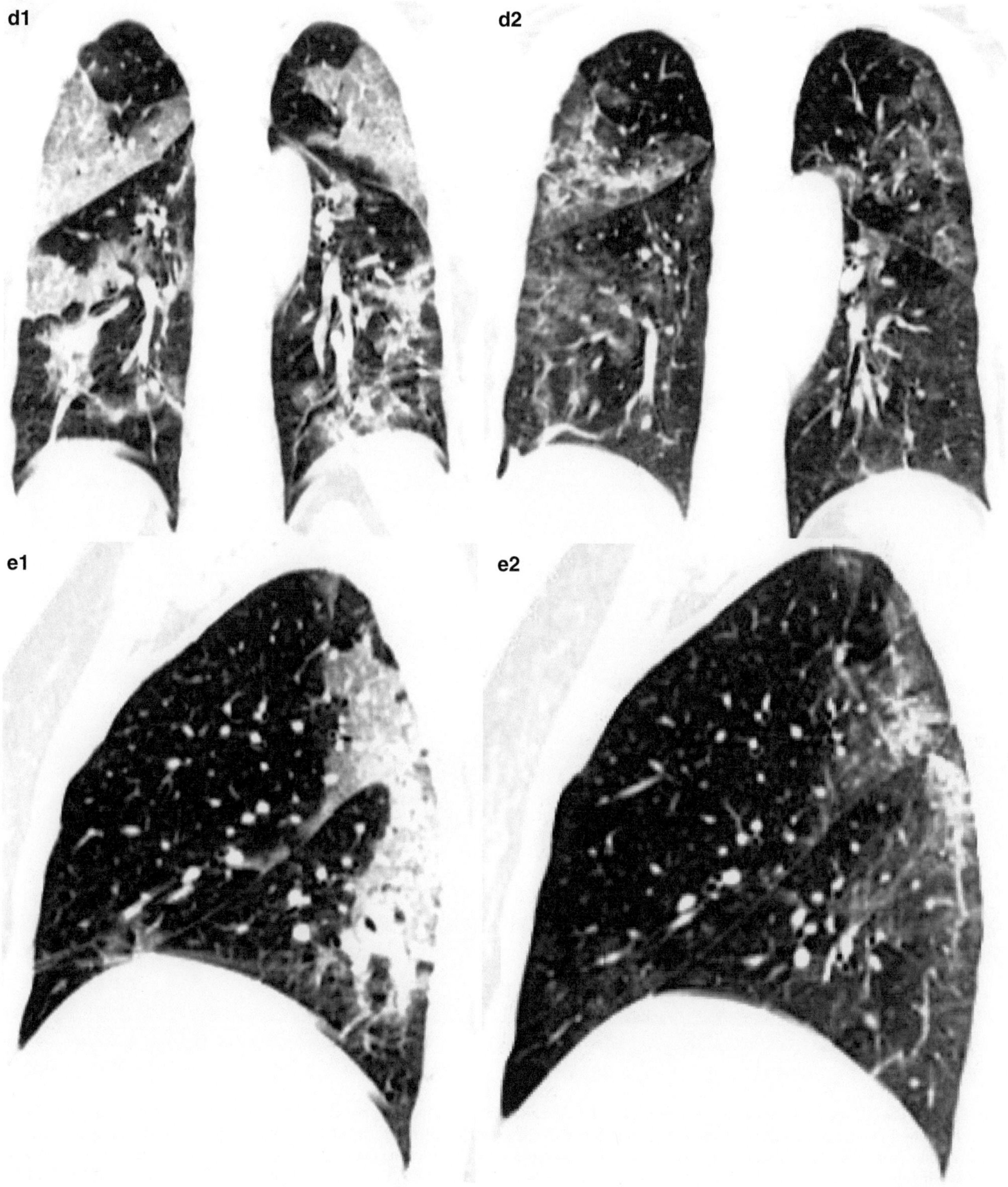

Fig. 5.1 (continued)

the real-time fluorescence polymerase chain reaction of the patient's pharyngeal swab was negative for two consecutive times of COVID-19 nucleic acid. On day 21 after the onset of symptoms, chest CT images (Fig. 5.2a2–e2) demonstrated most of the lesions in the bilateral lung decreased and disappeared, compared with previous images.

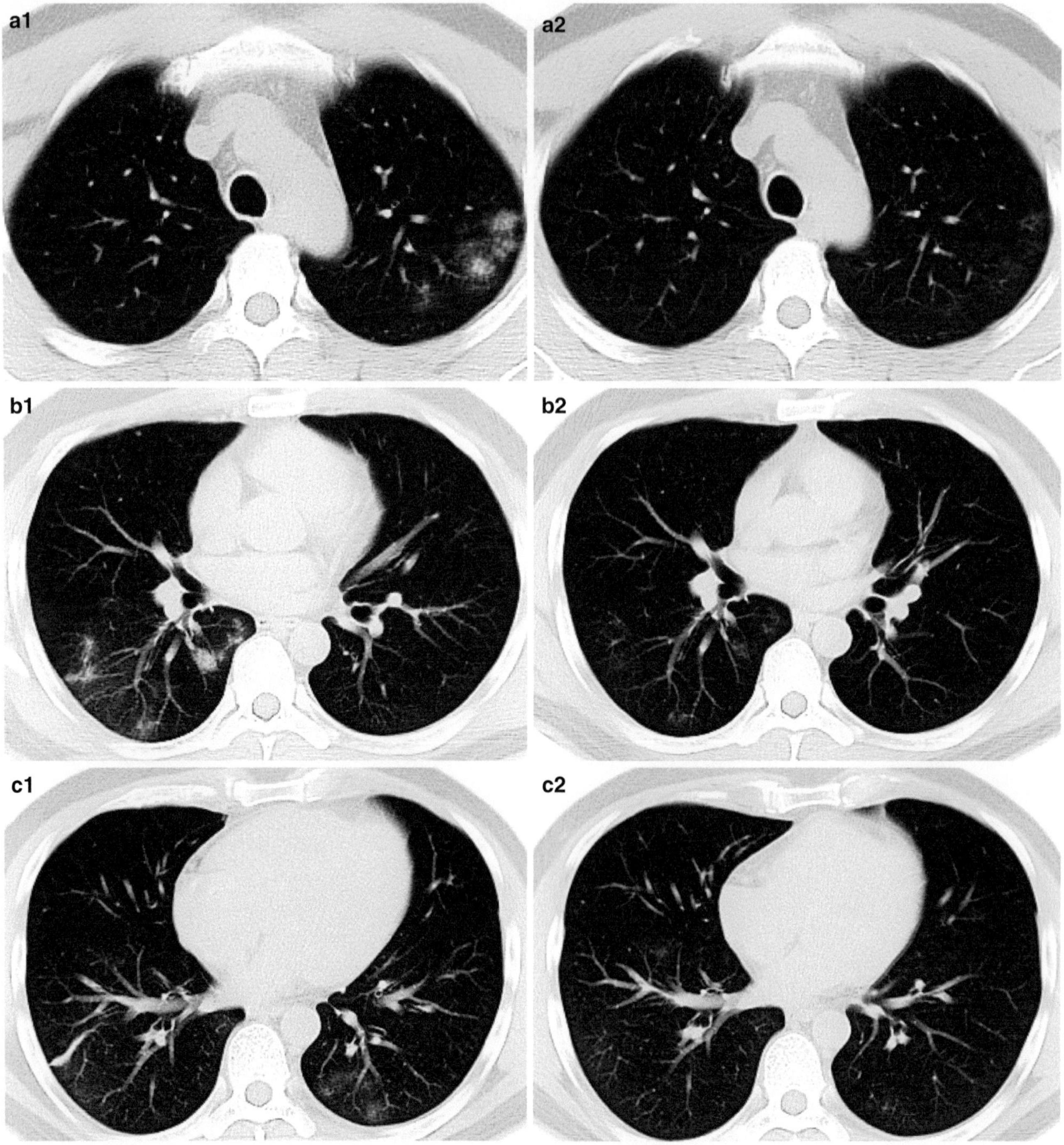

Fig. 5.2 On day 10 after the onset of symptoms, chest CT images (**a**1–**e**1) showed that patchy ground-glass opacities were found in the bilateral lung. After antiviral, anti-infection, and anti-asthmatic therapy, phlegm elimination, and treatment with traditional Chinese medicine, the body temperature returned to normal for 10 days, the clinical symptoms of the patient were improved significantly, and the real-time fluorescence polymerase chain reaction of the patient's pharyngeal swab was negative for two consecutive times of COVID-19 nucleic acid. On day 21 after the onset of symptoms, chest CT images (**a**2–**e**2) demonstrated most of the lesions in the bilateral lung decreased and disappeared, compared with previous images

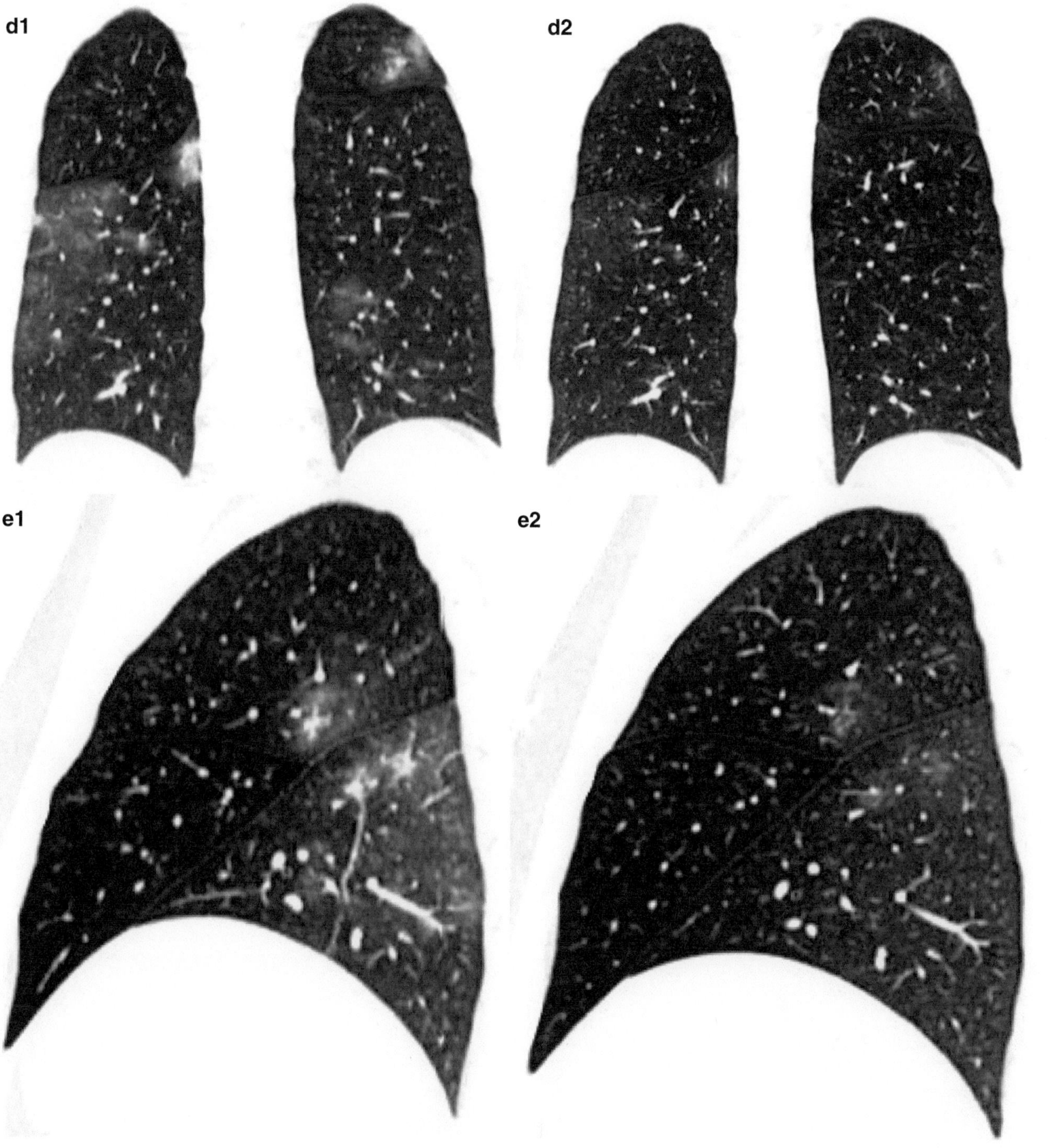

Fig. 5.2 (continued)

5.4 Case 3 (Fig. 5.3a1–e1, a2–e2)

A 35-year-old male with fever for 2 days, accompanied by cough and expectoration, was admitted, and he was exposed to confirmed cases with novel coronavirus pneumonia. The body temperature at admission was 39.1 °C. White blood cell count, neutrophil count, lymphocyte count, and C-reactive protein were 5.62×10^9/L, 1.31×10^9/L, 0.3×10^9/L, and 18.04 mg/L, respectively. The patient was laboratory confirmed by novel coronavirus nucleic acid throat swab test in Guangzhou CDC. Chest CT examination was performed 5 days and 20 days after the onset of symptoms (Fig. 5.3a1–e1, a2–e2).

On day 5 after the onset of symptoms, chest CT images (Fig. 5.3a1–e1) showed that patchy ground-glass opacities were found in the bilateral lung, accompanied by partial consolidation and linear opacities. After antiviral

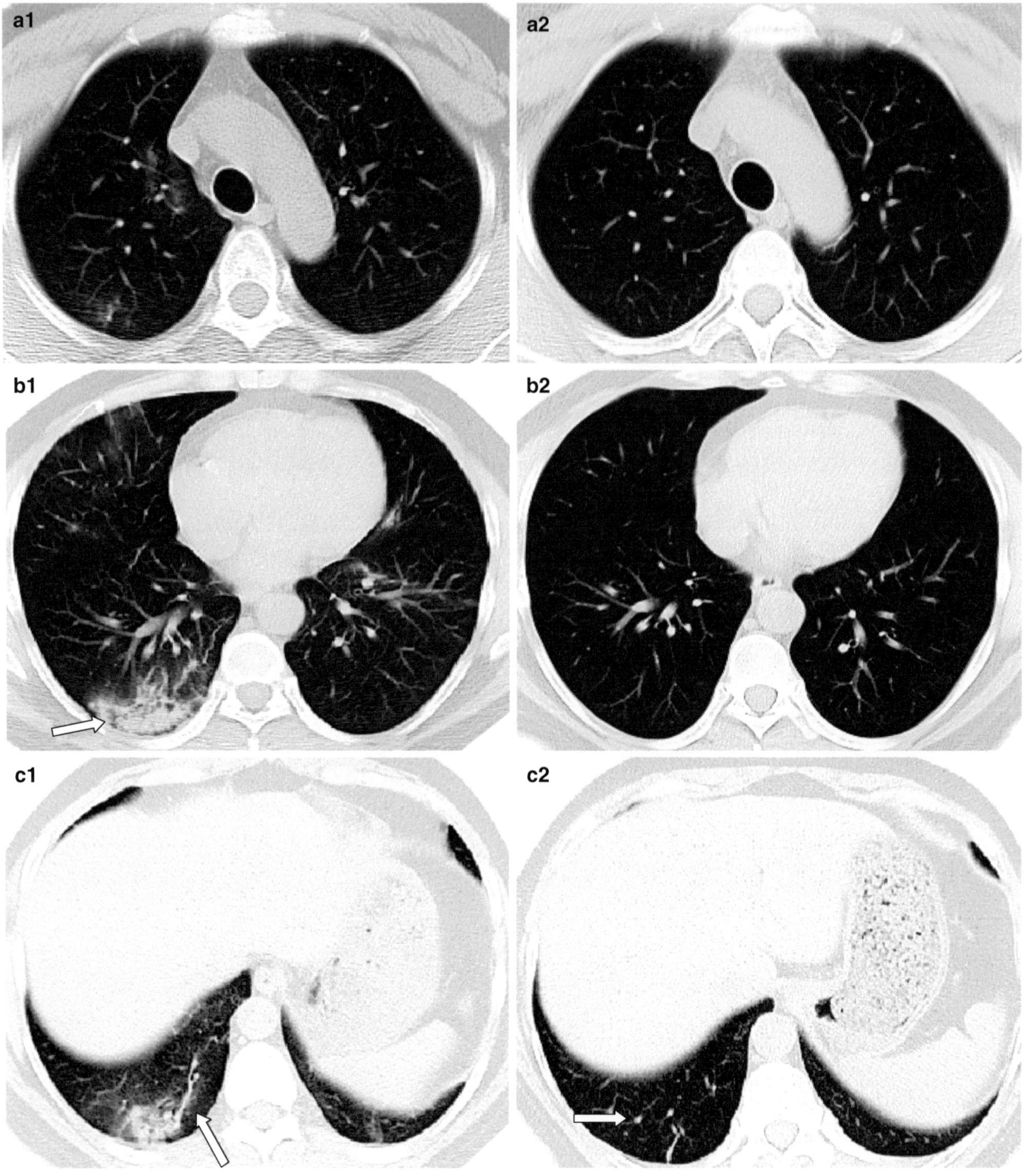

Fig. 5.3 On day 5 after the onset of symptoms, chest CT images (**a**1–**e**1) showed that patchy ground-glass opacities were found in the bilateral lung, accompanied by partial consolidation and linear opacities. After antiviral and anti-infection therapy and treatment with traditional Chinese medicine, the body temperature returned to normal for 2 weeks, the clinical symptoms of the patient were improved significantly, and the real-time fluorescence polymerase chain reaction of the patient's pharyngeal swab was negative for two consecutive times of COVID-19 nucleic acid. On day 20 after the onset of symptoms, chest CT images (**a**2–**e**2) demonstrated most of the lesions in the bilateral lung decreased and disappeared, but a few linear opacities remained, compared with previous images (**c**2)

and anti-infection therapy and treatment with traditional Chinese medicine, the body temperature returned to normal for 2 weeks, the clinical symptoms of the patient were improved significantly, and the real-time fluorescence polymerase chain reaction of the patient's pharyngeal swab was negative for two consecutive times of COVID-

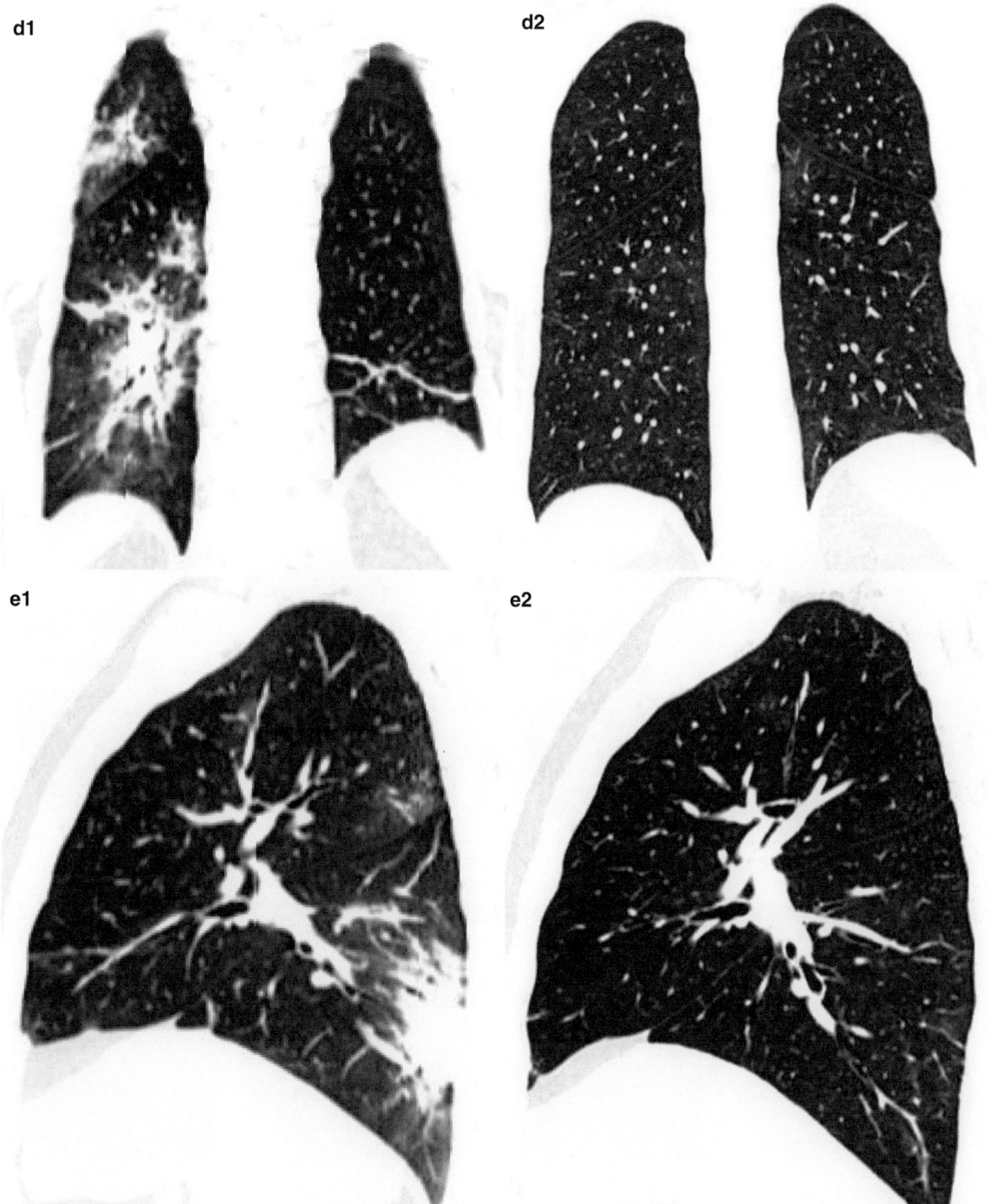

Fig. 5.3 (continued)

19 nucleic acid. On day 20 after the onset of symptoms, chest CT images (Fig. 5.3a2–e2) demonstrated most of the lesions in the bilateral lung decreased and disappeared, but a few linear opacities remained, compared with previous images (Fig. 5.3c2).

5.5 Case 4 (Fig. 5.4a1–e1, a2–e2)

A 28-year-old male with cough, phlegm, and fatigue for 8 days and fever for 3 days was admitted. He had no exposure to an infected patient or epidemic area. The body tempera-

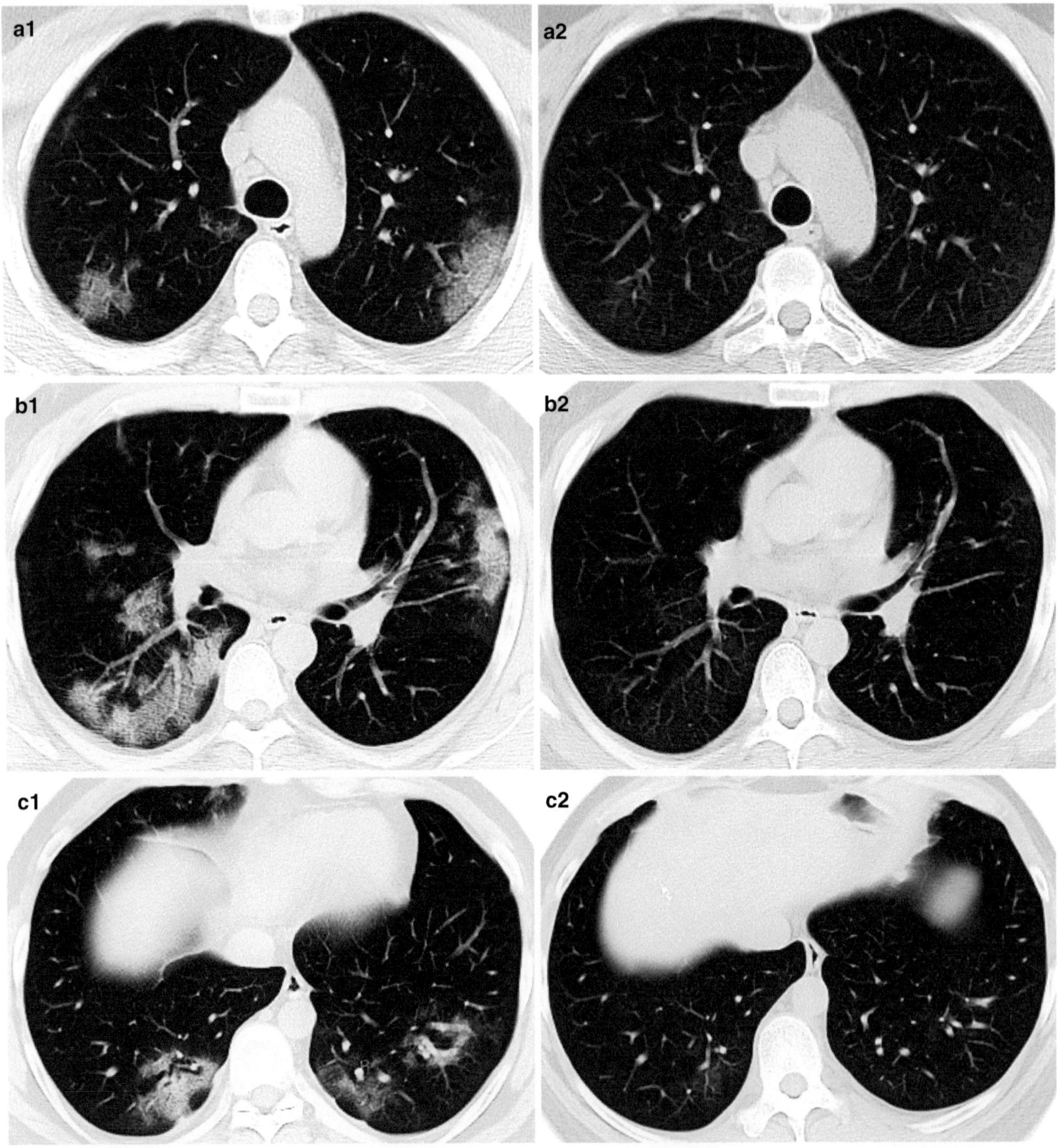

Fig. 5.4 On day 8 after the onset of symptoms, chest CT images (**a**1–**e**1) showed that patchy ground-glass opacities with thickening of the interlobular septa were found in the bilateral lung, representing a crazy-paving pattern. The body temperature returned to normal the next day after admission, after "oxygen therapy, anti-infection therapy, phlegm elimination, cough relieving, and immune enhancement"; the clinical symptoms of the patient were improved significantly, and the real-time fluorescence polymerase chain reaction of the patient's pharyngeal swab was negative for two consecutive times of COVID-19 nucleic acid. On day 26 after the onset of symptoms, chest CT images (**a**2–**e**2) demonstrated the lesions in the bilateral lung decreased, compared with previous images

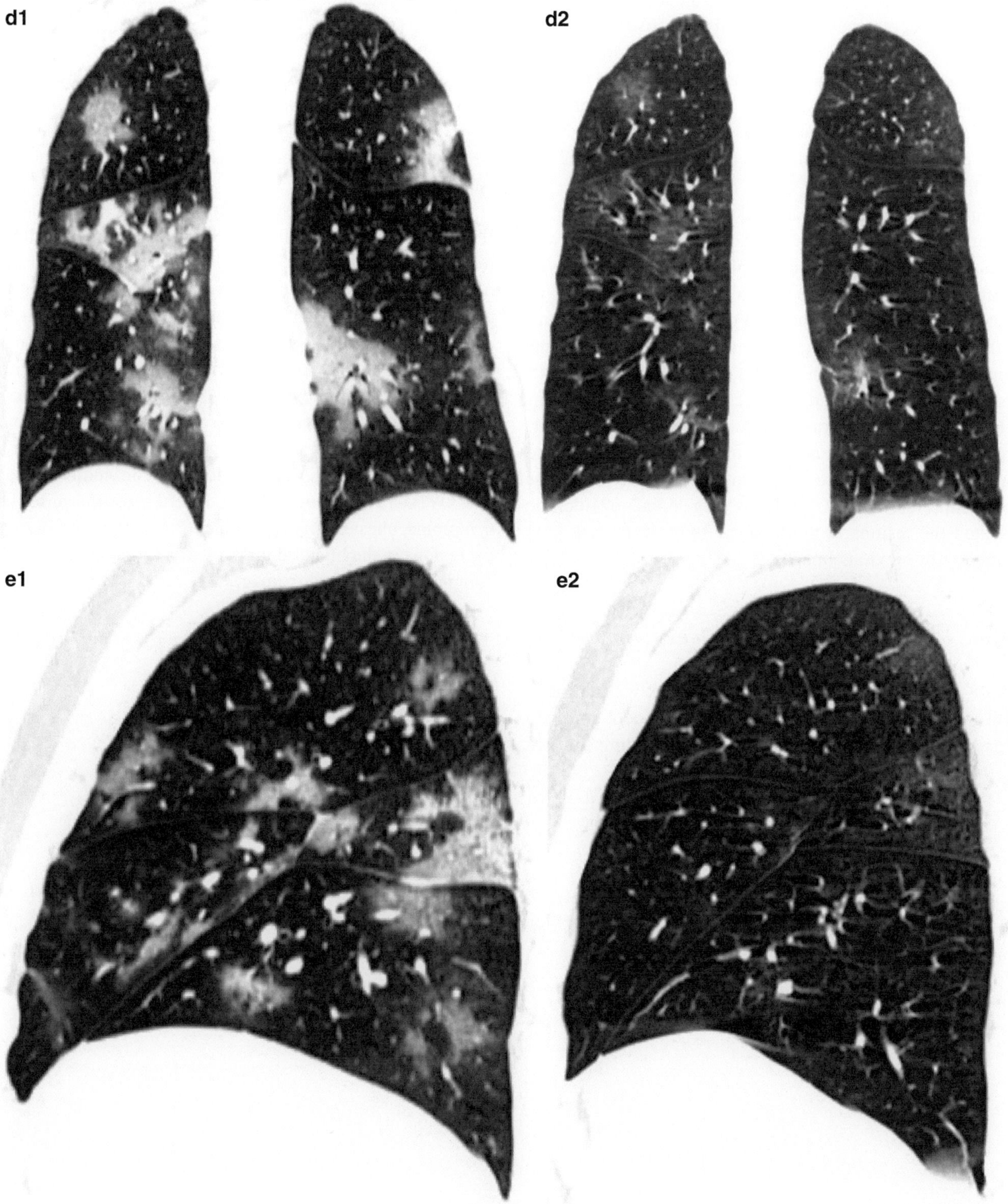

Fig. 5.4 (continued)

ture at admission was 39.6 °C. White blood cell count, neutrophil count, lymphocyte count, and C-reactive protein were 2.20 × 10^9/L, 1.48 × 10^9/L, 0.64 × 10^9/L, and 46.63 mg/L, respectively. The patient was laboratory confirmed by novel coronavirus nucleic acid throat swab test in Guangzhou CDC. Chest CT examination was performed 8 days and 26 days after the onset of symptoms (Fig. 5.4a1–e1, a2–e2).

On day 8 after the onset of symptoms, chest CT images (Fig. 5.4a1–e1) showed that patchy ground-glass opacities with thickening of the interlobular septa were found in the bilateral lung, representing a crazy-paving pattern. The body temperature returned to normal the next day after admission, after "oxygen therapy, anti-infection therapy, phlegm elimination, cough relieving, and immune enhancement"; the clinical symptoms of the patient were improved significantly, and the real-time fluorescence polymerase chain reaction of the patient's pharyngeal swab was negative for two consecutive times of COVID-19 nucleic acid. On day 26 after the onset of symptoms, chest CT images (Fig. 5.4a2–e2) demonstrated the lesions in the bilateral lung decreased, compared with previous images.

5.6 Case 5 (Fig. 5.5a1–e1, a2–e2)

A 48-year-old male with fever for 1 week was admitted. He was exposed to confirmed cases with novel coronavirus pneumonia. The body temperature at admission was 38.5 °C. White blood cell count, neutrophil count, lymphocyte count, and C-reactive protein were 3.76 × 10^9/L, 1.71 × 10^9/L, 1.71 × 10^9/L, and 22.48 mg/L, respectively. The patient was laboratory confirmed by novel coronavirus nucleic acid throat swab test in Guangzhou CDC. Chest CT examination was performed 7 days and 20 days after the onset of symptoms (Fig. 5.5a1–e1, a2–e2).

On day 7 after the onset of symptoms, chest CT images (Fig. 5.5a1–e1) showed that patchy ground-glass opacities with thickening of the interlobular septa and linear opacities were found in the bilateral lung, mainly distributed under the pleura. After antiviral and anti-infection therapy, phlegm elimination, cough relieving, and treatment with traditional Chinese medicine, the body temperature returned to normal the next day after admission, the clinical symptoms improved significantly, and the real-time fluorescence polymerase chain reaction of the patient's pharyngeal swab was negative for two consecutive times of COVID-19 nucleic acid. On day 20 after the onset of symptoms, chest CT images (Fig. 5.5a2–e2) demonstrated the lesions in the bilateral lung decreased and disappeared, compared with previous images.

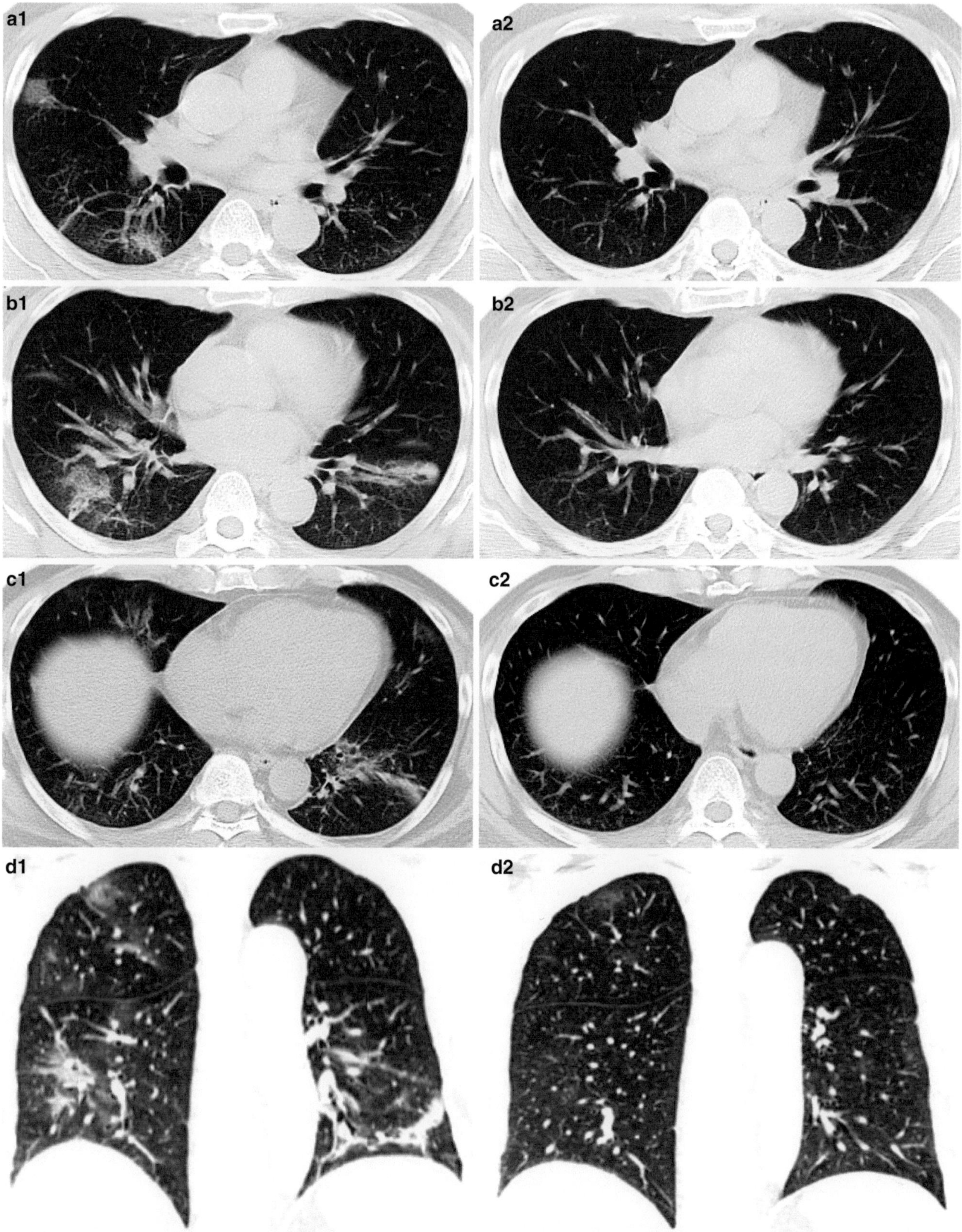

Fig. 5.5 On day 7 after the onset of symptoms, chest CT images (**a**1–**e**1) showed that patchy ground glass opacities with thickening of the interlobular septa and linear opacities were found in the bilateral lung, mainly distributed under the pleura. After antiviral and anti-infection therapy, phlegm elimination, cough relieving, and treatment with traditional Chinese medicine, the body temperature returned to normal the next day after admission, the clinical symptoms improved significantly, and the real-time fluorescence polymerase chain reaction of the patient's pharyngeal swab was negative for two consecutive times of COVID-19 nucleic acid. On day 20 after the onset of symptoms, chest CT images (**a**2–**e**2) demonstrated the lesions in the bilateral lung decreased and disappeared, compared with previous images

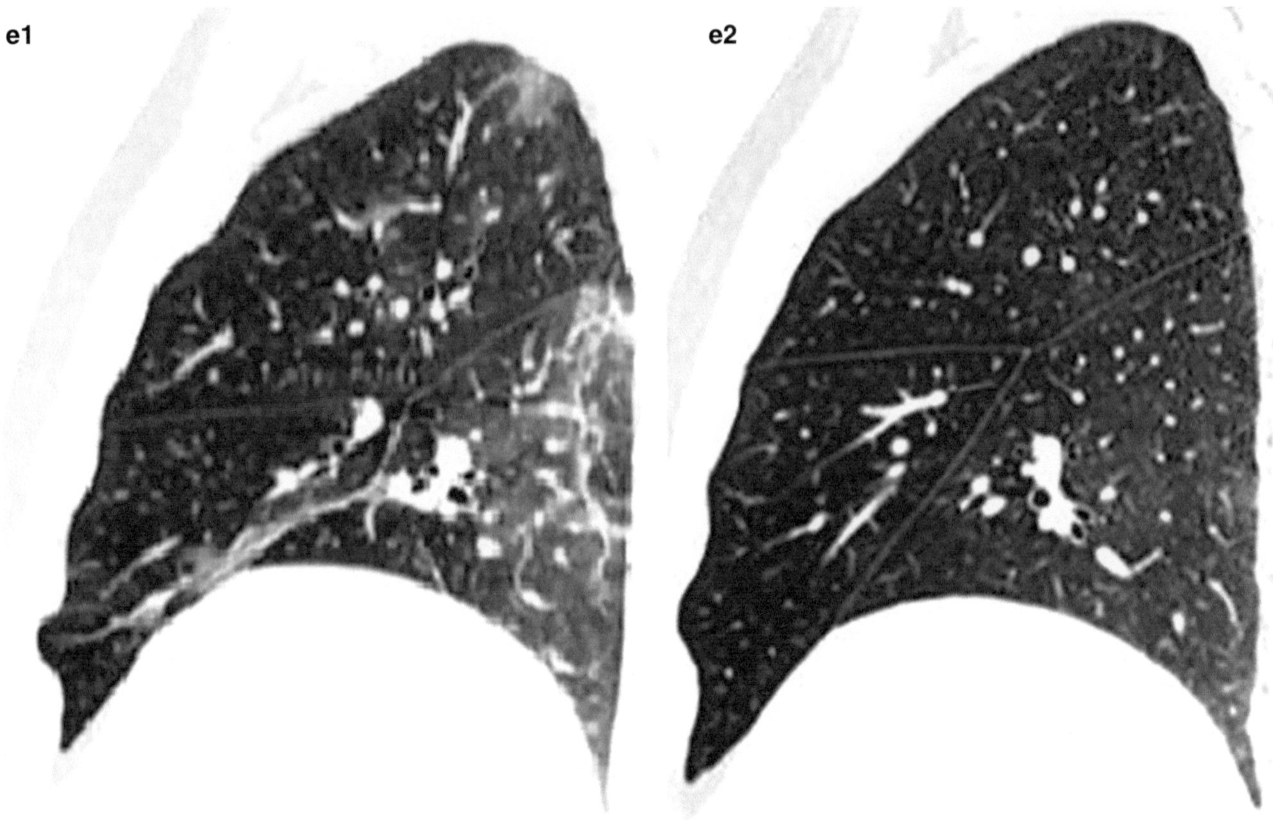

Fig. 5.5 (continued)

5.7 Case 6 (Fig. 5.6a1–e1, a2–e2)

A 37-year-old female with fever for 7 days and diarrhea and chest tightness for 3 days was admitted. She was exposed to confirmed cases with novel coronavirus pneumonia. The body temperature at admission was 38.2 °C. White blood cell count, neutrophil count, lymphocyte count, and C-reactive protein were 6.31×10^9/L, 4.93×10^9/L, 1.07×10^9/L, and 57.32 mg/L, respectively. The patient was laboratory confirmed by novel coronavirus nucleic acid throat swab test in Guangzhou CDC. Chest CT examination was performed 7 days and 14 days after the onset of symptoms (Fig. 5.6a1–e1, a2–e2).

On day 7 after the onset of symptoms, chest CT images (Fig. 5.6a1–e1) showed that patchy ground-glass opacities in the bilateral lung were mainly distributed under the pleura, accompanied by partial consolidation (Fig. 5.6c1), and subpleural curvilinear line was found in the bilateral lung (Fig. 5.6a1). After oxygen therapy and antiviral and anti-infection therapy, the body temperature returned to normal for 7 days, the clinical symptoms of the patient were improved significantly, and the real-time fluorescence polymerase chain reaction of the patient's pharyngeal swab was negative for two consecutive times of COVID-19 nucleic acid. On day 14 after the onset of symptoms, chest CT images (Fig. 5.6a2–e2) demonstrated the lesions in the bilateral lung decreased, compared with previous images.

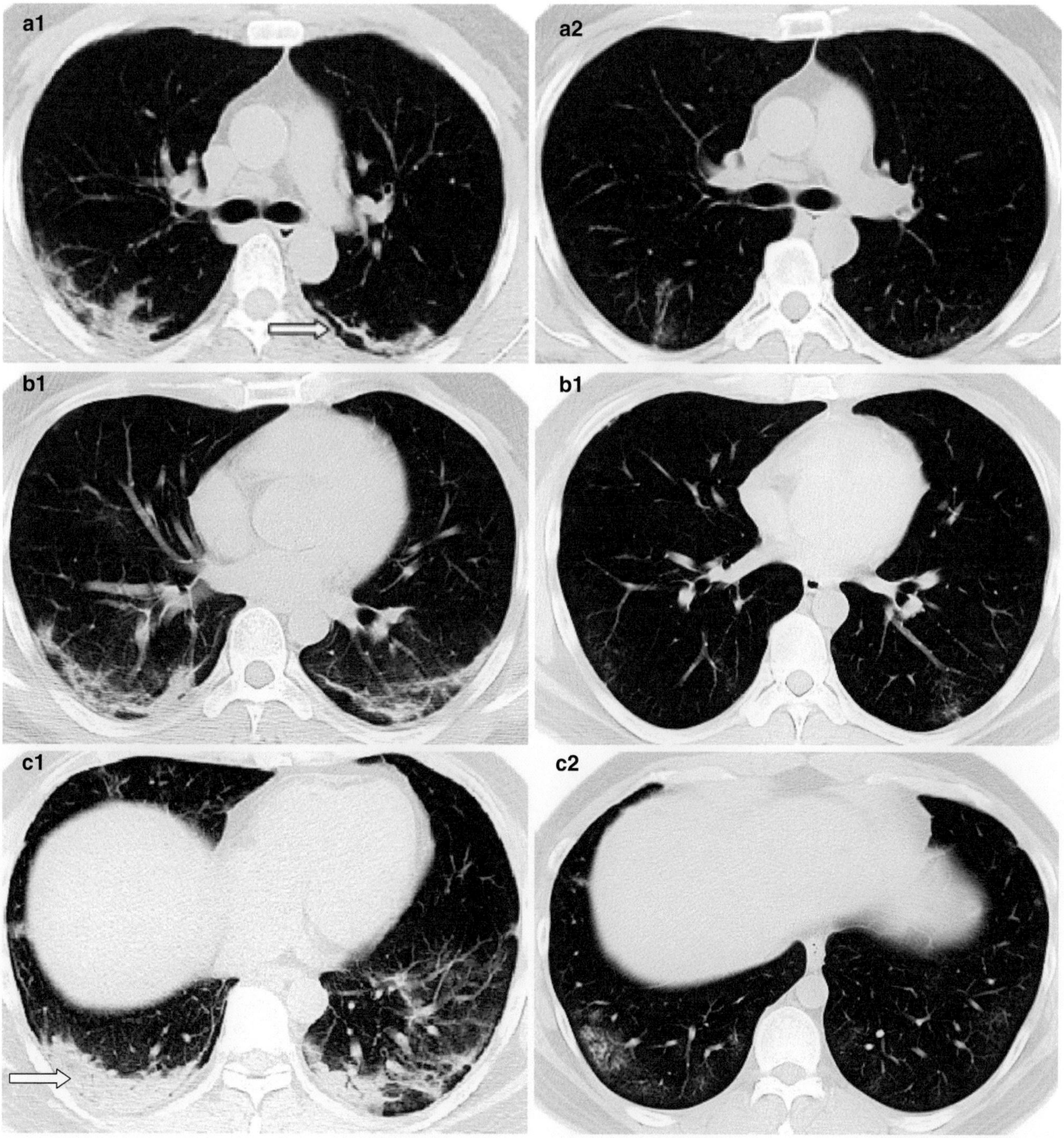

Fig. 5.6 On day 7 after the onset of symptoms, chest CT images (**a**1–**e**1) showed that patchy ground glass opacities in the bilateral lung were mainly distributed under the pleura, accompanied by partial consolidation (**c**1), and subpleural curvilinear line was found in the bilateral lung (**a**1). After oxygen therapy and antiviral and anti-infection therapy, the body temperature returned to normal for 7 days, the clinical symptoms of the patient were improved significantly, and the real-time fluorescence polymerase chain reaction of the patient's pharyngeal swab was negative for two consecutive times of COVID-19 nucleic acid. On day 14 after the onset of symptoms, chest CT images (**a**2–**e**2) demonstrated the lesions in the bilateral lung decreased, compared with previous images

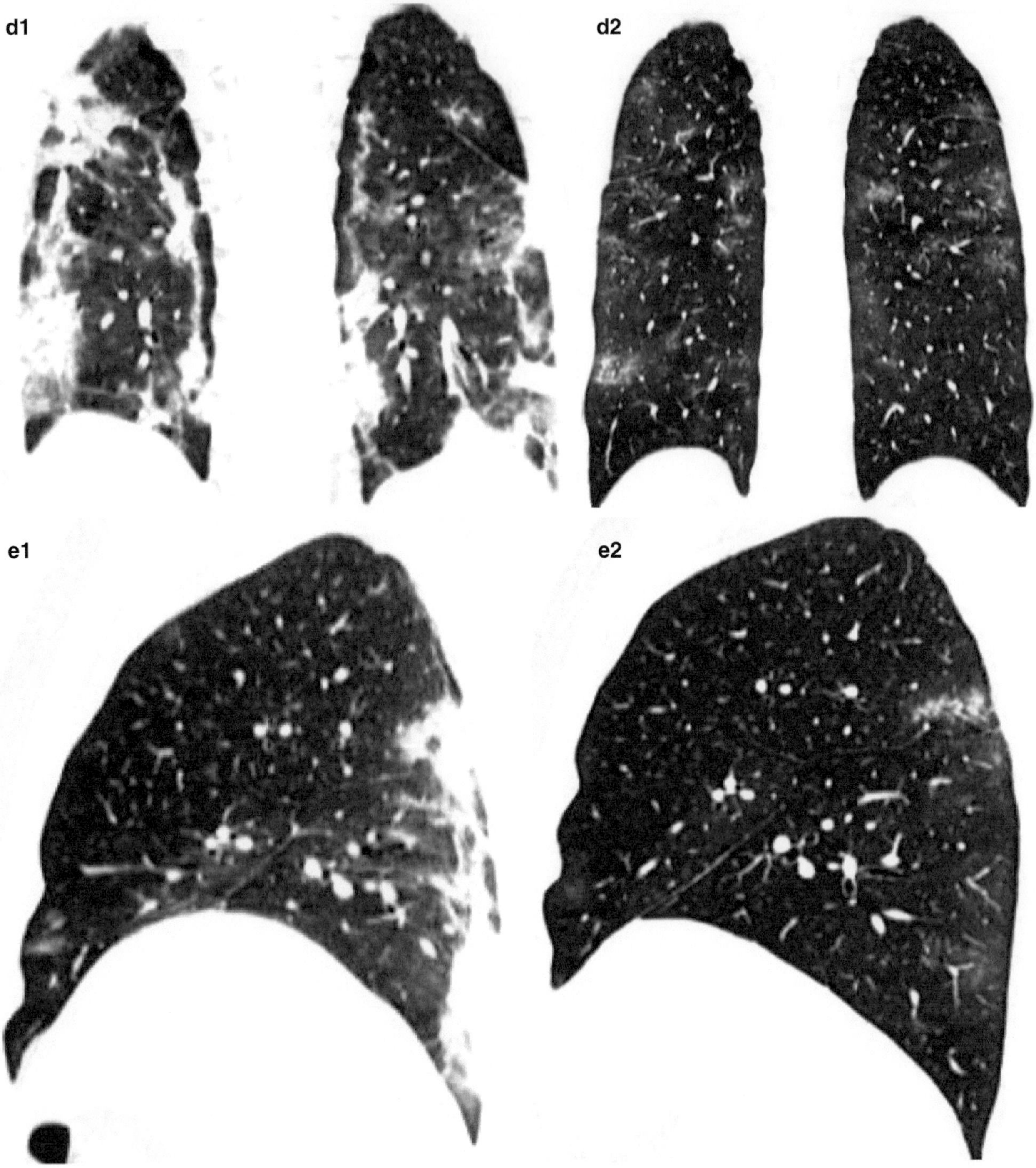

Fig. 5.6 (continued)

5.8 Case 7 (Fig. 5.7a1–e1, a2–e2)

A 30-year-old male with fever and cough for 4 days, accompanied by chills, muscle soreness, dizziness, and poor appetite, was admitted. He was exposed to confirmed cases with novel coronavirus pneumonia. The body temperature at admission was 39.1 °C. White blood cell count, neutrophil count, lymphocyte count, and C-reactive protein were 4.13×10^9/L, 2.42×10^9/L, 1.33×10^9/L, and 51.12 mg/L, respectively. The patient was laboratory confirmed by novel coronavirus nucleic acid throat swab test in Guangzhou CDC. Chest CT examination was performed 4 days and 15 days after the onset of symptoms (Fig. 5.7a1–e1, a2–e2).

On day 4 after the onset of symptoms, chest CT images (Fig. 5.7a1–e1) showed that patchy consolidation was

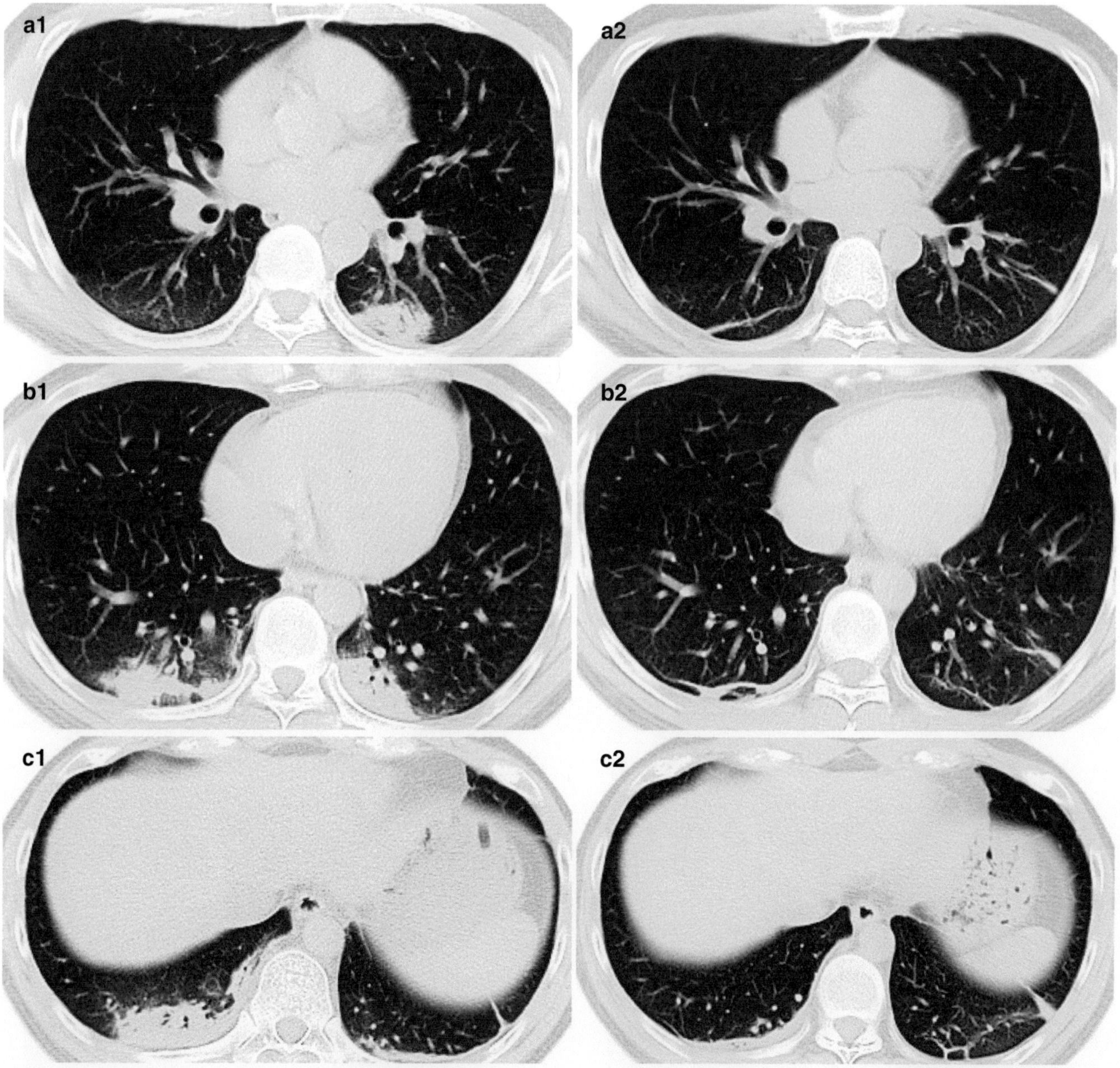

Fig. 5.7 On day 4 after the onset of symptoms, chest CT images (**a**1–**e**1) showed that patchy consolidation was found in the bilateral lung, with air bronchogram signs. After antiviral, anti-infection, and anti-inflammatory therapy and reinforcing immunity, the body temperature returned to normal for 9 days, the clinical symptoms of the patient were improved significantly, and the real-time fluorescence polymerase chain reaction of the patient's pharyngeal swab was negative for two consecutive times of COVID-19 nucleic acid. On day 15 after the onset of symptoms, chest CT images (**a**2–**e**2) demonstrated most of the lesions in the bilateral lung disappeared, but a few linear opacities remained, compared with previous images

found in the bilateral lung, with air bronchogram signs. After antiviral, anti-infection, and anti-inflammatory therapy and reinforcing immunity, the body temperature returned to normal for 9 days, the clinical symptoms of the patient were improved significantly, and the real-time fluorescence polymerase chain reaction of the patient's pharyngeal swab was negative for two consecutive times of COVID-19 nucleic acid. On day 15 after the onset of symptoms, chest CT images (Fig. 5.7a2–e2) demonstrated most of the lesions in the bilateral lung disappeared, but a few linear opacities remained, compared with previous images.

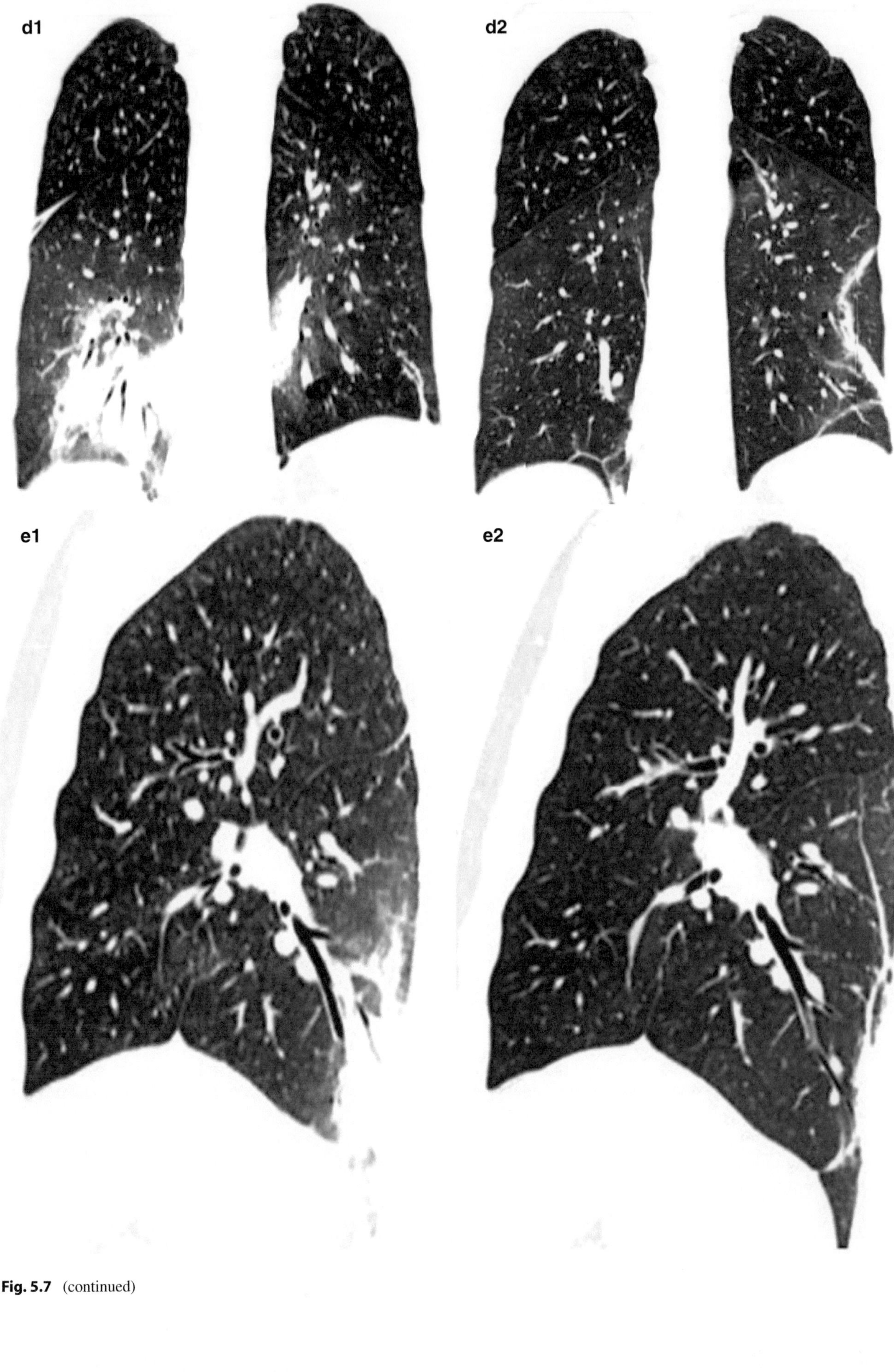

Fig. 5.7 (continued)

5.9 Case 8 (Fig. 5.8a1–e1, a2–e2)

A 33-year-old male was admitted with fever and cough for 5 days. He was exposed to confirmed cases with novel coronavirus pneumonia. The body temperature at admission was 37.9 °C. White blood cell count, neutrophil count, lymphocyte count, and C-reactive protein were 3.73×10^9/L, 2.60×10^9/L, 0.8×10^9/L, and<10 mg/L, respectively. The patient was laboratory confirmed by novel coronavirus nucleic acid throat swab test in Guangzhou CDC. Chest CT examination was performed 7 days and 20 days after the onset of symptoms (Fig. 5.8a1–e1, a2–e2).

On day 7 after the onset of symptoms, chest CT images (Fig. 5.8a1–e1) showed that patchy ground-glass opacities

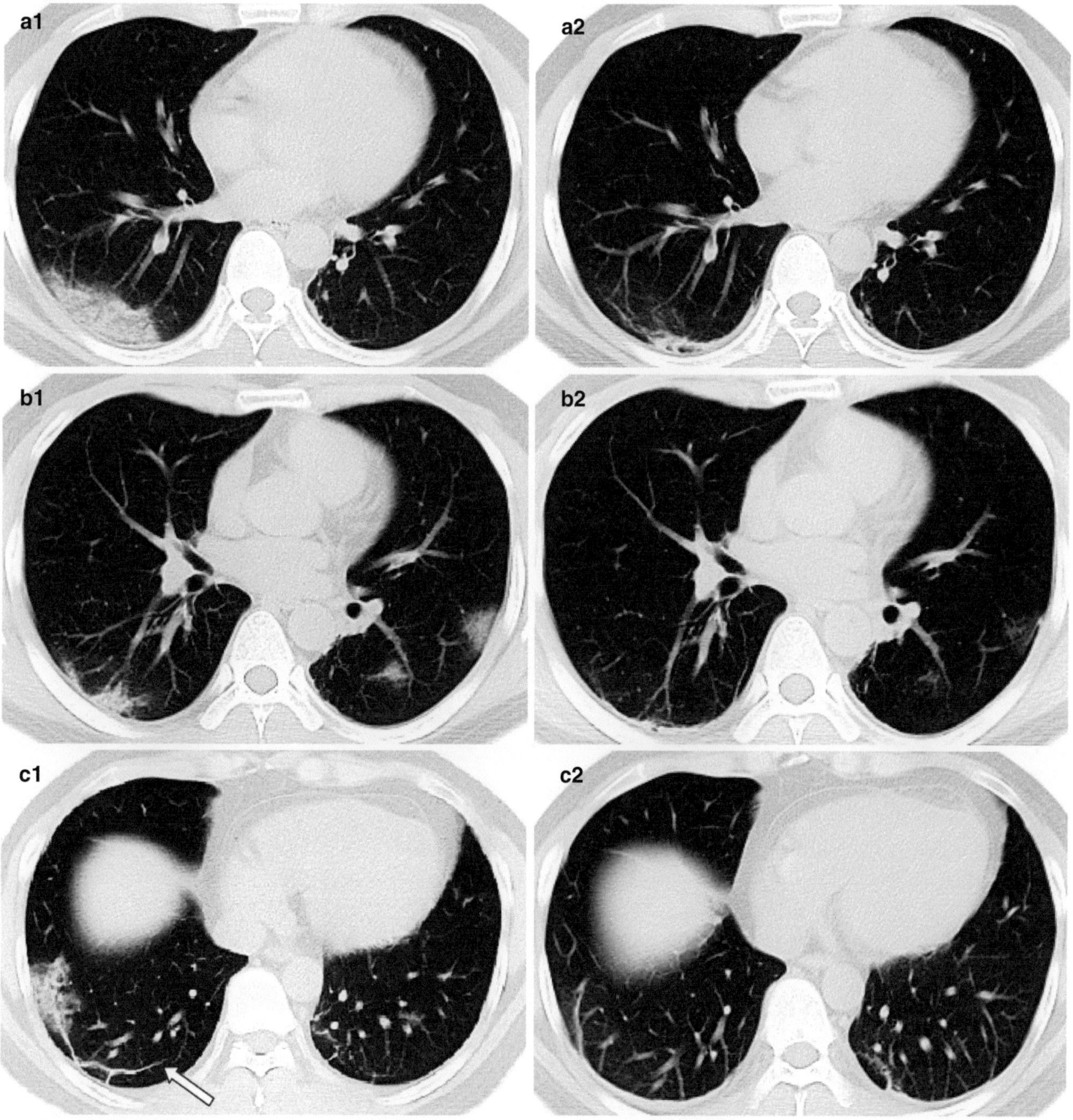

Fig. 5.8 On day 7 after the onset of symptoms, chest CT images (**a**1–**e**1) showed that patchy ground-glass opacities with thickening of the interlobular septa were found in the bilateral lung, accompanied by partial consolidation (**c**1). After antiviral and anti-infection therapy, the body temperature returned to normal for 7 days, the clinical symptoms of the patient were improved significantly, and the real-time fluorescence polymerase chain reaction of the patient's pharyngeal swab was negative for two consecutive times of COVID-19 nucleic acid. On day 20 after the onset of symptoms, chest CT images (**a**2–**e**2) demonstrated the lesions in the bilateral lung decreased, compared with previous images

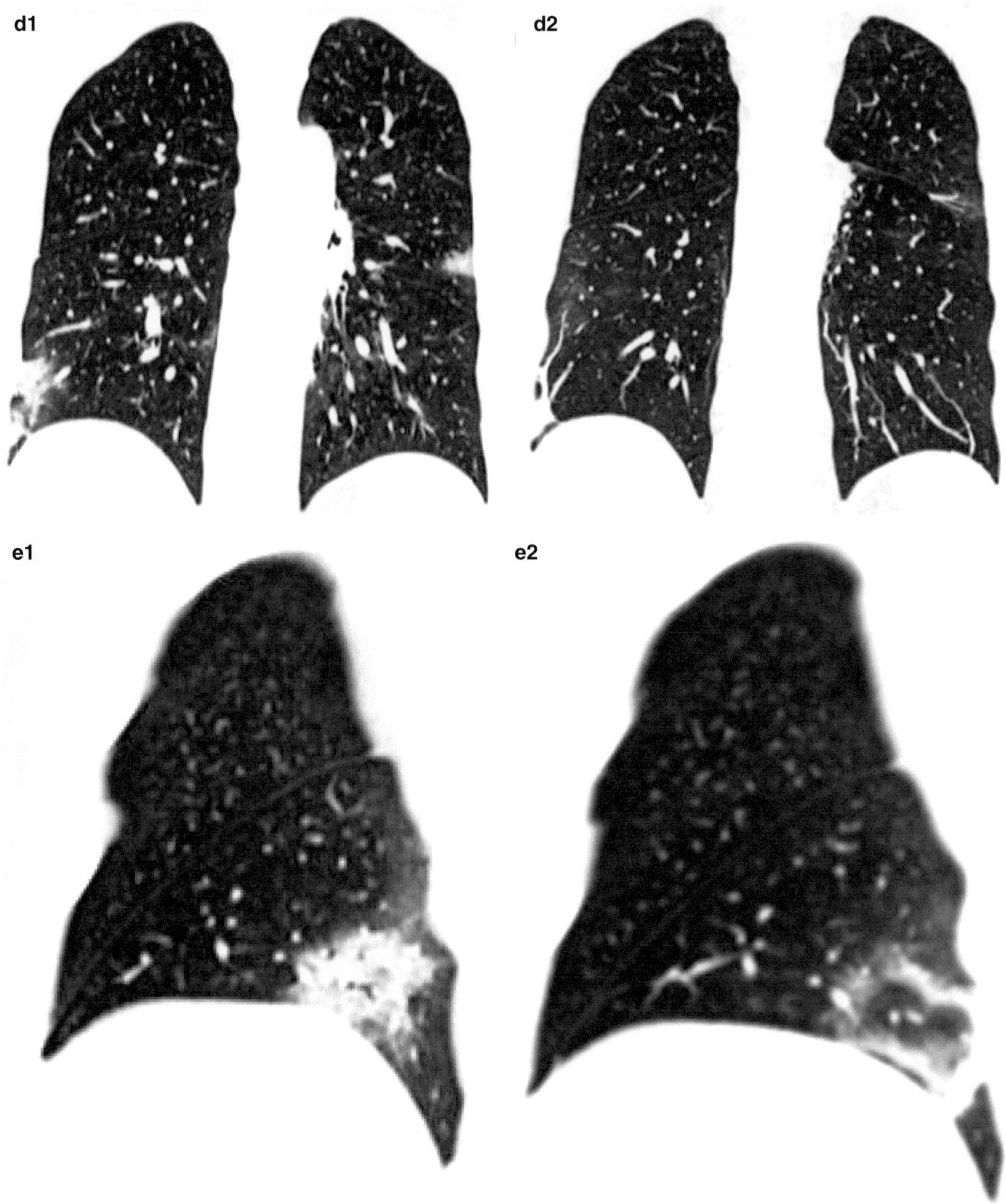

Fig. 5.8 (continued)

with thickening of the interlobular septa were found in the bilateral lung, accompanied by partial consolidation (Fig. 5.8c1). After antiviral and anti-infection therapy, the body temperature returned to normal for 7 days, the clinical symptoms of the patient were improved significantly, and the real-time fluorescence polymerase chain reaction of the patient's pharyngeal swab was negative for two consecutive times of COVID-19 nucleic acid. On day 20 after the onset of symptoms, chest CT images (Fig. 5.8a2–e2) demonstrated the lesions in the bilateral lung decreased, compared with previous images.

References

1. Pan F, Ye T, Sun P, et al. Time course of lung changes on chest CT during recovery from 2019 novel coronavirus (COVID-19) pneumonia. Radiology. 2020; [Epub ahead of print]
2. Das KM, Lee EY, Al Jawder SE, et al. Acute Middle East respiratory syndrome coronavirus: temporal lung changes observed on the chest radiographs of 55 patients. AJR. 2015:W267–74. [web]
3. Müller NL, Ooi GC, Khong PL, et al. High-resolution CT findings of severe acute respiratory syndrome at presentation and after admission. AJR. 2004;182:39–44.
4. Ooi GC, Khong PL, Müller NL, et al. Severe acute respiratory syndrome: temporal lung changes at thin-section CT in 30 patients. Radiology. 2004;230:836–44.

Chest Features of Severe and Critical Patients with COVID-19 Pneumonia

6

Jing Qu, Xilong Deng, and Yanqing Ding

6.1 Introduction

In some COVID-19 patients, the disease progresses rapidly, resulting in respiratory failure, multiple organ dysfunction or failure, and even death sometimes.

According to the novel coronavirus pneumonia treatment strategies [1]:

1. *Any one of the following conditions is considered as severe type:*
   (a) Respiratory distress, RR $\geq$ 30 times/min.
   (b) At rest, oxygen saturation $\leq$93%.
   (c) Arterial partial oxygen pressure (PaO_2)/oxygen absorption concentration (FiO_2) $\leq$300 mmHg.
   (d) Chest images showed significant progression of lesions more than 50% within 24–48 h.
2. *Any of the following conditions are considered as critical type:*
   (a) Respiratory failure, requiring mechanical ventilation.
   (b) Shock.
   (c) Patients with other organ failure should be treated in the intensive care unit (ICU).

This chapter aims to improve the understanding of chest imaging features in severe and critical COVID-19 by presenting clinical characteristics and dynamic chest CT images of relevant cases.

Chest CT imaging features of severe and critical cases:

1. Multiple ground-glass opacities and consolidative opacities in bilateral lungs.
2. The thickened vascular profile can be seen in ground-glass opacities, and "air bronchi signs" may be present, which can be accompanied by bronchiectasis.
3. Interlobular septum and subpleural interstitium thickening is common. In severe cases, most of the bilateral lung may be affected, presenting as "white lung"-like or "white lung."
4. A small amount of pleural effusion can be seen in very few patients [2–4].

3. *Individuals at increased risk of severe and critical illness*
   (a) People over 65
   (b) People with cardiovascular and cerebrovascular diseases (including hypertension), chronic lung diseases (chronic obstructive pulmonary disease, moderate to severe asthma), diabetes, chronic liver and kidney diseases, tumors, and other basic diseases
   (c) People with immunodeficiencies (e.g., in AIDS patients, long-term use of corticosteroids or other immunosuppressive drugs)
   (d) Obese people (body mass index $\geq$30)
   (e) Women in the third trimester of pregnancy and perinatal period
   (f) Heavy smokers
4. *Prognostic factors for deteriorated conditions*
   (a) Adults

If one or a combination of the following signs shows up, the COVID-19 patients should be closely monitored and pre-treated in cases of disease deterioration: (1) progressive aggravation of hypoxemia or respiratory distress; (2) tissue oxygenation index deteriorates or lactic acid increases progressively; (3) peripheral blood lymphocyte count reduces progressively or peripheral blood inflammatory markers such as IL-6, CRP, and ferritin are progressively increased; (4) indexes related to coagulation function, such as D-dimer,

J. Qu (✉) · X. Deng
Guangzhou Eighth People's Hospital, Guangzhou Medical University, Guangzhou, China

Y. Ding
Nanfang Hospital, Southern Medical University, Guangzhou, China

J. Liu et al. (eds.), *Atlas of Chest Imaging in COVID-19 Patients*, https://doi.org/10.1007/978-981-16-1082-0_6

increases significantly; (5) chest images show significant progression of pulmonary lesions.

(b) Children
- Increased respiratory rate.
- Poor mental reaction and lethargy.
- Progressive increase of lactic acid.
- Inflammatory markers such as CRP, PCT, and ferritin are significantly increased.
- Chest CT images demonstrate bilateral and multiple opacities, pleural effusion, or rapid progression of lesions in a short period.
- Underlying diseases (congenital heart disease, bronchopulmonary dysplasia, respiratory malformations, abnormal hemoglobin, severe malnutrition, etc.), immunodeficiency (long-term use of immunosuppressive agents), or hypoxia and neonates.

6.2 Case 1 (Fig. 6.1a–l)

A 60-year-old woman was admitted to the hospital with repeated fever and cough for 7 days. She had no exposure to an infected patient or epidemic area. The body temperature at admission was 38.6 °C, and the highest temperature in the course of the disease was 39 °C. Laboratory examination: white blood cell count in peripheral blood was 4.58×10^9/L, the lymphocyte count was 1.05×10^9/L, the C-reactive protein was 30.75 mg/L, and the oxygenation index was 245 mmHg. The patient was laboratory confirmed by novel coronavirus nucleic acid throat swab test in Guangzhou CDC. Chest CT examination was performed on day 2 (8 days after the onset of symptoms), day 7 (13 days after the onset of symptoms), and day 14 of admission (20 days after the onset of symptoms) (Fig. 6.1a–l).

On day 2 of admission, chest CT images showed multiple ground-glass opacities in the bilateral lungs, with subpleural distribution (Fig. 6.1a–d).

On day 7 of admission, after anti-infection and antipyretic treatment, low-flow oxygen inhalation through a nasal catheter, and other treatments, the patient had heavier symptoms than before. Chest CT images showed increased density of multiple lesions and thickened interlobular septum (Fig. 6.1e–h).

On day 14 of admission, after anti-infection therapy and maintenance of electrolyte acid-base balance, the patient's condition was further aggravated. Chest CT images showed increased and enlarged lesions of bilateral lungs (Fig. 6.1i–l).

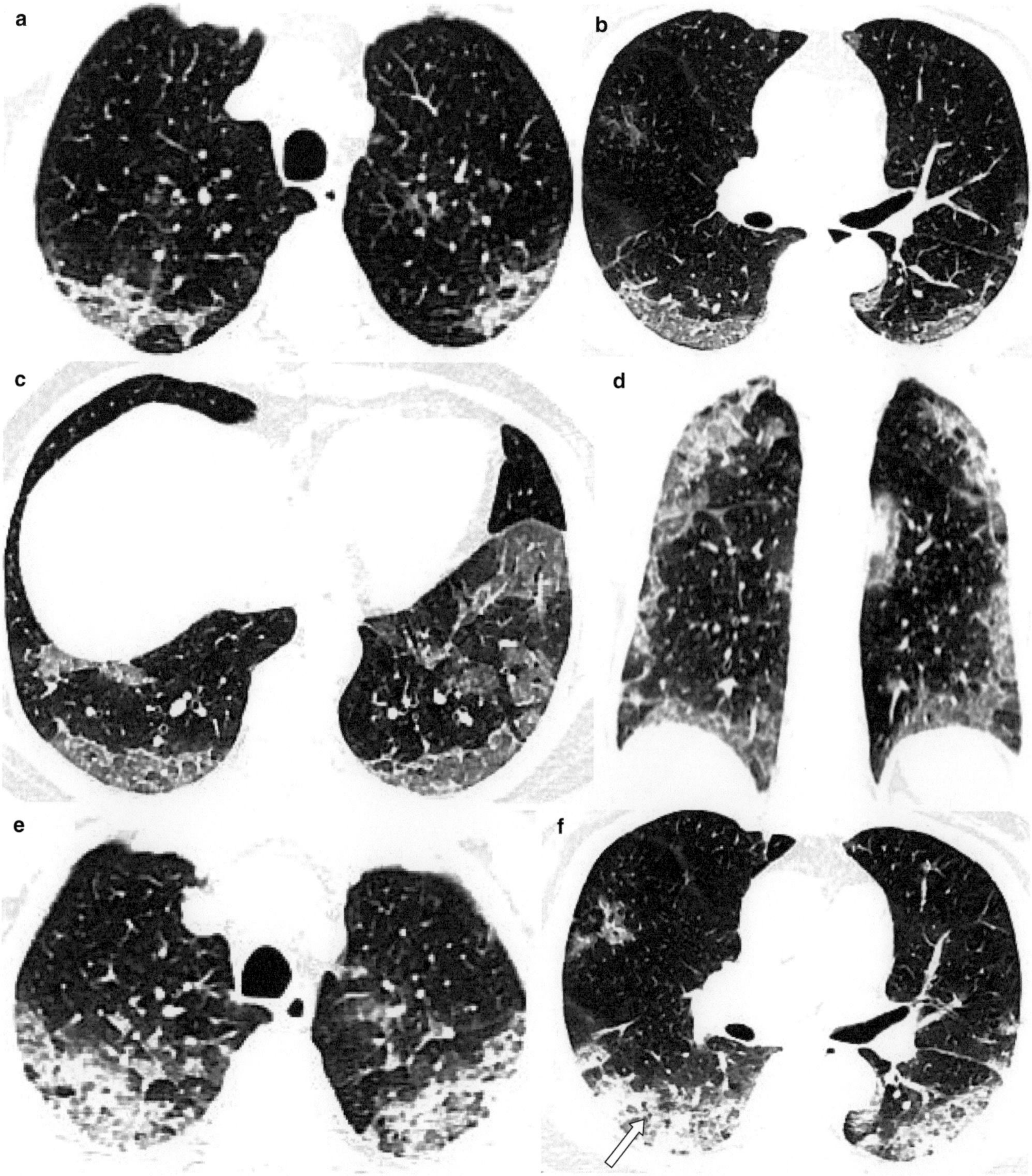

Fig. 6.1 On day 2 of admission, chest CT images showed multiple ground-glass opacities in the bilateral lungs, with subpleural distribution (**a–d**). On day 7 of admission, after anti-infection and antipyretic treatment, low-flow oxygen inhalation through a nasal catheter, and other treatments, the patient had heavier symptoms than before. Chest CT images showed increased density of multiple lesions and thickened interlobular septum (**e–h**). On day 14 of admission, after anti-infection treatment and maintenance of electrolyte acid-base balance, the patient's condition was further aggravated. Chest CT images showed increased and enlarged lesions of bilateral lungs (**i–l**)

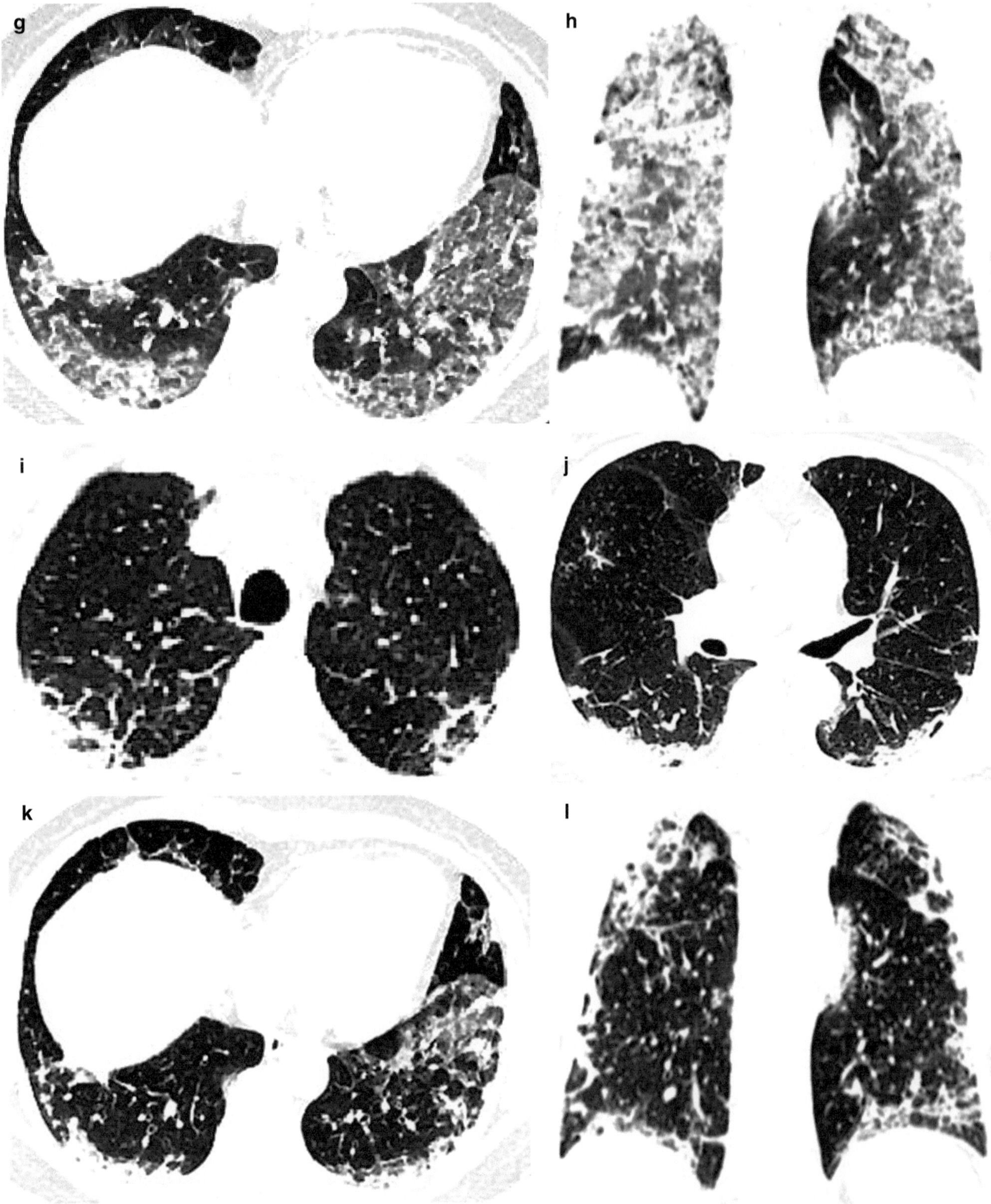

Fig. 6.1 (continued)

6.3 Case 2 (Fig. 6.2a–l)

A 59-year-old male got a fever for 4 days, and he was exposed in the epidemic area. The body temperature at admission was 37.9 °C. Laboratory examination: white blood cell count in peripheral blood was 4.26×10^9/L, the lymphocyte count was 1.36×10^9/L, and the C-reactive protein was 12.33 mg/L. The patient was laboratory con-

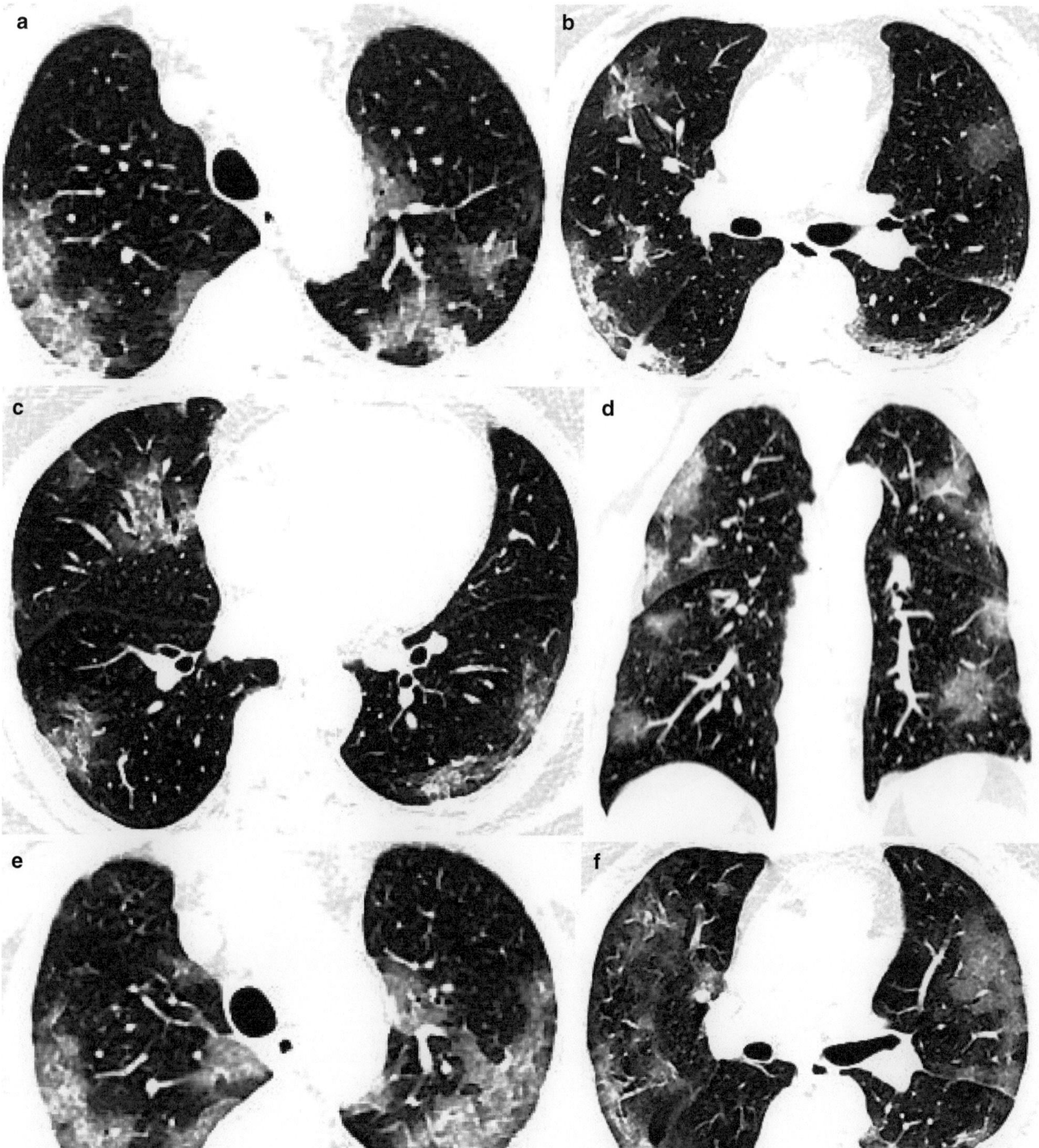

Fig. 6.2 On day 4 of admission, chest CT images showed multiple ground-glass opacities and consolidations in subpleural regions of both lungs (**a**–**d**). On day 6 of admission, after high-frequency humidification-assisted ventilation and anti-infection, anti-inflammatory, and nutritional support treatment, the patient's symptoms did not improve significantly. Chest CT images showed increased density of multiple lesions and thickened interlobular septum (**e**–**h**). On day 16 of admission, the patient underwent anti-infection and antivirus treatment, immunity enhancement, and high-frequency humidification-assisted ventilation treatment; subsequently, his symptoms improved significantly. The range of multifocal lesions was reduced. However, the local density increased, the interlobular septum was thickened, and the subpleural line (hollow arrow) was present (**i**–**l**)

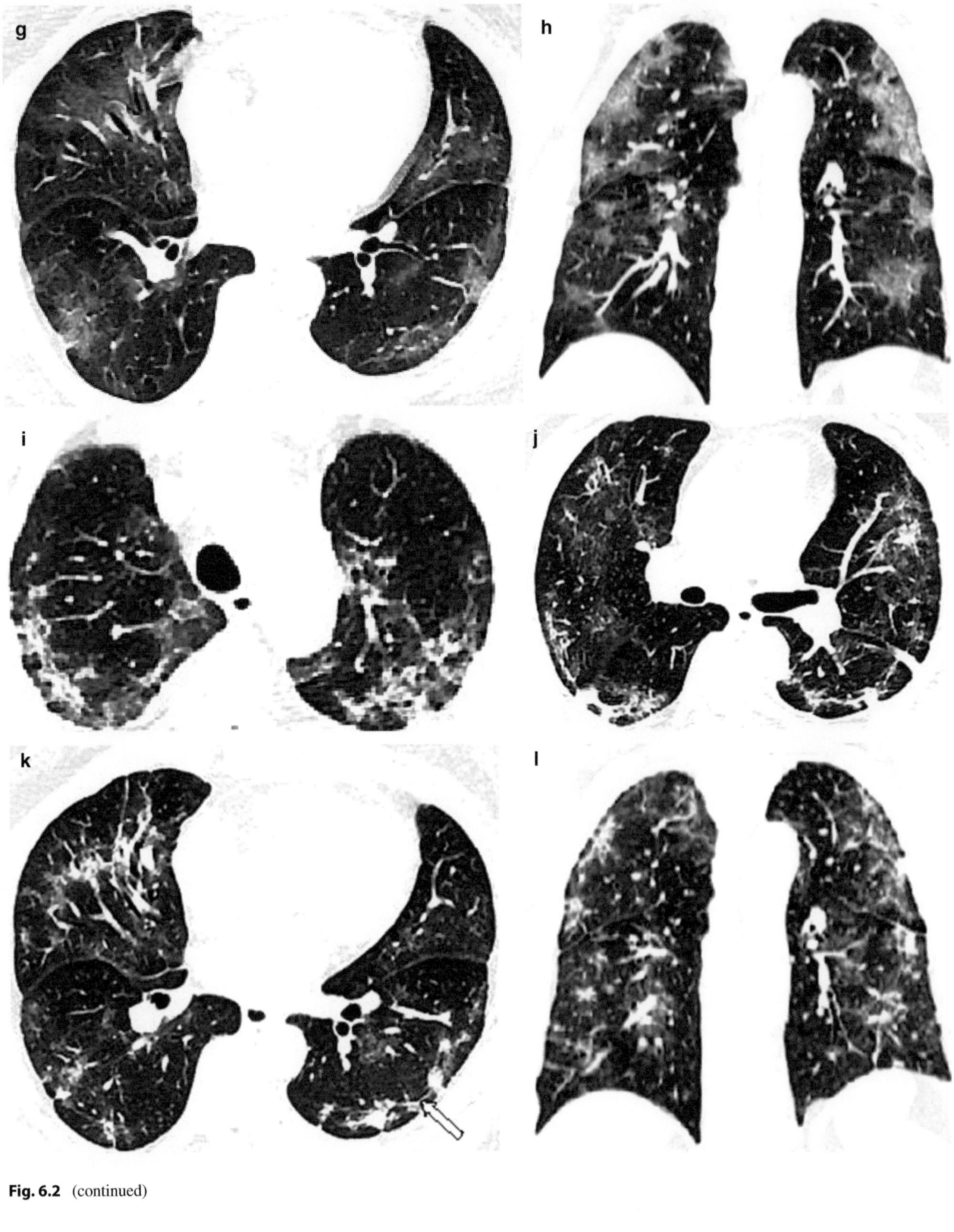

Fig. 6.2 (continued)

firmed by novel coronavirus nucleic acid throat swab test in Guangzhou CDC. Chest CT examination was performed on day 4 (7 days after the onset of symptoms), day 6 (9 days after the onset of symptoms), and day 16 of admission (19 days after the onset of symptoms), as shown in Fig. 6.2a–l.

On day 4 of admission, chest CT images showed multiple ground-glass opacities and consolidations in subpleural regions of both lungs (Fig. 6.2a–d).

On day 6 of admission, after high-frequency humidification-assisted ventilation and anti-infection, anti-inflammatory, and nutritional support treatment, the patient's symptoms did not improve significantly. Chest CT images showed increased density of multiple lesions and thickened interlobular septum (Fig. 6.2e–h).

On day 16 of admission, the patient underwent anti-infection and antivirus treatment, immunity enhancement, and high-frequency humidification-assisted ventilation treatment; subsequently, his symptoms improved significantly. The range of multifocal lesions was reduced. However, the local density increased, the interlobular septum was thickened, and the subpleural line (hollow arrow) was present (Fig. 6.2i–l).

6.4 **Case 3** (Fig. 6.3a–l)

A 62-year-old male was admitted with fever, cough, and expectoration for more than 10 days. He was exposed in the epidemic area. The body temperature at admission was 37.9 °C, and the highest temperature in the course of the disease was 39 °C. Laboratory examination: white blood cell count in peripheral blood was 8.91×10^9/L, the lymphocyte count was 0.48×10^9/L, the C-reactive protein was 50.27 mg/L, and the D-dimer was 1870 μg/L. The patient was laboratory confirmed by novel coronavirus nucleic acid throat swab test in Guangzhou CDC. Chest CT examination was performed on day 2, day 7, and day 15 of admission (19 days after the onset of symptoms), as shown in Fig. 6.3a–l.

On day 2 of admission, CT images exhibited multiple ground-glass opacities in the right upper lobe. The interlobular septum and the right oblique fissure were thickened (Fig. 6.3a–d).

On day 7 of admission, after high-frequency humidification and antiviral therapy, the clinical symptoms of the patient improved. Chest CT images showed reduced lesions, but the local density was increased (Fig. 6.3e–h).

On day 15 of admission, after high-frequency humidification and antiviral therapy, the clinical symptoms of the patients improved. CT scan showed decreased lesions, compared with previous images (Fig. 6.3i–l).

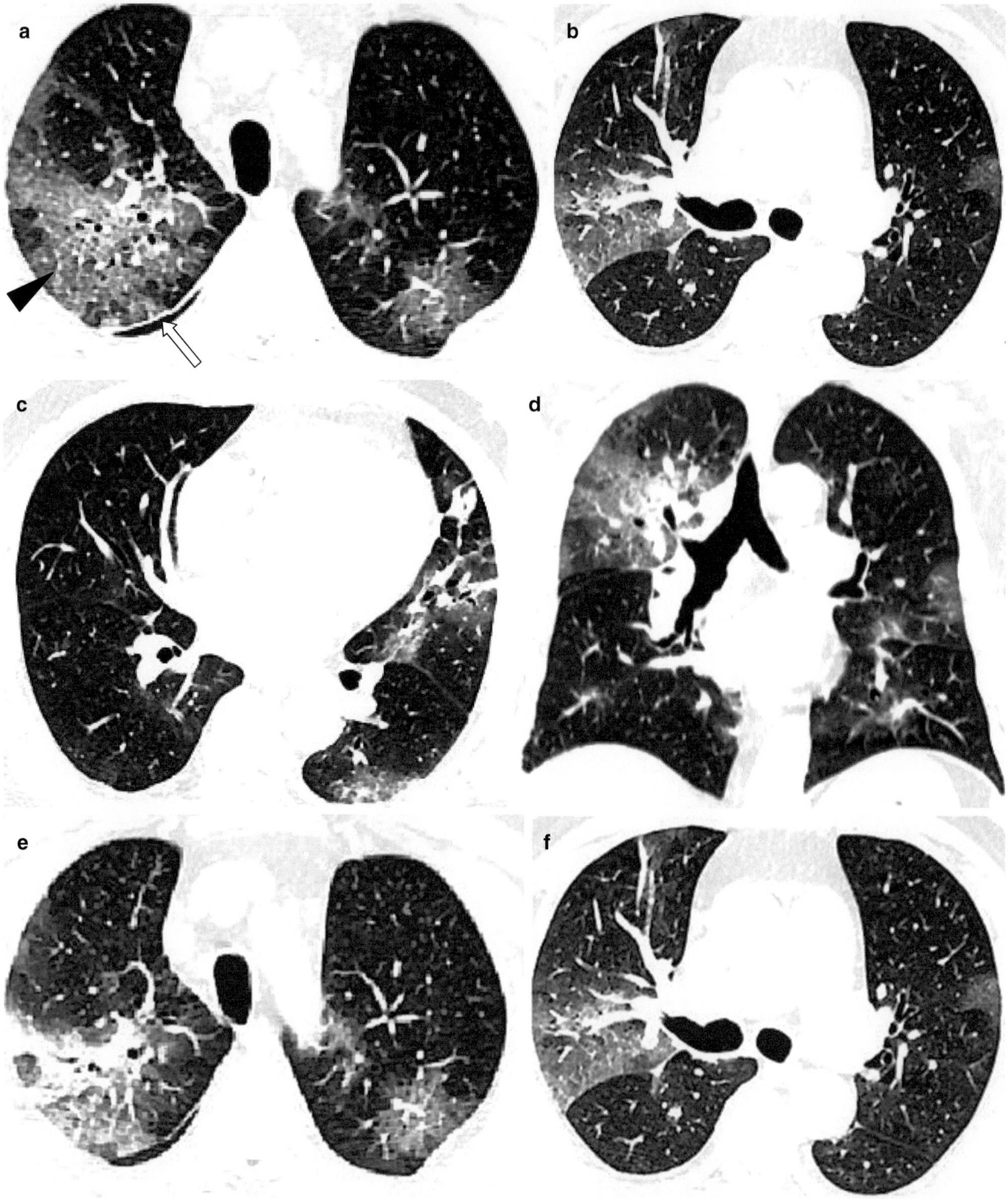

Fig. 6.3 On day 2 of admission, CT images exhibited multiple ground-glass opacities in the right upper lobe. The interlobular septum and the right oblique fissure were thickened (**a**–**d**). On day 7 of admission, after high-frequency humidification and antiviral therapy, the clinical symptoms of the patient improved. Chest CT images showed reduced lesions, but the local density was increased (**e**–**h**). On day 15 of admission, after high-frequency humidification and antiviral therapy, the clinical symptoms of the patients improved. CT scan showed decreased lesions, compared with previous images (**i**–**l**)

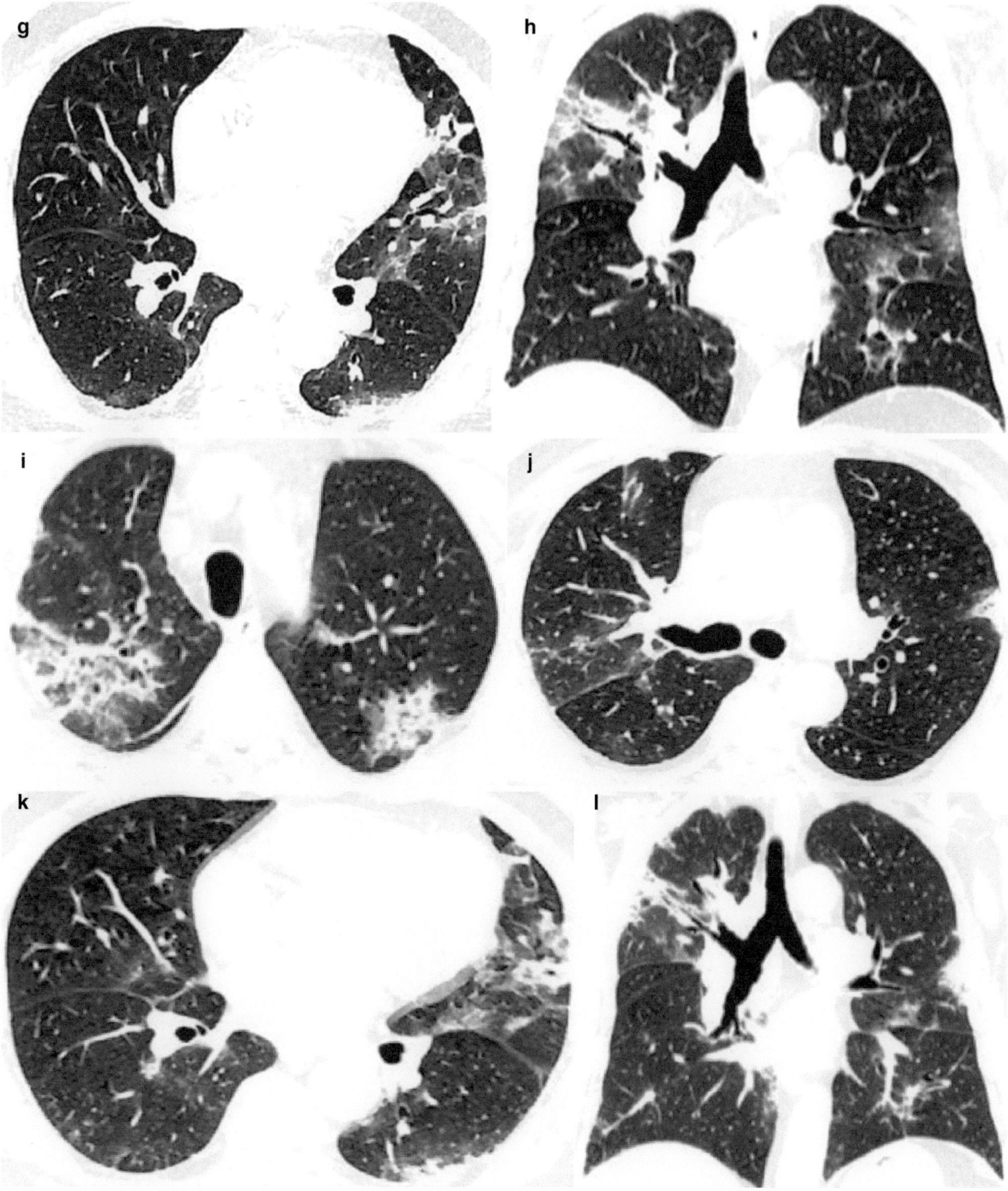

Fig. 6.3 (continued)

6.5 Case 4 (Fig. 6.4a–j)

A 72-year-old male was admitted to the hospital for 5 days, and he was exposed to suspected cases with novel coronavirus pneumonia. His body temperature at admission was 37.7 °C. Laboratory examination: white blood cell count in peripheral blood was 11.5 × 10^9/L, the lymphocyte count was 0.89 × 10^9/L, the C-reactive protein was 34.2 mg/L, and the D-dimer was 1520 μg/L. The patient was laboratory confirmed by novel coronavirus nucleic acid throat swab test in

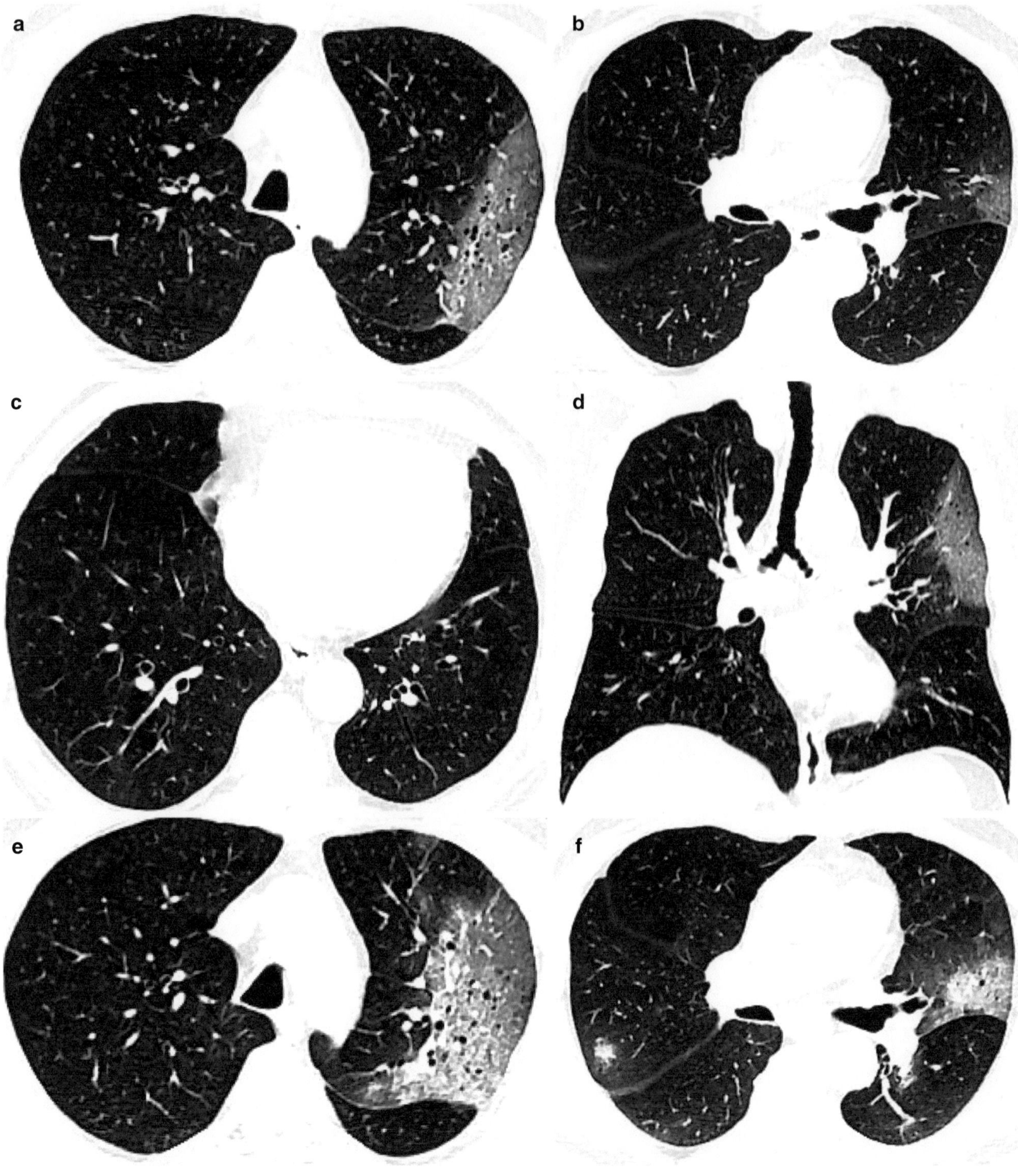

Fig. 6.4 On day 2 of admission, CT images showed ground-glass opacities in the subpleural regions of the left upper lobe (**a**–**d**). On day 7 of admission, after high-flow oxygen therapy, combined anti-infection, anti-inflammatory, and anti-shock therapy, and symptomatic treatment, the symptoms were aggravated. Chest CT images showed new multiple ground-glass opacities and consolidation in the upper and lower lobes of both lungs. The volume of the upper left lobe reduced (**e**–**j**)

Guangzhou CDC. Chest CT examination was performed on day 2 and day 7 of admission, as shown in Fig. 6.4a–j.

On day 2 of admission, CT images showed ground-glass opacities in the subpleural regions of the left upper lobe (Fig. 6.4a–d).

On day 7 of admission, after high-flow oxygen therapy, combined anti-infection, anti-inflammatory, and anti-shock therapy, and symptomatic treatment, the symptoms were aggravated. Chest CT images showed new multiple ground-glass opacities and consolidation in the upper and lower

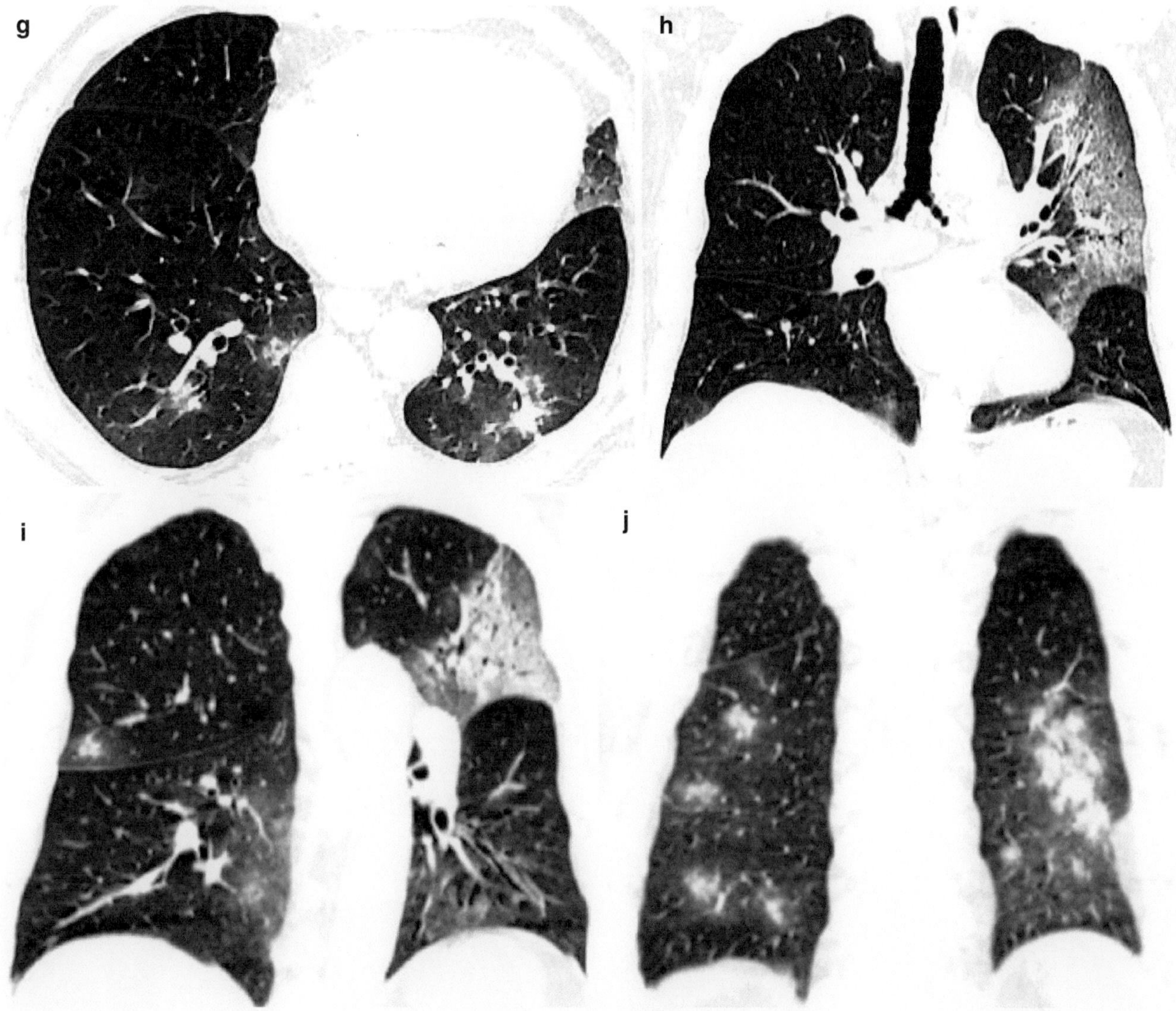

Fig. 6.4 (continued)

lobes of both lungs. The volume of the upper left lobe reduced (Fig. 6.4e–j).

6.6 Case 5 (Fig. 6.5a–l)

A 58-year-old male was admitted to the hospital for 9 days, and he was exposed to suspected cases with novel coronavirus pneumonia. The body temperature at admission was 38 °C. Laboratory examination: white blood cell count in peripheral blood was 6.69×10^9/L, the lymphocyte count was 2.14×10^9/L, and the C-reactive protein was 25.1 mg/L. The patient was laboratory confirmed by novel coronavirus nucleic acid throat swab test in Guangzhou CDC. Chest CT examination was performed on day 3, day 6, and day 9 of admission, as shown in Fig. 6.5a–l.

On day 3 of admission, chest CT images showed ground-glass opacities in subpleural regions of bilateral lungs (Fig. 6.5a–d).

On day 6 of admission, the patient was treated with a low-flow nasal catheter for oxygen inhalation and anti-infection, anti-inflammatory, and immune-enhancing treatment. The symptoms of the patient were aggravated. Chest CT images showed increased and enlarged lesions of both lungs, the interlobular septum thickened, and the subpleural line was present. (Fig. 6.5e–h).

On day 9 of admission, the patient was transferred to the ICU. After treatment with high-flow humidified oxygen therapy instrument-assisted breathing and adjustment of anti-infection strategy, the condition was further aggravated. Chest CT images showed that the lung lesions increased and enlarged, and the intralobular septa and interlobular septa thickening were more obviously than before (Fig. 6.5i–l).

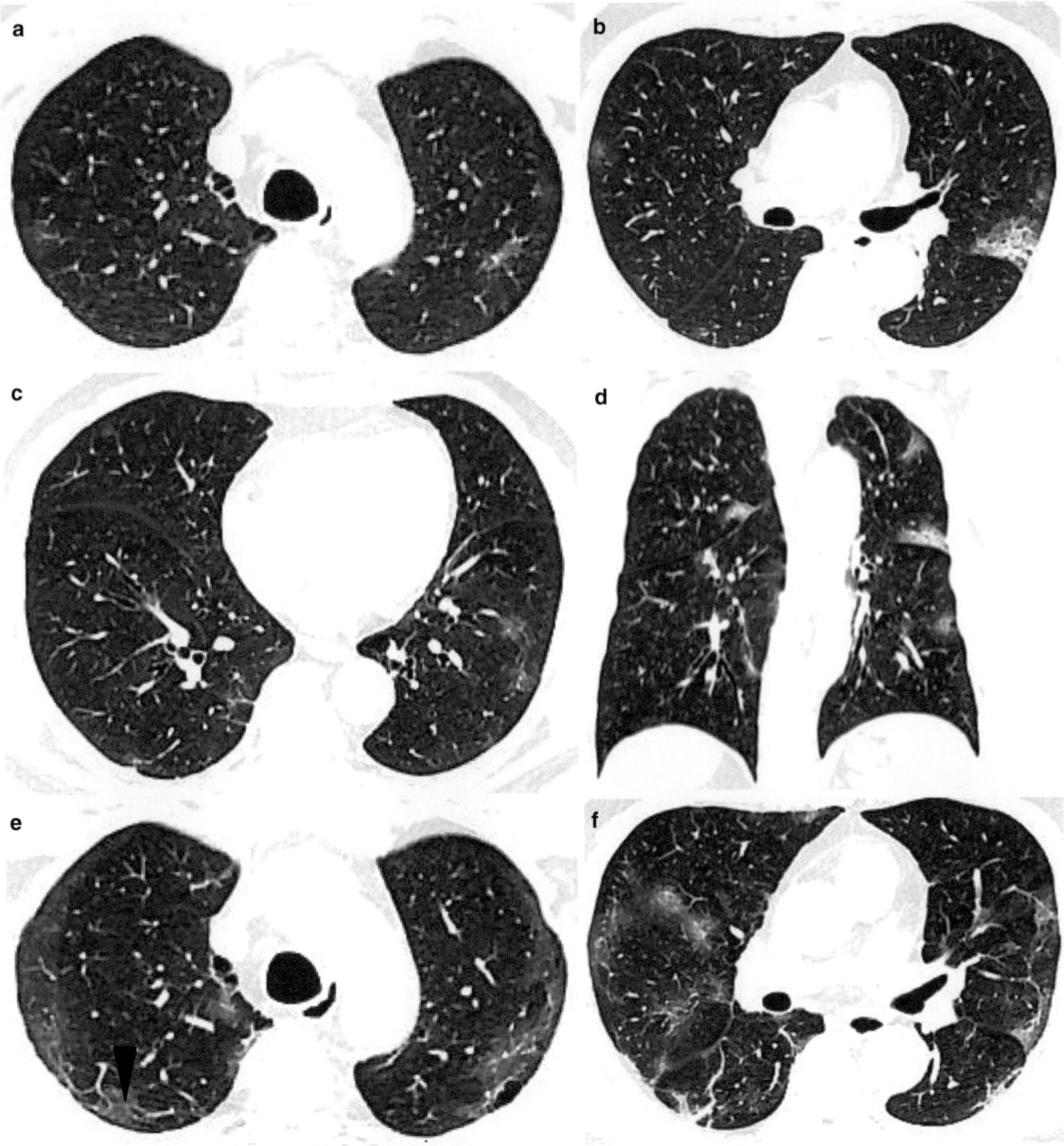

Fig. 6.5 On day 3 of admission, chest CT images showed ground-glass opacities in subpleural regions of bilateral lungs (**a–d**). On day 6 of admission, the patient was treated with a low-flow nasal catheter for oxygen inhalation and anti-infection, anti-inflammatory, and immune-enhancing treatment. The symptoms of the patient were aggravated. Chest CT images showed increased and enlarged lesions of both lungs, the interlobular septum thickened, and the subpleural line was present (**e–h**). On day 9 of admission, the patient was transferred to the ICU. After treatment with high-flow humidified oxygen therapy instrument-assisted breathing and adjustment of anti-infection strategy, the condition was further aggravated. Chest CT images showed that the lung lesions increased and enlarged, and the intralobular septa and interlobular septa thickening were more obviously than before (**i–l**)

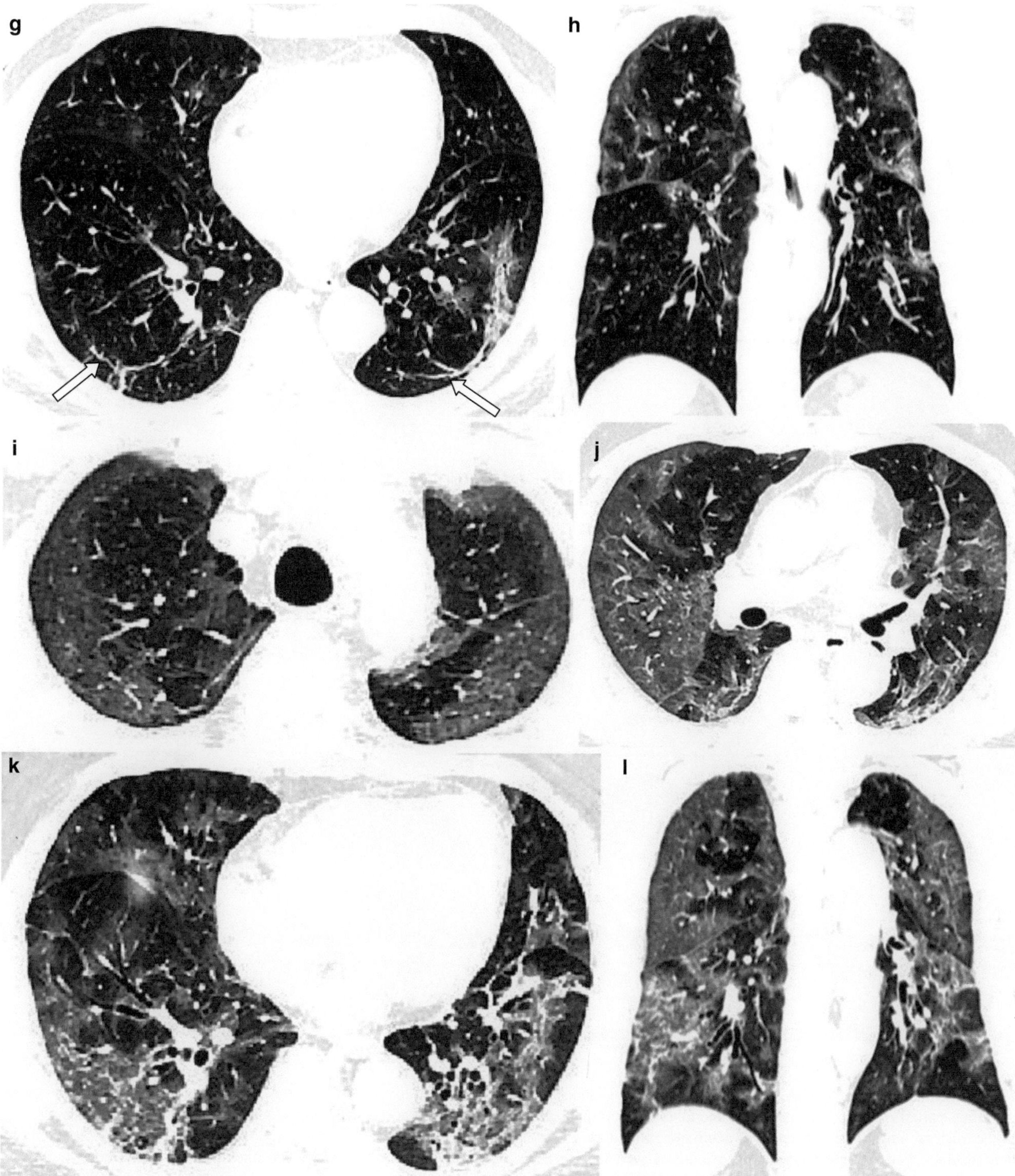

Fig. 6.5 (continued)

6.7 Case 6 (Fig. 6.6a–l)

A 61-year-old female was admitted to the hospital with cough and sputum for 11 days and fever for 2 days. The body temperature at admission was 36.5 °C, and the highest temperature in the course of the disease was 38.4 °C. Laboratory examination: white blood cell count in peripheral blood was 4.29×10^9/L, the lymphocyte count was 1.07×10^9/L, the C-reactive protein was 63.66 mg/L, and the D-dimer was 1460 μg/L. The patient was laboratory confirmed by novel

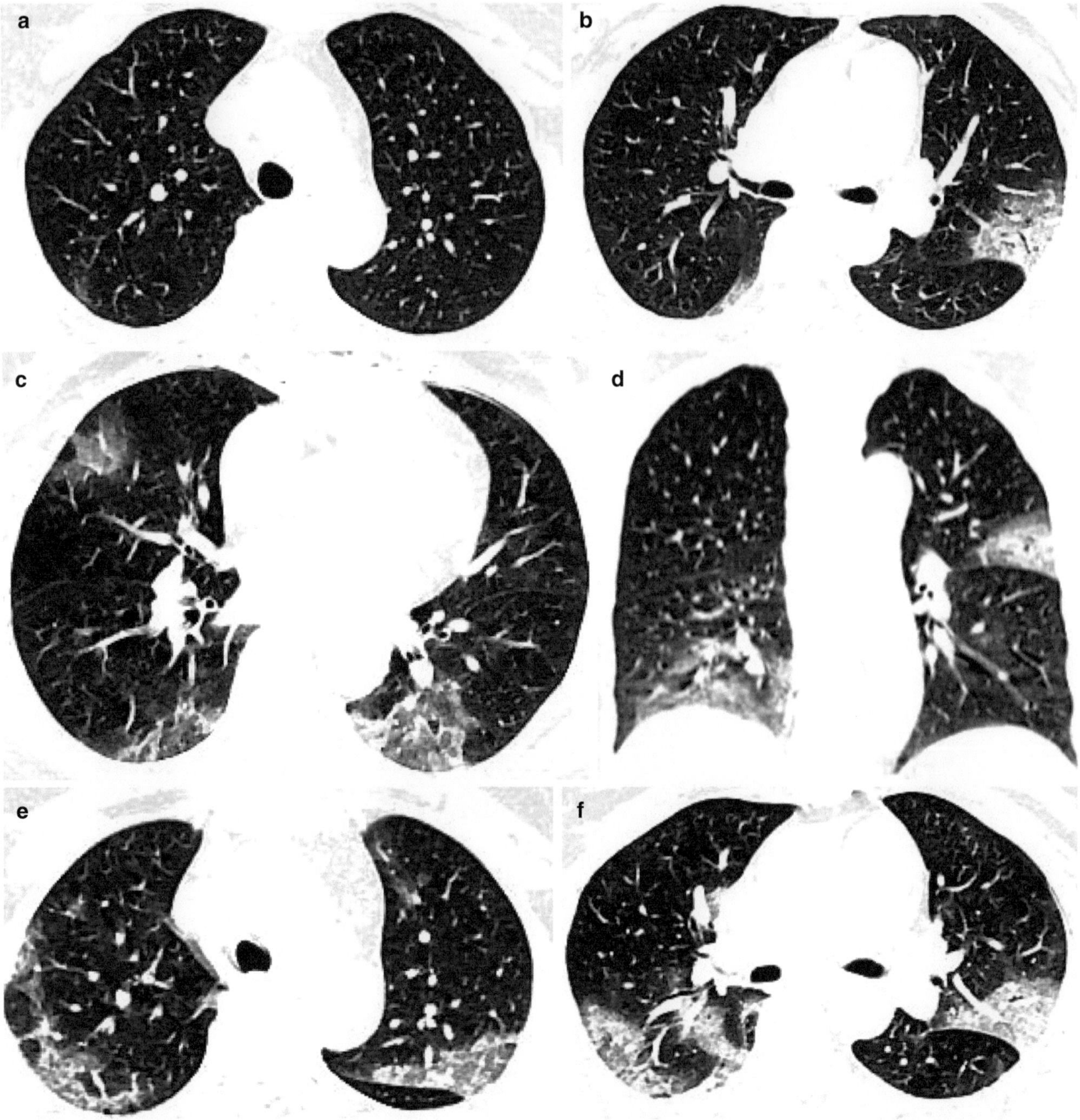

Fig. 6.6 On day 1 of admission, chest CT scan showed ground-glass opacities, partial consolidation, and local interlobular septal thickening in the bilateral lungs (**a**–**d**). On day 5 of admission, after anti-infection and medium-flow oxygen therapy, the symptoms were worse than before. Chest CT scan showed increased and enlarged lung lesions in the bilateral lobes (**e**–**h**). On day 12 of admission, after anti-infection, anti-inflammation, and high-to-medium-flow oxygen therapy, the patient's symptoms improved. Chest CT scan showed decreased multiple lung lesions and thickening of the interlobular septum (**i**–**l**)

coronavirus nucleic acid throat swab test in Guangzhou CDC. Chest CT examination was performed on day 1 (5 days after the onset of symptoms), day 5 (9 days after the onset of symptoms), and day 12 (16 days after the onset of symptoms) of admission, as shown in Fig. 6.6a–l.

On day 1 of admission, chest CT scan showed ground-glass opacities, partial consolidation, and local interlobular septal thickening in the bilateral lungs (Fig. 6.6a–d).

On day 5 of admission, after anti-infection and medium-flow oxygen therapy, the symptoms were worse than before.

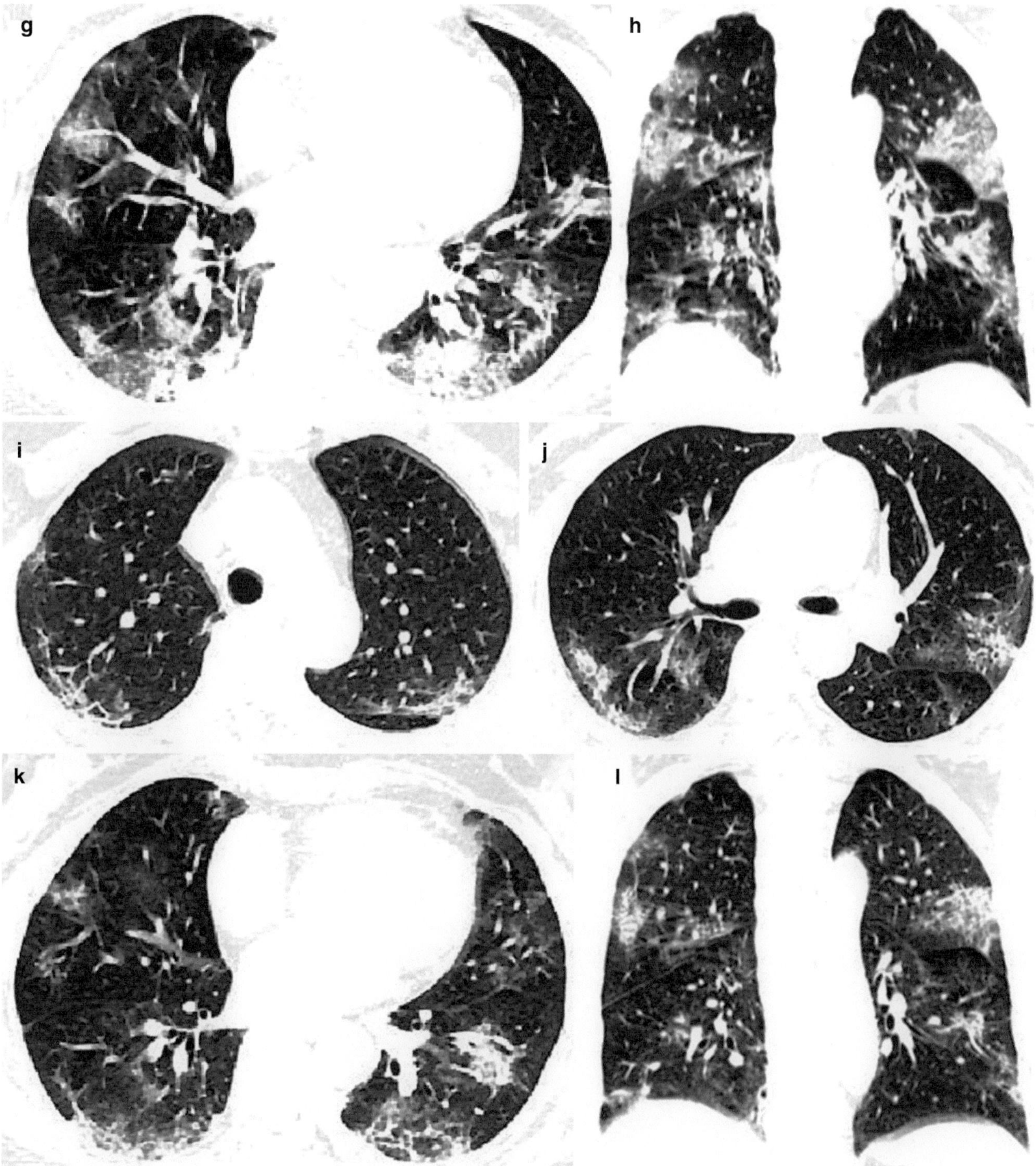

Fig. 6.6 (continued)

Chest CT scan showed increased and enlarged lung lesions in the bilateral lobes (Fig. 6.6e–h).

On day 12 of admission, after anti-infection, anti-inflammation, and high-to-medium-flow oxygen therapy, the patient's symptoms improved. Chest CT scan showed decreased multiple lung lesions and thickening of the interlobular septum (Fig. 6.6i–l).

6.8 Case 7 (Fig. 6.7a–l)

A 61-year-old female was admitted to the hospital with cough and sputum for 11 days and fever for 2 days. The body temperature at admission was 36.5 °C, and the highest temperature in the course of the disease was 38.4 °C. Laboratory examination: white blood cell count in

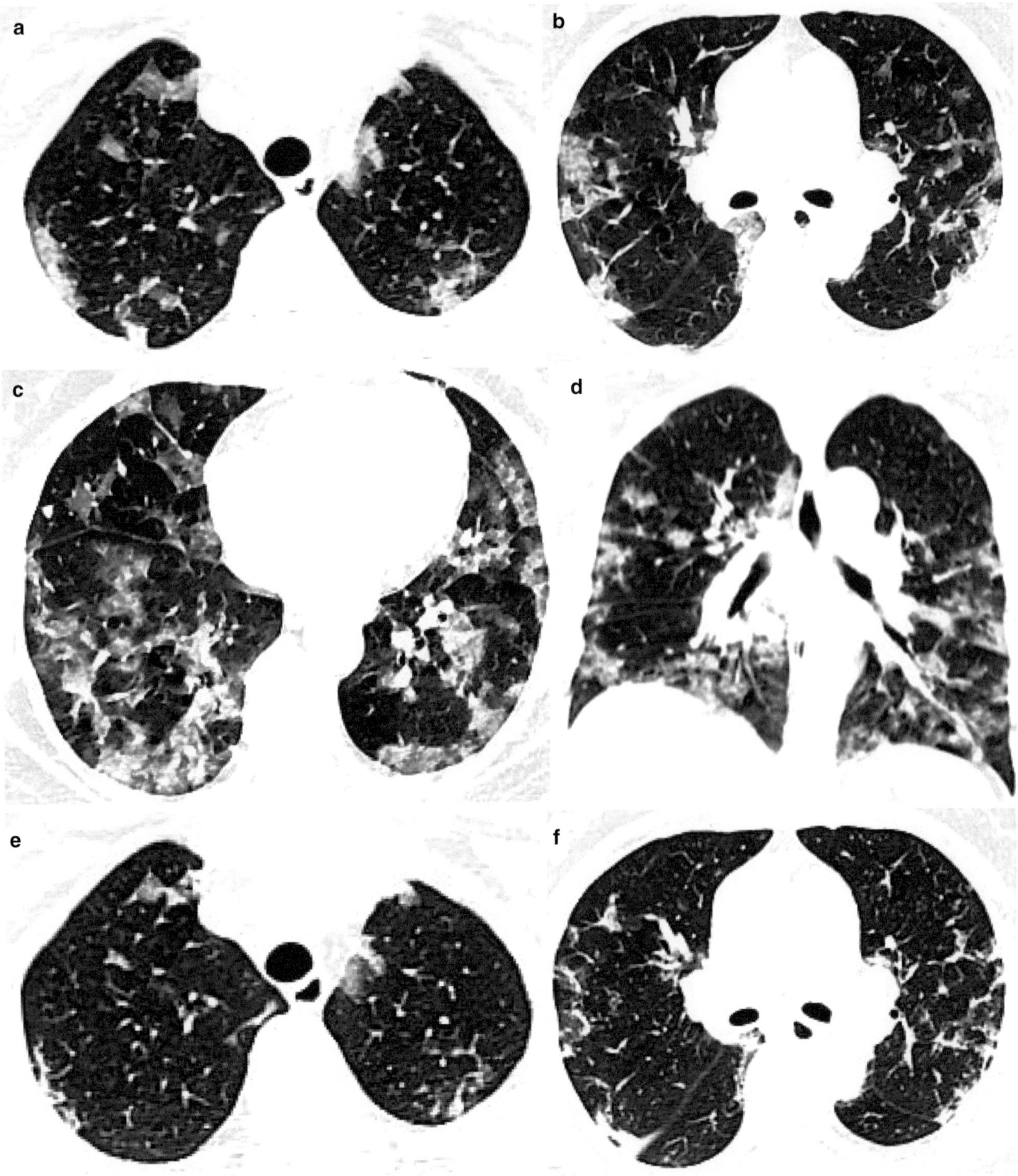

Fig. 6.7 On day 2 of admission, chest CT scan showed multiple ground-glass opacities, partial consolidation, and local interlobular septal thickening in the bilateral lungs (**a**–**d**). On day 8 of admission, after high-frequency humidification-assisted ventilation and anti-infection, anti-fungus, anti-inflammatory, and antivirus treatment, the patient's symptoms improved. Chest CT scan showed decreased lesions in the bilateral lungs (**e**–**h**). On day 17 of admission, the patient underwent the same treatment as before, and the symptoms turned better than before. The chest CT images showed that the bilateral lung lesions decreased, compared with previous images (**i**–**l**)

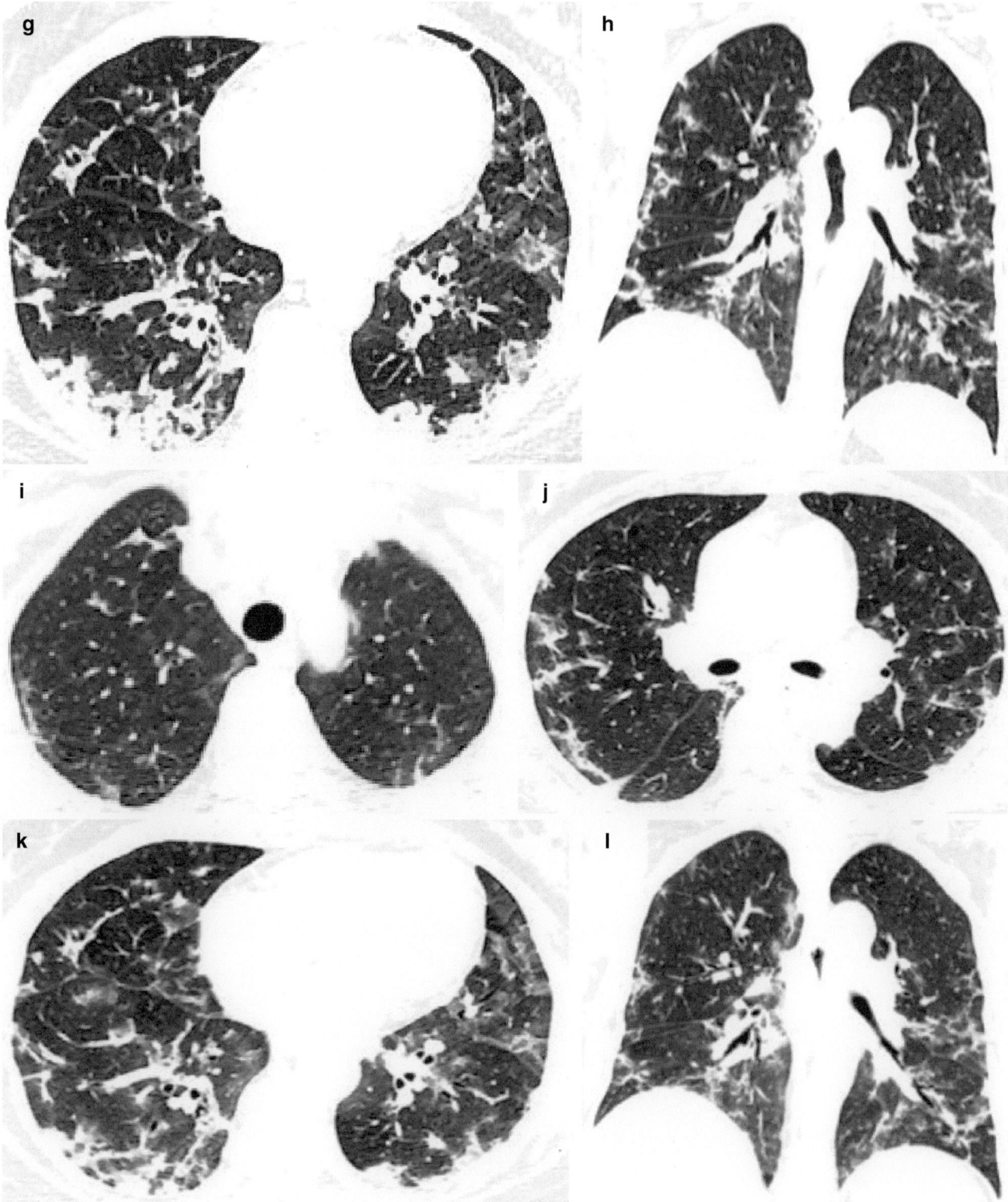

Fig. 6.7 (continued)

peripheral blood was 4.29×10^9/L, the lymphocyte count was 1.07×10^9/L, the C-reactive protein was 63.66 mg/L, and the D-dimer was 1460 μg/L. The patient was laboratory confirmed by novel coronavirus nucleic acid throat swab test in Guangzhou CDC. Chest CT examination was performed on day 2 (13 days after the onset of symptoms), day 8 (19 days after the onset of symptoms), and day 17 (28 days after the onset of symptoms) of admission, as shown in Fig. 6.7a–l.

On day 2 of admission, chest CT scan showed multiple ground-glass opacities, partial consolidation, and local interlobular septal thickening in the bilateral lungs (Fig. 6.7a–d).

On day 8 of admission, after high-frequency humidification-assisted ventilation and anti-infection, anti-fungus, anti-inflammatory, and antivirus treatment, the patient's symptoms improved. Chest CT scan showed decreased lesions in the bilateral lungs (Fig. 6.7e–h).

On day 17 of admission, the patient underwent the same treatment as before, and the symptoms turned better than before. The chest CT images showed that the bilateral lung lesions decreased, compared with previous images (Fig. 6.7i–l).

6.9 Case 8 (Fig. 6.8a–k)

A 65-year-old male was admitted to the hospital with fever for 11 days, diarrhea for 5 days, and shortness of breath for 3 days. The body temperature at admission was 37.5 °C, and the highest temperature in the course of the disease was 39.2 °C. Laboratory examination: white blood cell count in peripheral blood was 4.39×10^9/L, the lymphocyte count was 0.47×10^9/L, and the C-reactive protein was 108.8 mg/L. The patient was laboratory confirmed by novel coronavirus nucleic acid throat swab test in Guangzhou CDC. Chest CT examination was performed on day 4 (15 days after the onset of symptoms) and day 12 (23 days after the onset of symptoms). Bedside chest radiographs were taken on day 16 (27 days after the onset of symptoms), day 18 (29 days after the onset of symptoms), and day 24 (35 days after the onset of symptoms), shown in Fig. 6.8a–k.

On day 4 of admission, chest CT images showed extensive ground-glass opacities and consolidation (with air bronchogram sign) of bilateral lungs and thickening of the interlobular septa, forming a "crazy-paving pattern" (hollow arrow), and subpleural subline was present (Fig. 6.8a–d).

On day 12 of admission, after assisted ventilation and anti-infection treatment, the symptoms of the patients were worse than before. Chest CT scan showed the increased density of bilateral lung lesions (Fig. 6.8e–h).

On day 16 of admission, bedside chest radiograph of the patient showed multiple ground-glass opacities in bilateral lungs, especially in the lower lobes (Fig. 6.8i).

On day 18 of admission, the patient's symptoms were worse than before, and the reexamination of the bedside chest radiograph showed enlarged lesions and progressive ground-glass opacities in both lower lobes, indicating disease progression (Fig. 6.8j).

On day 24 of admission, the patient's symptoms improved, and the bedside chest radiograph showed that lesions were reduced (Fig. 6.8k).

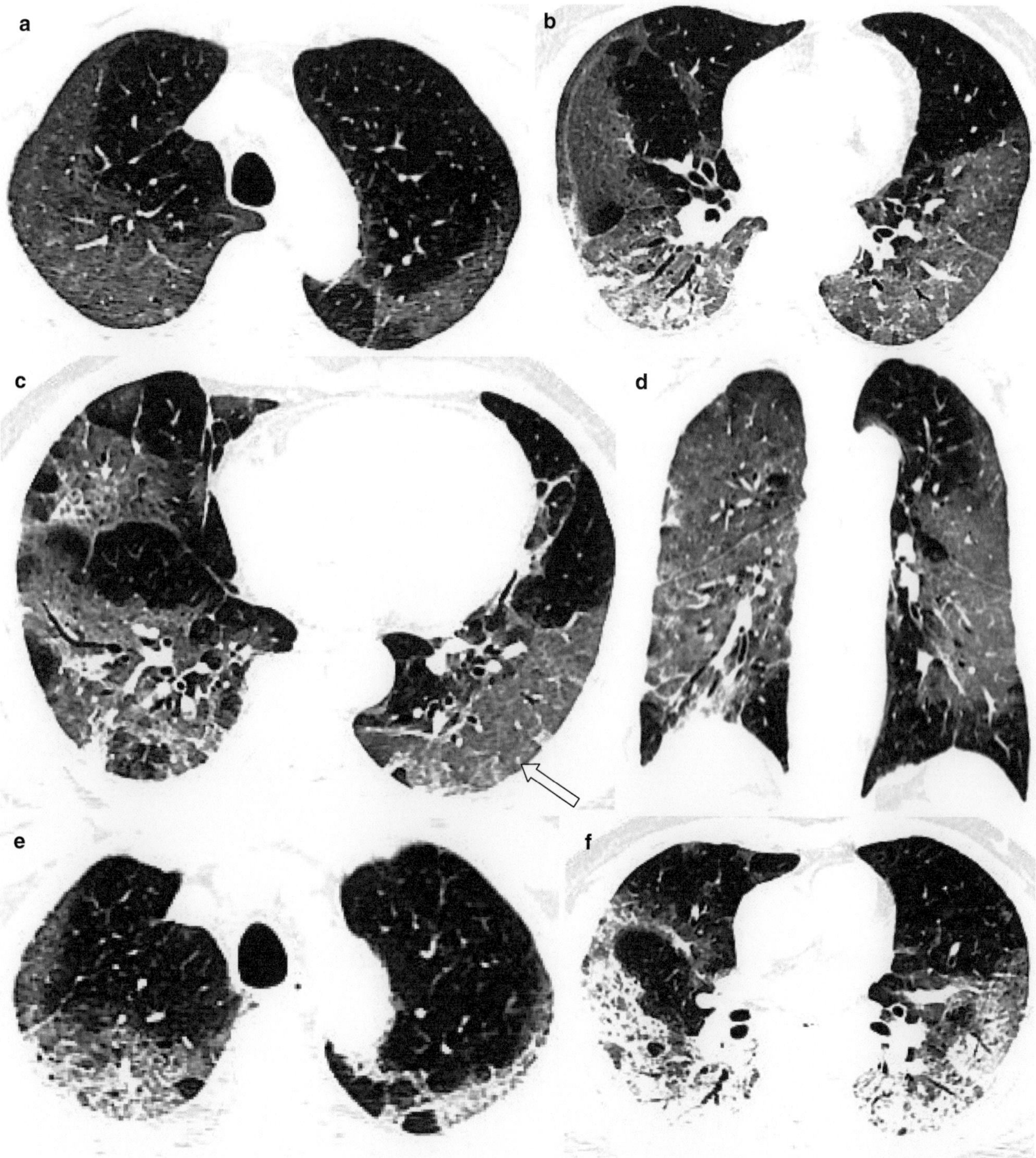

Fig. 6.8 On day 4 of admission, chest CT images showed extensive ground-glass opacities and consolidation (with air bronchogram sign) of bilateral lungs and thickening of the interlobular septa, forming a "crazy-paving pattern" (hollow arrow), and subpleural subline was present (**a**–**d**). On day 12 of admission, after assisted ventilation and anti-infection treatment, the symptoms of the patients were worse than before. Chest CT scan showed the increased density of bilateral lung lesions (**e**–**h**). On day 16 of admission, bedside chest radiograph of the patient showed multiple ground-glass opacities in bilateral lungs, especially in the lower lobes (**i**). On day 18 of admission, the patient's symptoms were worse than before, and the reexamination of the bedside chest radiograph showed enlarged lesions and progressive ground-glass opacities in both lower lobes, indicating disease progression (**j**). On day 24 of admission, the patient's symptoms improved, and the bedside chest radiograph showed that lesions were reduced (**k**)

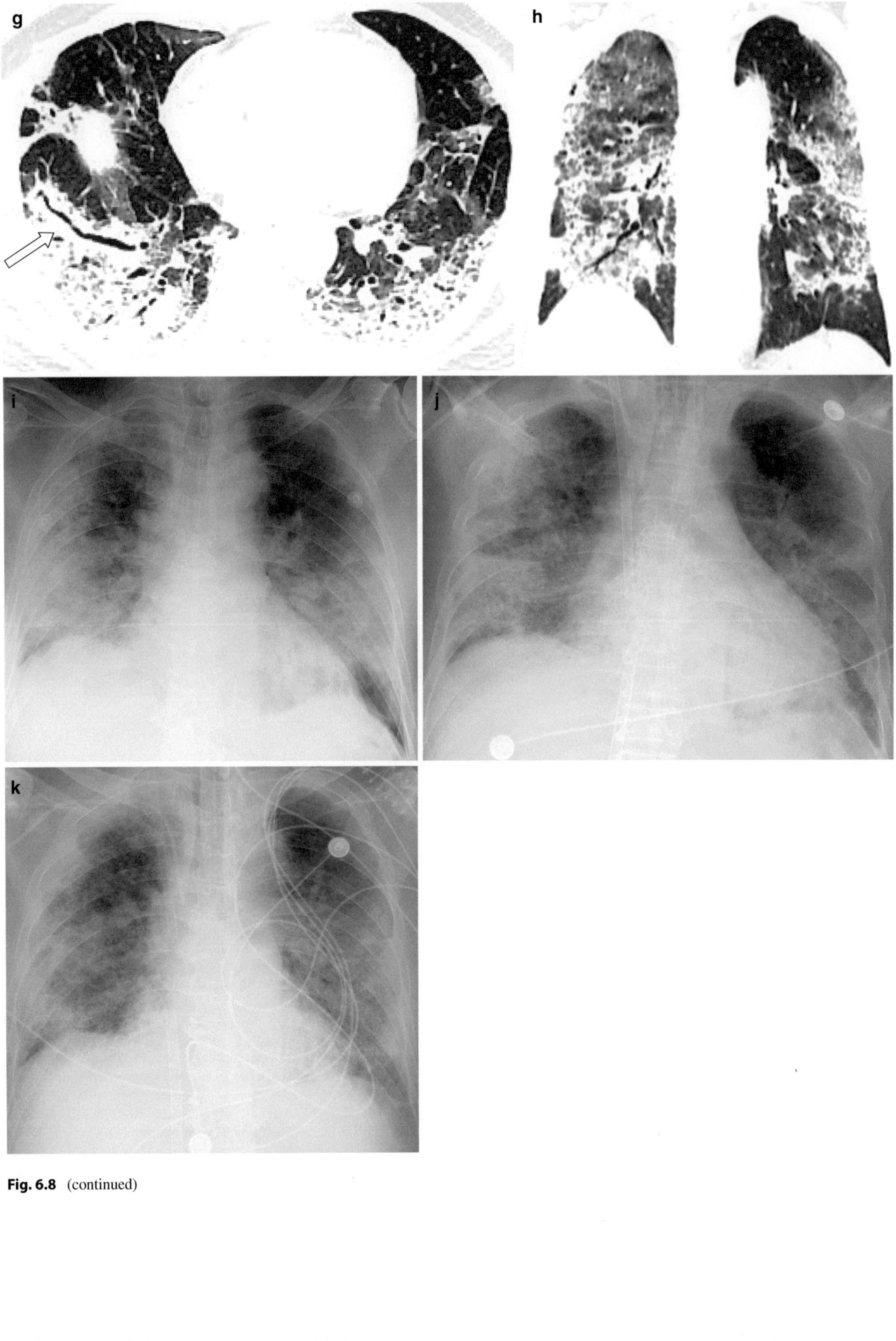

Fig. 6.8 (continued)

6.10 Case 9 (Fig. 6.9a–k)

A 55-year-old female was admitted to the hospital with fever for 2 days. The body temperature at admission was 38 °C, and the highest temperature in the course of the disease was 38.1 °C. Laboratory examination: white blood cell count in peripheral blood was 6.29 × 10^9/L, the lymphocyte count was 2.09 × 10^9/L, the C-reactive protein was 20.37 mg/L, and the D-dimer was 1090 μg/L. The patient was laboratory confirmed by novel coronavirus nucleic acid throat swab test in Guangzhou CDC. Chest CT examination was performed on day 1 (3 days after the onset of symptoms) and day 6 (8 days after the onset of symptoms). Bedside chest radiographs were taken on day 9 (11 days after the onset of symptoms), day 14 (16 days after the onset of symptoms), and day 17 (19 days after the onset of symptoms), shown in Fig. 6.9a–k.

On day 1 of admission, chest CT scan showed ground-glass opacities in multiple lobes (Fig. 6.9a–d).

On day 6 of admission, the patient was admitted to ICU after high-flow mask oxygen inhalation and antiviral, anti-infection, and anti-inflammatory treatment, and the symptoms were more severe than before. Chest CT images showed that the bilateral lung lesions increased and enlarged, with the range increased by more than 50%, and the interlobular septum thickened; "crazy-paving pattern" (hollow arrow) was observed (Fig. 6.9e–h).

On day 9 of admission, the patient's symptoms were aggravated; bedside chest radiograph of the patient showed multiple ground-glass opacities in the bilateral lungs (Fig. 6.9i).

On day 14 of admission, the patient's symptoms improved, and the bedside chest radiograph showed progressive lesions in both lower lobes compared with previous images (Fig. 6.9j).

On day 17 of admission, the patient's symptoms did not improve significantly, and the bedside chest radiograph showed that lesions were more aggravated than before, and the bilateral lung showed like "white lung" (Fig. 6.9k).

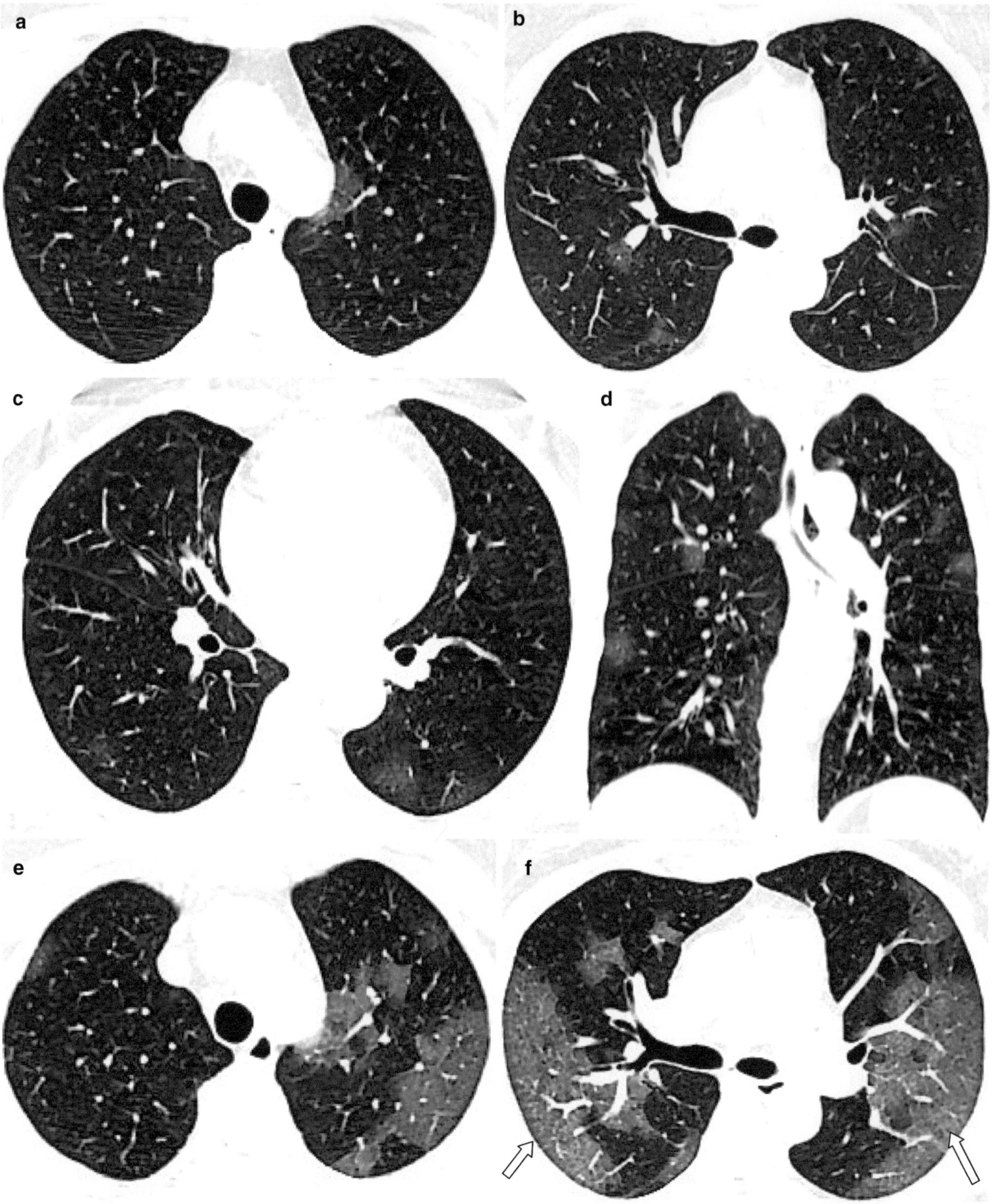

Fig. 6.9 On day 1 of admission, chest CT scan showed ground-glass opacities in multiple lobes (**a**–**d**). On day 6 of admission, the patient was admitted to ICU after high-flow mask oxygen inhalation and antiviral, anti-infection, and anti-inflammatory treatment, and the symptoms were more severe than before. Chest CT images showed that the bilateral lung lesions increased and enlarged, with the range increased by more than 50%, and the interlobular septum thickened; a "crazy-paving pattern" (hollow arrow) was observed (**e**–**h**). On day 9 of admission, the patient's symptoms were aggravated; bedside chest radiograph of the patient showed multiple ground-glass opacities in the bilateral lungs (**i**). On day 14 of admission, the patient's symptoms improved, and the bedside chest radiograph showed progressive lesions in both lower lobes compared with previous images (**j**). On day 17 of admission, the patient's symptoms did not improve significantly, and the bedside chest radiograph showed that lesions were more aggravated than before, and the bilateral lung showed like "white lung" (**k**)

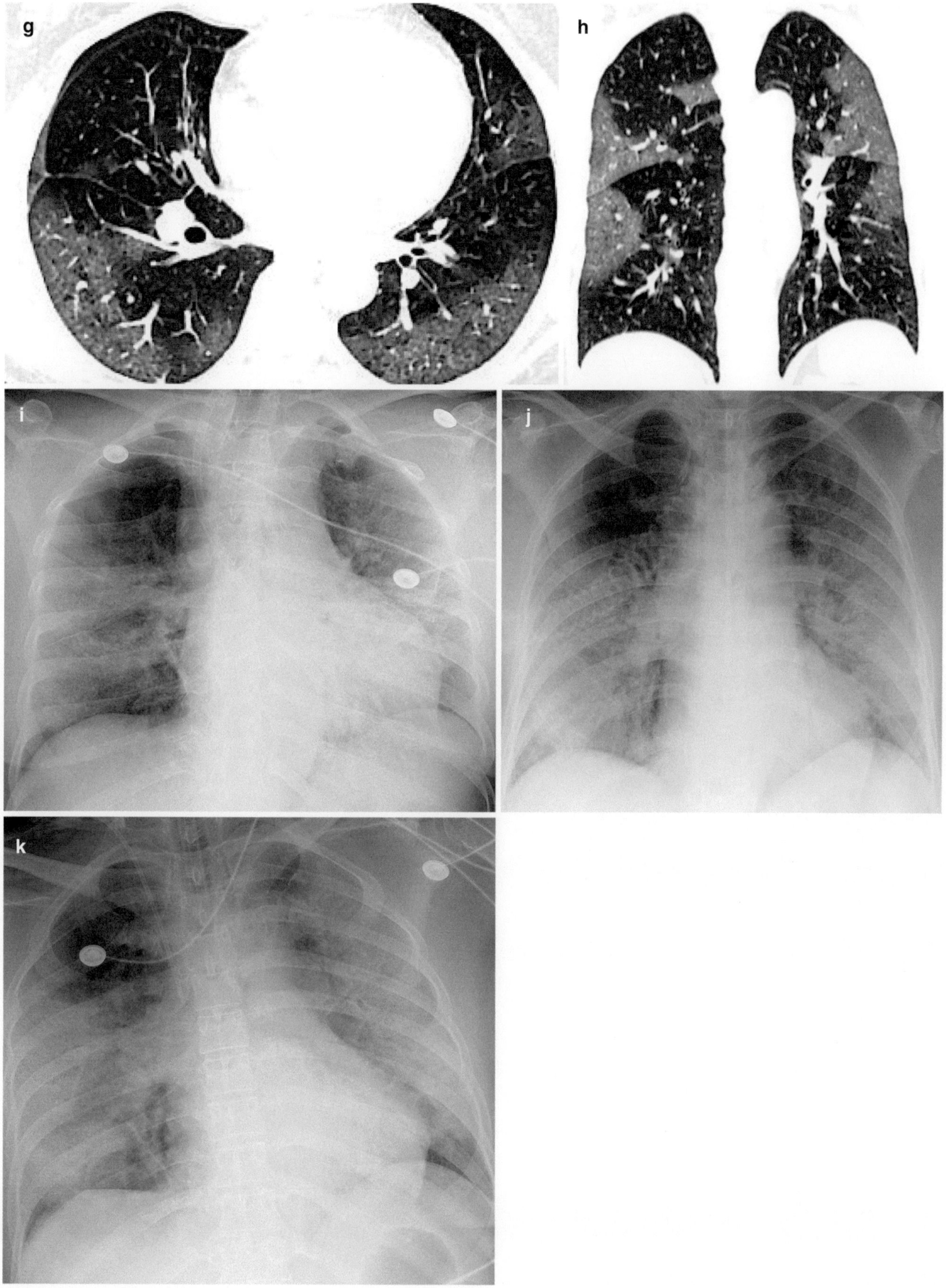

Fig. 6.9 (continued)

References

1. Huang C, Wang Y, Li X, et al. Clinical features of patients infected with 2019 novel coronavirus in Wuhan, China. Lancet. 2020;395:497–506. https://doi.org/10.1016/S0140-6736(20)30183-5.
2. Ooi GC, Daqing M. SARS: radiological features. Respirology. 2003;8(Suppl):S15–9. https://doi.org/10.1046/j.1440-1843.2003.00519.x.
3. Das KM, Lee EY, Langer RD, Larsson SG. Middle East respiratory syndrome coronavirus: what does a radiologist need to know? AJR Am J Roentgenol. 2016;206:1193–201. https://doi.org/10.2214/AJR.15.15363.
4. Chung M, Bernheim A, Mei X, et al. CT imaging features of 2019 novel coronavirus (2019-nCoV). Radiology. 2020; https://doi.org/10.1148/radiol.2020200230.

7 Role of CT and CT Features of Suspected COVID-19 Patients (PCR Negative)

Qingxin Gan, Tianli Hu, and Songfeng Jiang

7.1 Introduction

The COVID-19 pneumonia is a specific infectious disease caused by severe acute respiratory syndrome coronavirus 2 (SARS-COV-2) which is a single-stranded positive-strand RNA virus and has not been found in humans previously [1–3]. Since the outbreak of COVID-19 in January 2020, it has spread rapidly among general population through respiratory droplets and indirect or direct contact, especially in middle-aged and elderly people [4–6]. The incubation period of COVID-19 pneumonia is 1–14 days, usually 3–7 days. The main clinical manifestations are fever, fatigue, dry cough, and muscle soreness, a few accompanied by nasal congestion, runny nose, diarrhea, and so on [7]. Most patients present with mild clinical symptoms initially, while for some severe or critically ill patients, symptoms can manifest as dyspnea and hypoxemia within a week and progress to respiratory failure and death [8, 9].

At present, the detection of SARS-CoV-2 viral RNA by RT-PCR is the gold standard for confirmation of COVID-19. Unfortunately, the rate of detectable viral RNA in upper respiratory swab samples is only 30–50%, which is much lower than 76.4% of CT [10]. The main reason is that virus is not detectable in nasal and pharynx swabs even when virus replicates in the lung. At this time, the suspected patients should have chest CT examination to exclude the infection of COVID-19 pneumonia. If the chest CT images of suspected patient show evidence of progressive COVID-19 pneumonia, they should be admitted to the hospital for isolation and treatment immediately and take multiple nucleic acid tests for subsequent confirmation. Therefore, diagnosis of COVID-19 pneumonia should be based on a combination of clinical features, the results of chest CT and nucleic acid test.

Q. Gan (✉) · T. Hu · S. Jiang
Guangzhou Eighth People's Hospital, Guangzhou Medical University, Guangzhou, China

For most of suspected patients, the common features on chest CT are single or multiple, nodular or patchy ground-glass opacities with or without blurred margin; most of the lesions are located in the peripheral region of the lung, especially in the lower lobes. In few cases, chest CT images show patchy ground-glass opacities in the bilateral lung with focal consolidation shadows. In this chapter, we aim to describe the CT features of suspected COVID-19 pneumonia patients with negative finding of PCR to improve the detection rate of the disease in detail.

7.2 Case 1 (Fig. 7.1a–j)

A 64-year-old female patient, who had no exposure to epidemic areas. On January 20, 2020, she went out for dinner with her family. The next day, she developed fever with a temperature of up to 38.5 °C, accompanied by headache and body aches, with no aversion to cold or shivering, no coughing or expectoration, and no tightness or shortness of breath. On January 21, 2020, CT examination was performed, and the chest CT images showed pneumonia. The clinical symptoms did not significantly improve after 1 week of treatment. Body temperature fluctuated from 37.5 °C to 38.5 °C. At the time of admission, the body temperature was 38.2 °C, the respiratory rate was 18 breaths per minute, total white blood cell count was 3.48×10^9/L, C-reactive protein was 25.68 mg/L, neutrophil count was 1.50×10^9/L, lymphocyte count was 1.56×10^9/L, platelet count was 134×10^9/L, and oxygen saturation was 97.5%. The viral RNA in throat swab was negative for three examinations. In her fourth examination, she was finally confirmed by Guangzhou CDC. On January 30, 2020, chest CT images showed multiple patchy ground-glass opacities in bilateral lungs.

CT images showed multiple patchy ground-glass opacities in bilateral lungs (Fig. 7.1a–j), mainly located in subpleural areas of the lung, accompanied with enlarged vessels (Fig. 7.1f, h), thickened interlobular septa and intralobular septa, and linear opacities (Fig. 7.1j).

J. Liu et al. (eds.), *Atlas of Chest Imaging in COVID-19 Patients*, https://doi.org/10.1007/978-981-16-1082-0_7

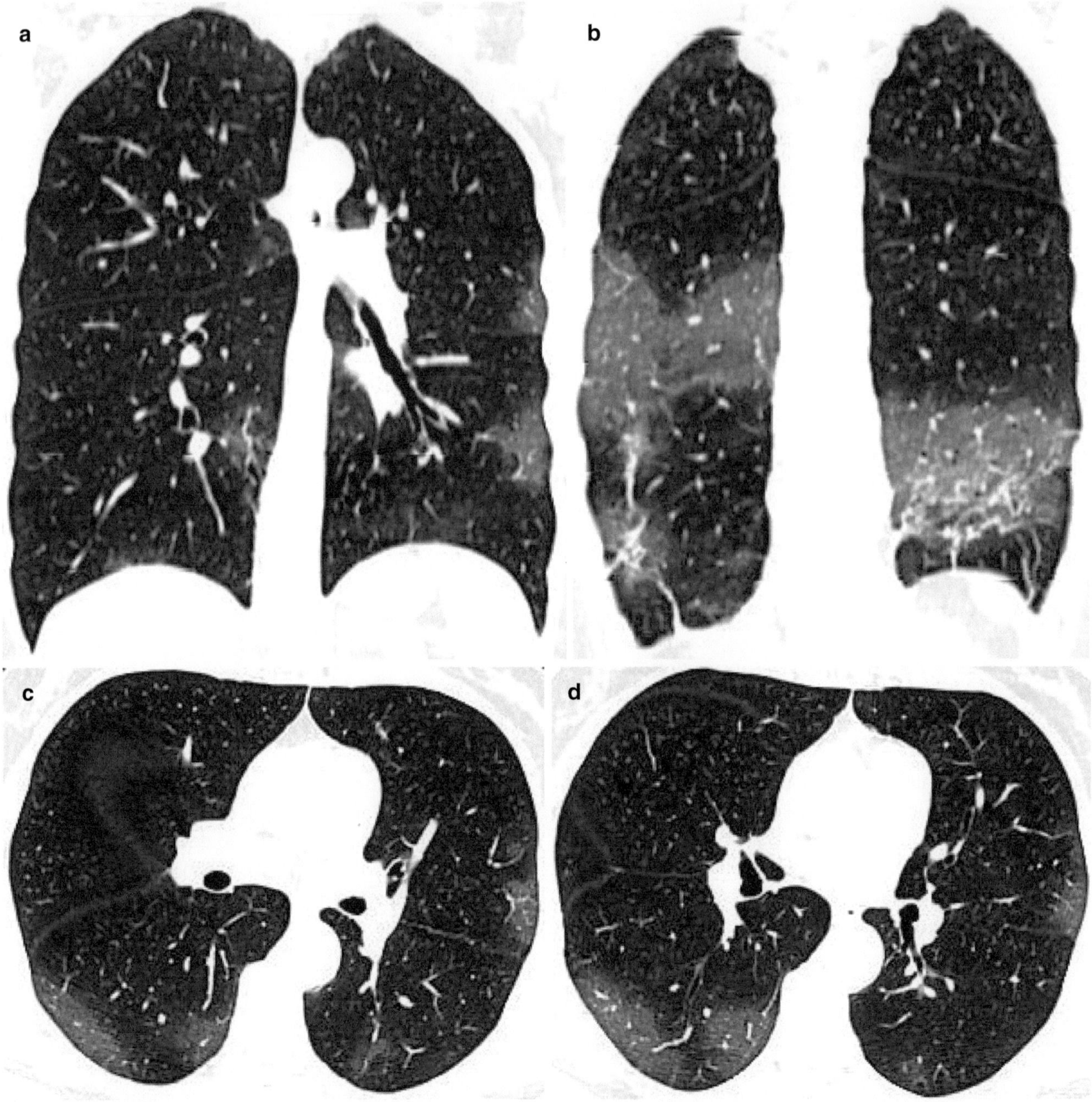

Fig. 7.1 CT images showed multiple patchy ground-glass opacities in bilateral lungs (**a**–**j**), mainly located in subpleural areas of the lung, accompanied with enlarged vessels (**f**, **h**), thickened interlobular septa and intralobular septa, and linear opacities (**a**–**j**)

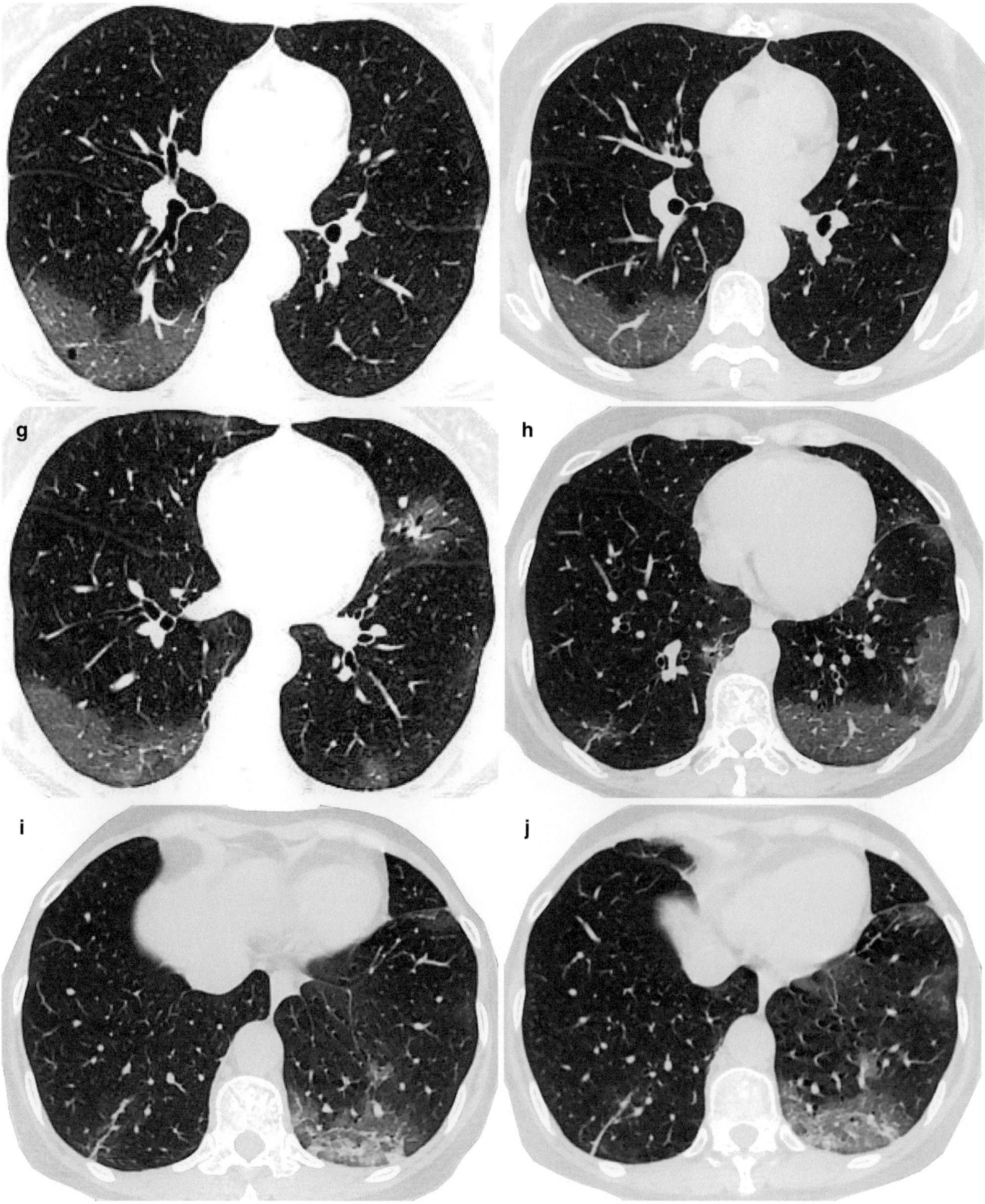

Fig. 7.1 (continued)

7.3 **Case 2** (Fig. 7.2a–j)

A 65-year-old female patient with a history of exposure to the epidemic area presented with fever and chills on January 24, 2020 without obvious inducement. She was admitted to the hospital on January 30, 2020. At the time of admission, the body temperature was 37.7 °C, the respiratory rate was 18 breaths per minute, total white blood cell count was

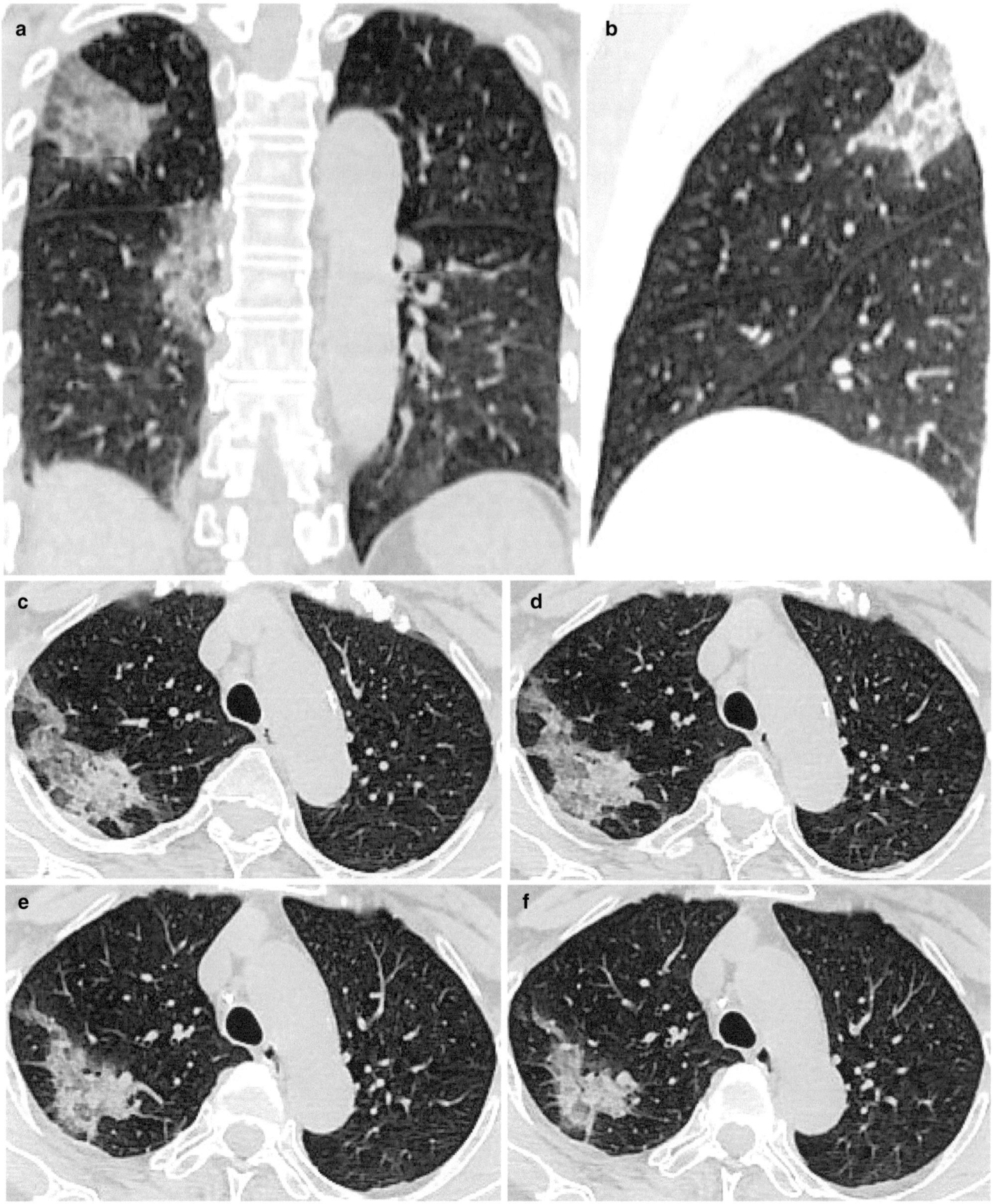

Fig. 7.2 CT images showed a segmental consolidation in the posterior segment of the upper lobe of the right lung with "air bronchogram" (**c**–**g**). There was a small patchy increase in the density of the basal segment of the right lower lobe (**h**–**j**)

2.54×10^9 L, C-reactive protein was 20.09 mg/L, neutrophil count was 1.25×10^9 L, lymphocyte count was 0.93×10^9 L, platelet count was 147×10^9 L, and oxygen saturation was 96.4%. The viral RNA in throat swab was negative in her first examination. In her second examination, she was finally confirmed by Guangzhou CDC. On January 31, 2020, chest

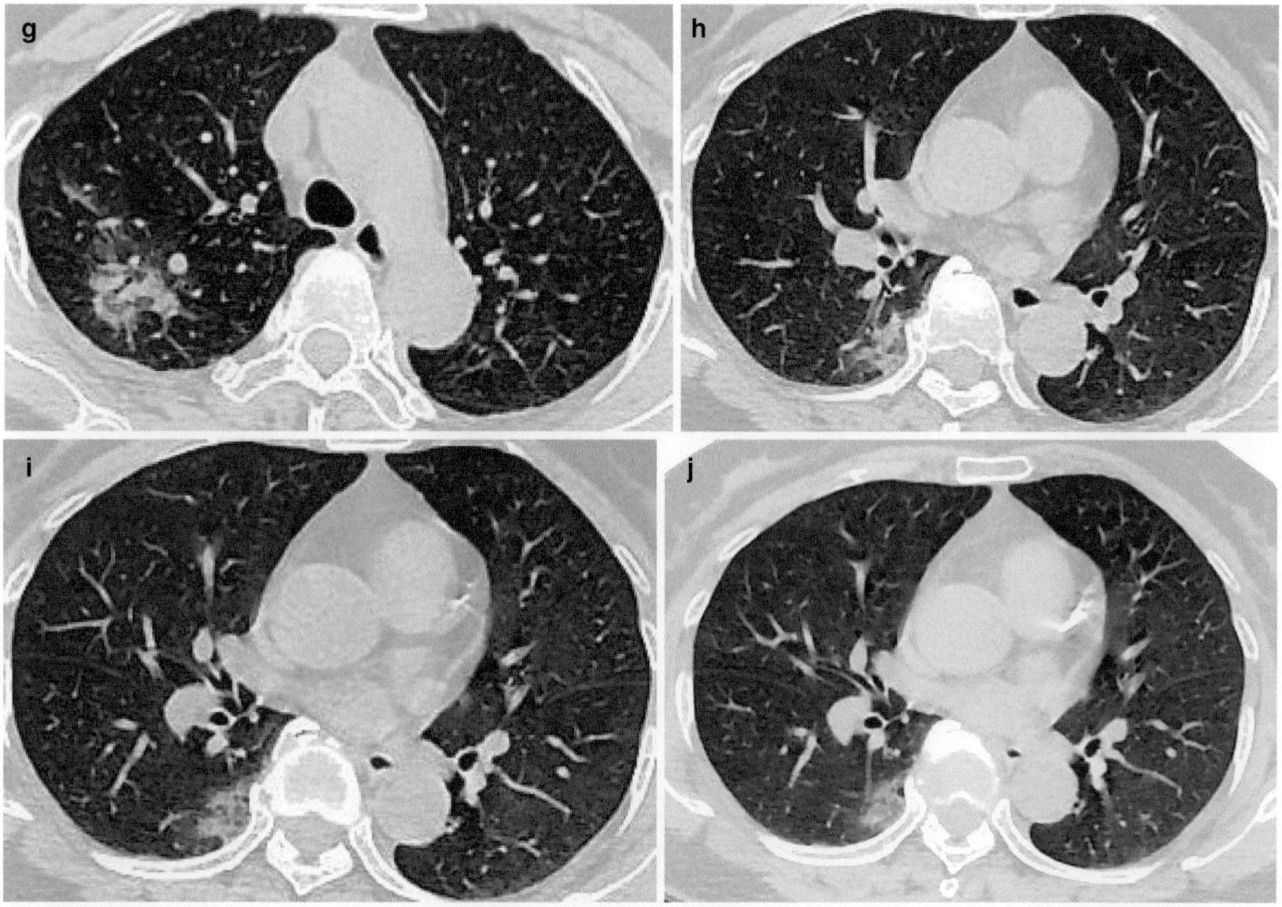

Fig. 7.2 (continued)

CT images revealed multiple patchy ground-glass opacities in bilateral lungs.

CT images showed a segmental consolidation in the posterior segment of the upper lobe of the right lung with "air bronchogram" (Fig. 7.2c–g). There was a small patchy increase in the density of the basal segment of the right lower lobe (Fig. 7.2h–j).

7.4 Case 3 (Fig. 7.3a–j)

A 63-year-old female patient had a history of exposure to epidemic areas. On January 28, 2020, she presented with pharynx discomfort and expectoration, with no fever, no chest tightness or shortness of breath, no nausea or vomiting, and no abdominal distension or abdominal pain. She was admitted to the hospital on January 30, 2020. At the time of admission, the body temperature was 36.6 °C, the respiratory rate was 18 breaths per minute, total white blood cell count was 5.08×10^9 L, C-reactive protein was 2.73 mg/L, neutrophil count was 2.54×10^9 L, lymphocyte count was 2.09×10^9 L, platelet count was 154×10^9 L, and oxygen saturation was 95.9%. The viral RNA in throat swab was negative in her first examination. In her second examination, she was finally confirmed by Guangzhou CDC. On January 31, 2020, chest CT images showed multiple ground-glass opacities in bilateral lungs.

CT images showed multiple ground-glass opacities (Fig. 7.3a–j) in the lower lobe of bilateral lungs (Fig. 7.3d), with thickening of the interlobular septa (Fig. 7.3e–i) and linear opacities (Fig. 7.3j) in the left lower lobe (Fig. 7.3j).

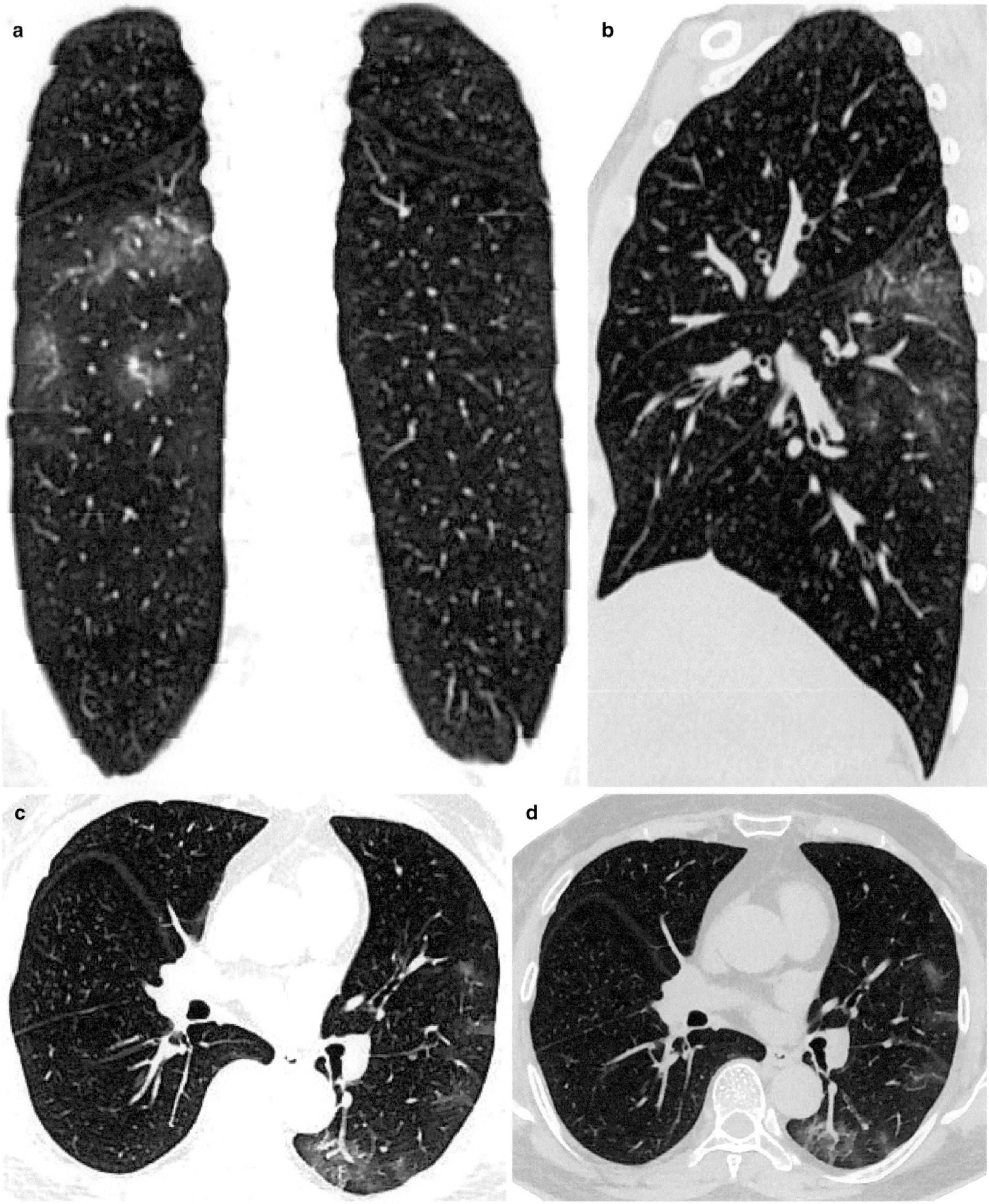

Fig. 7.3 CT images showed multiple ground-glass opacities (**a**–**j**) in the lower lobe of bilateral lungs (**d**), with thickening of the interlobular speta (**e**–**i**) and linear opacities (**j**) in the left lower lobe (**j**)

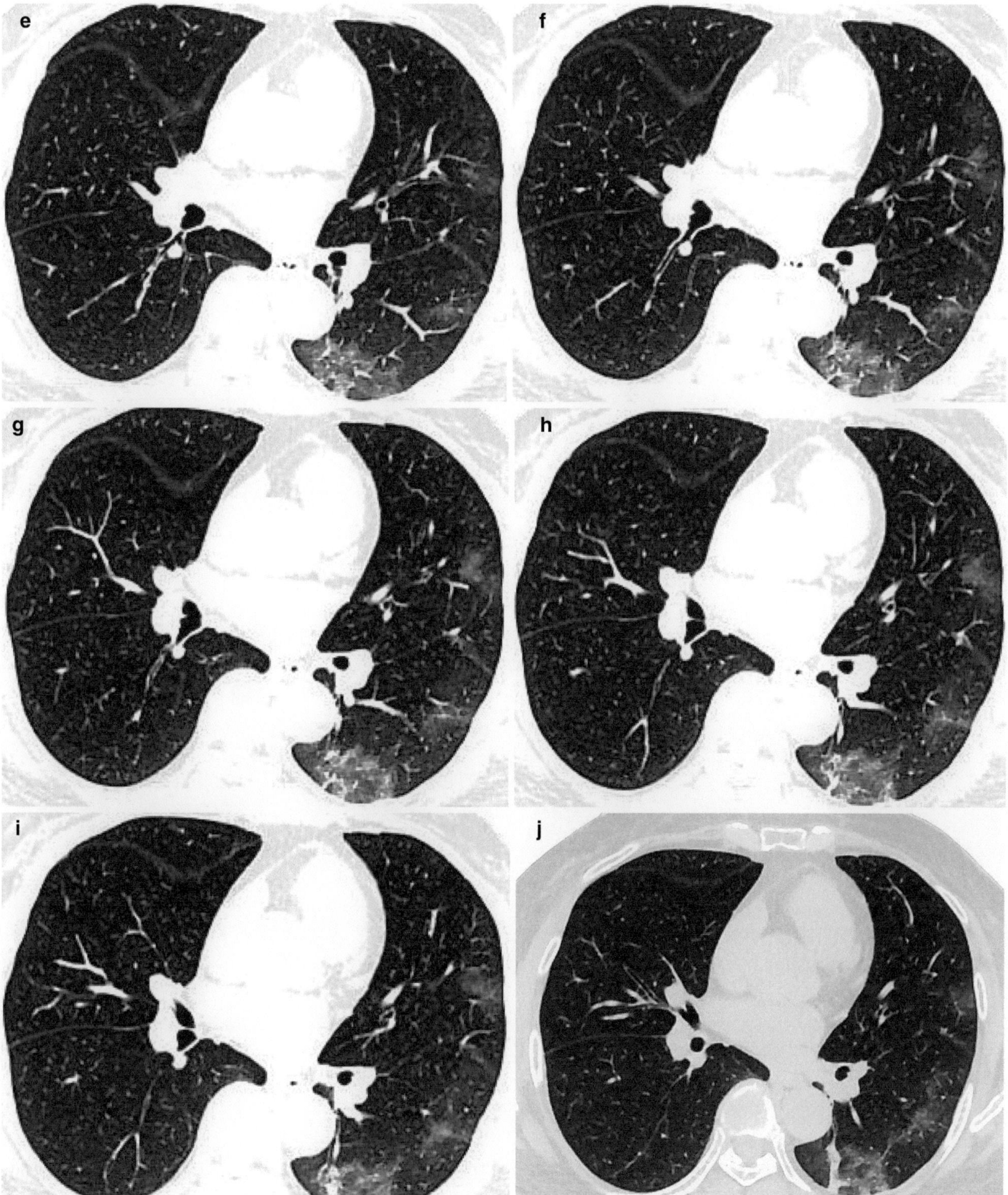

Fig. 7.3 (continued)

7.5 Case 4 (Fig. 7.4a–j)

A 26-year-old male patient had a history of exposure to epidemic areas. On January 20, 2020, he presented with fever and cough with no obvious inducement, and the clinical symptoms improved after treatment. The next week, he was readmitted with fever. At the time of admission, the body temperature was 38.5 °C, the respiratory rate was

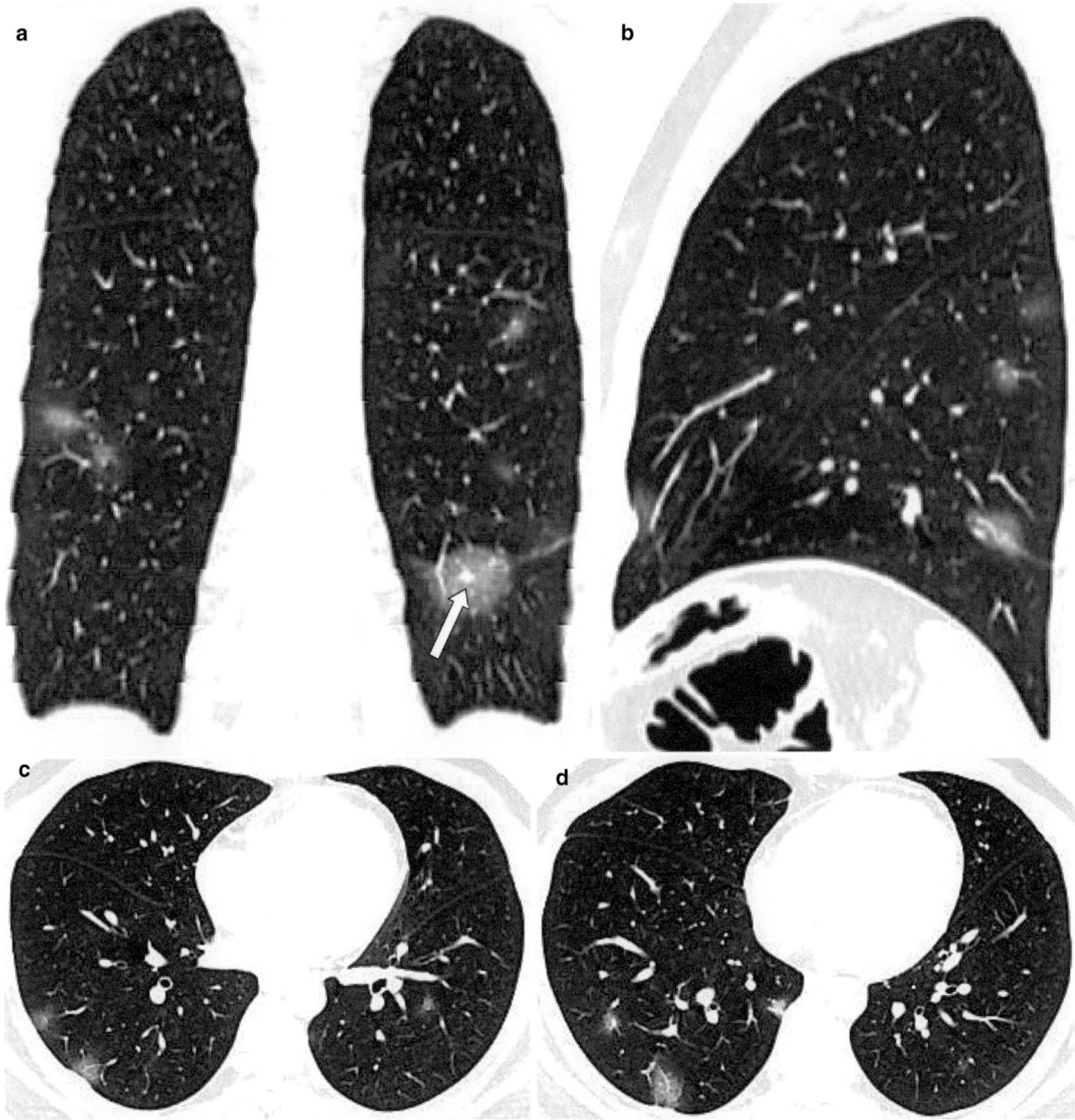

Fig. 7.4 CT images showed multiple nodular and patchy ground-glass opacities in both lungs, mainly located in the subpleural area of the lung (**a**–**j**). The central structure of lobules was thickened (**a** white arrow, **h** black arrow)

18 breaths per minute, total white blood cell count was 3.60×10^9 L, C-reactive protein was 5.3 mg/L, neutrophil count was 1.26×10^9 L, lymphocyte count was 1.98×10^9 L, platelet count was 191×10^9 L, and oxygen saturation was 97.6%. The viral RNA in throat swab was negative in his first examination. In his second examination, he was finally confirmed by Guangzhou CDC. On January 31, 2020, chest CT images showed multiple ground-glass opacities in bilateral lungs.

CT images showed multiple nodular and patchy ground-glass opacities in both lungs, mainly located in the subpleural area of the lung (Fig. 7.4a–j). The central structure of lobules was thickened (Fig. 7.4a, white arrow; Fig. 7.4h, black arrow).

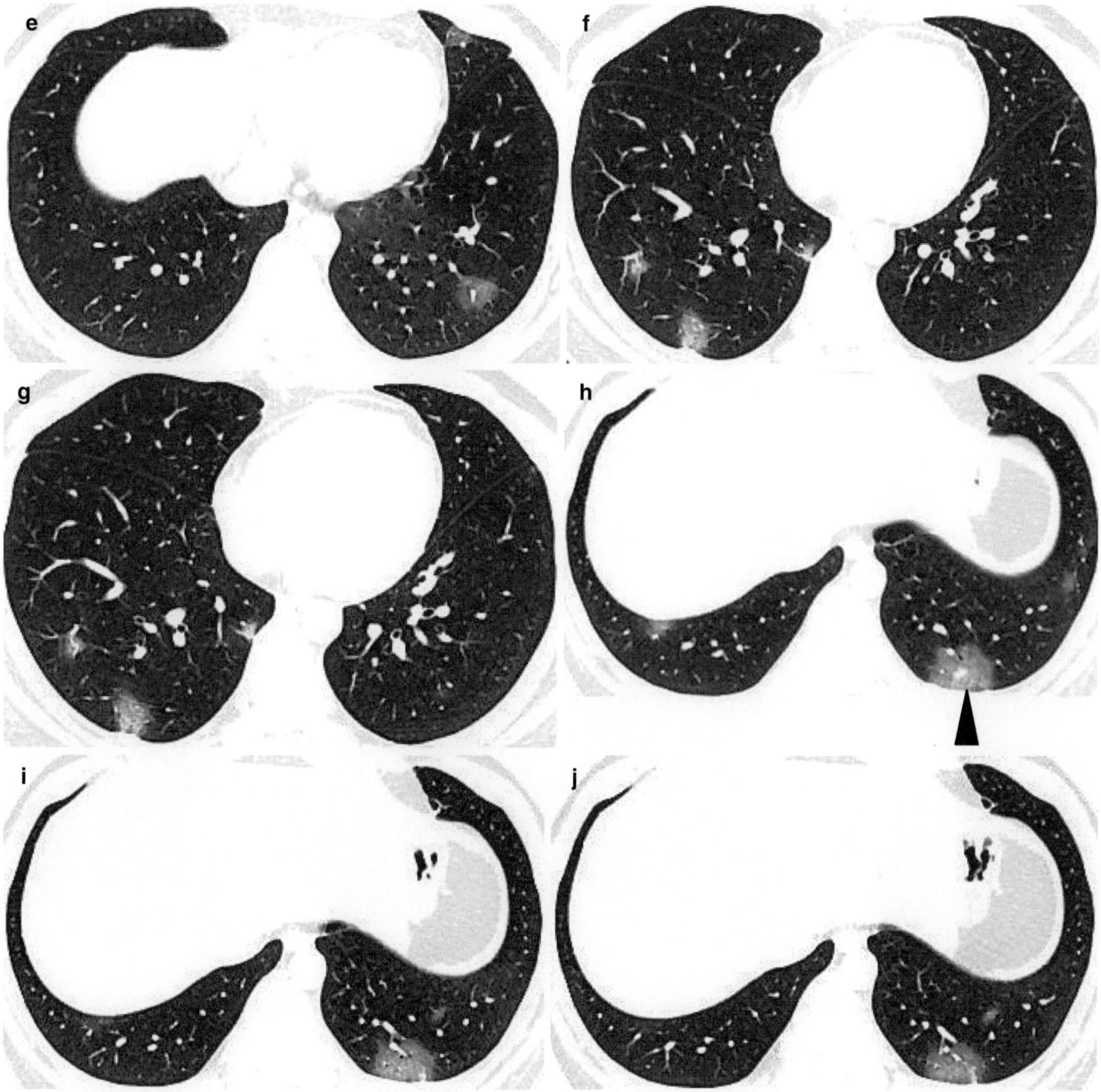

Fig. 7.4 (continued)

7.6 Case 5 (Fig. 7.5a–j)

A 54-year-old female patient had a history of exposure to an epidemic area. On January 22, 2020, she presented with fever and fatigue, accompanied by headache, muscle ache, cough, sputum, and slight shortness of breath after exercise. Chest x-ray showed pneumonia, and she was admitted to the hospital on January 24, 2020. At the time of admission, the body temperature was 36.1 °C, the respiratory rate was 21 breaths per minute, total white blood cell count was 6.77×10^9 L, C-reactive protein was 15.11 mg/L, neutrophil count was 3.88×10^9 L, lymphocyte count was 2.42×10^9 L, platelet count was 246×10^9 L, and oxygen saturation was 99%. The viral RNA in throat swab was negative in her first examination. In her second examination, she was finally confirmed by Guangzhou CDC. On January 25, 2020, chest CT images showed multiple ground-glass opacities in bilateral lungs.

CT images showed multiple patchy ground-glass opacities in bilateral lungs with enlarged vessels in the lesions (Fig. 7.5j).

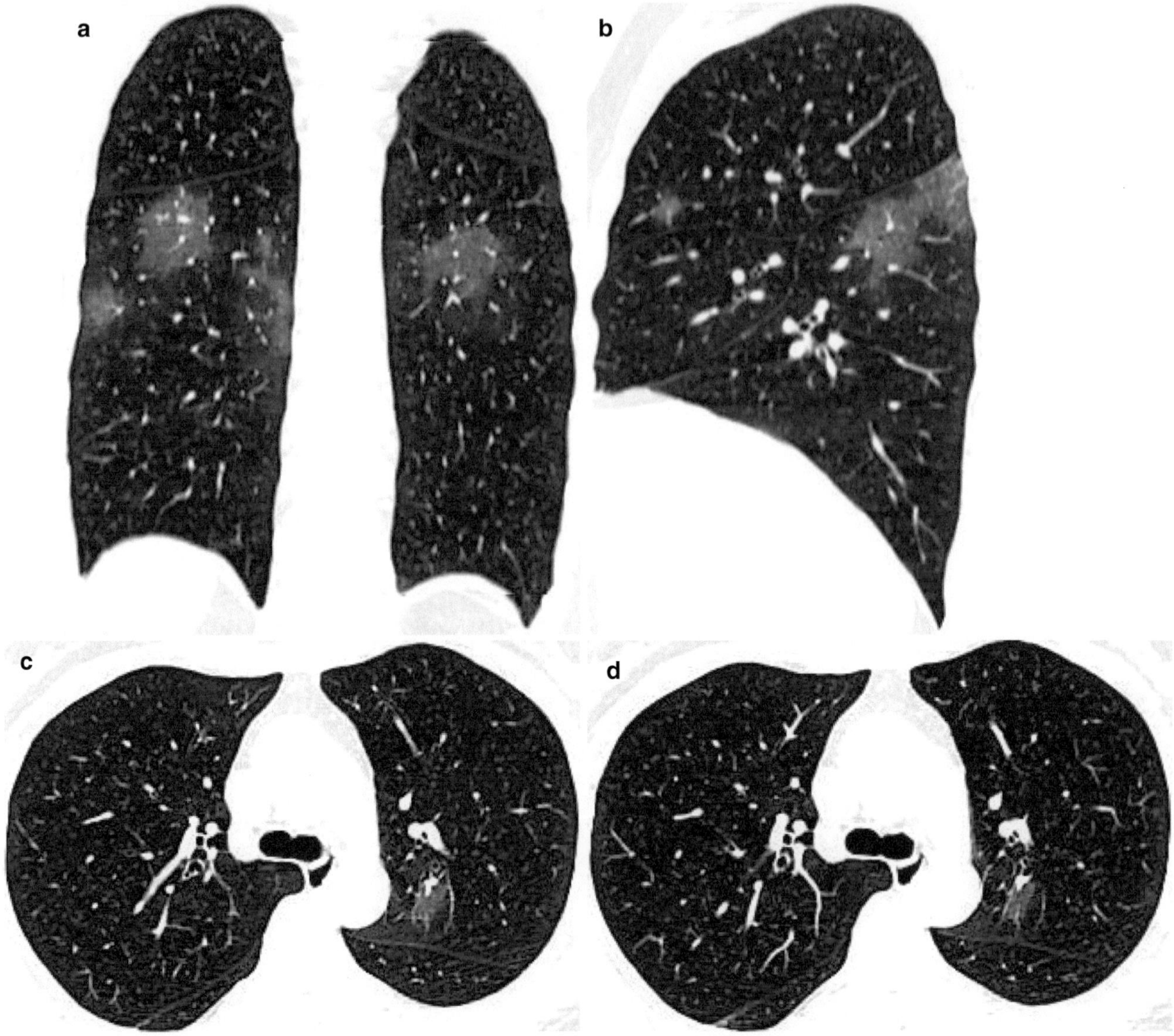

Fig. 7.5 CT images showed multiple patchy ground-glass opacities in bilateral lungs with enlarged vessels in the lesions (**j**)

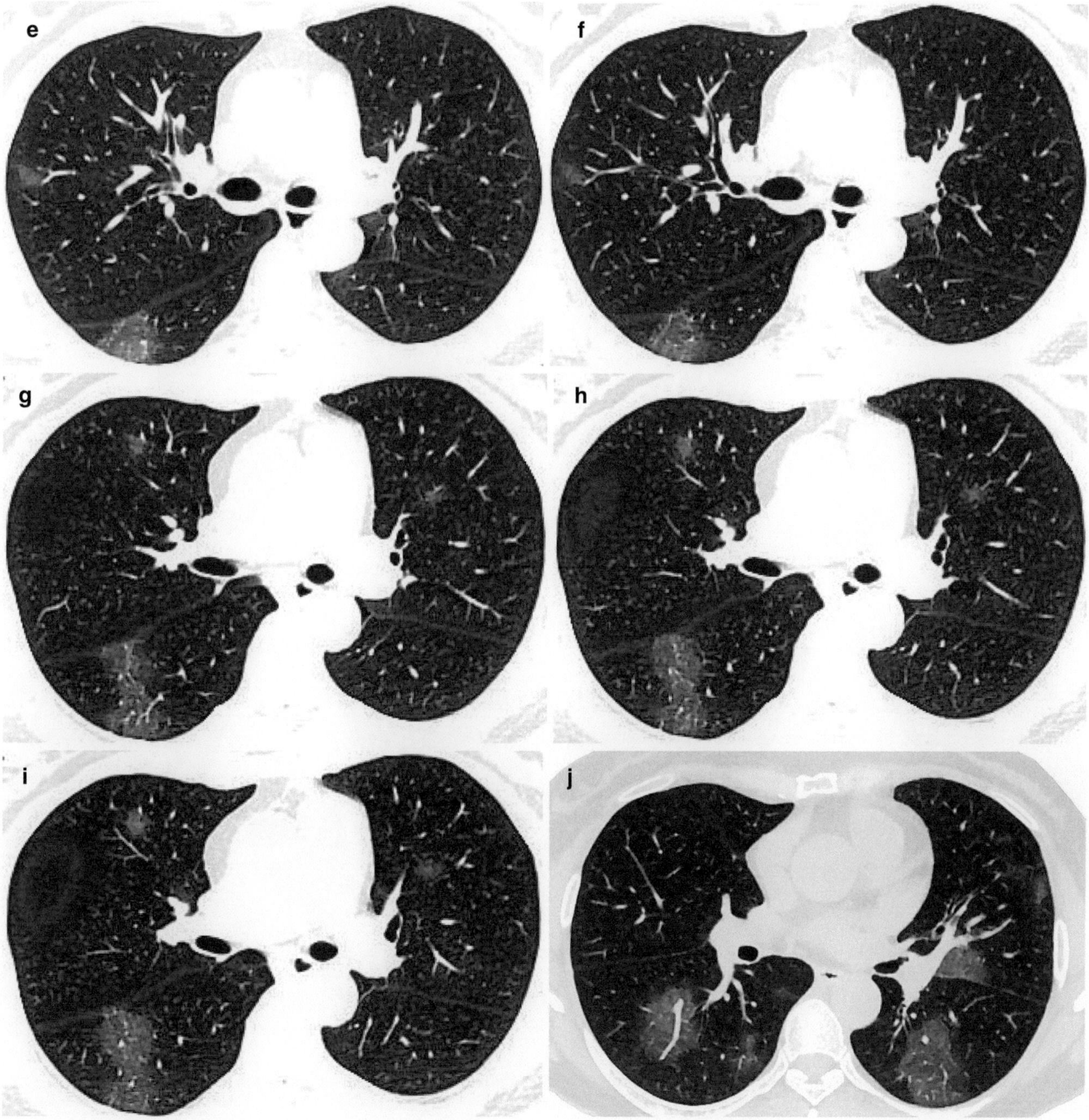

Fig. 7.5 (continued)

7.7 Case 6 (Fig. 7.6a–j)

A 57-year-old male patient with a history of exposure to epidemic areas presented with chills and fever on January 26, 2020. He was admitted to the hospital on February 1, 2020. At the time of admission, the body temperature was 37 °C, the respiratory rate was 20 breaths per minute, total white blood cell count was 6.77×10^9 L, C-reactive protein was 18.50 mg/L, neutrophil count was 5.28×10^9 L, lymphocyte count was 0.95×10^9 L, platelet count was 101×10^9 L, and oxygen saturation was 99.6%. The viral RNA in throat swab was negative in his first examination. In his second examination, he was finally confirmed by Guangzhou CDC. On February 5, 2020, chest CT images showed multiple ground-glass opacities in bilateral lungs.

CT images showed multiple patchy ground-glass opacities in bilateral lungs with enlarged vessels in the lesions (Fig. 7.6j).

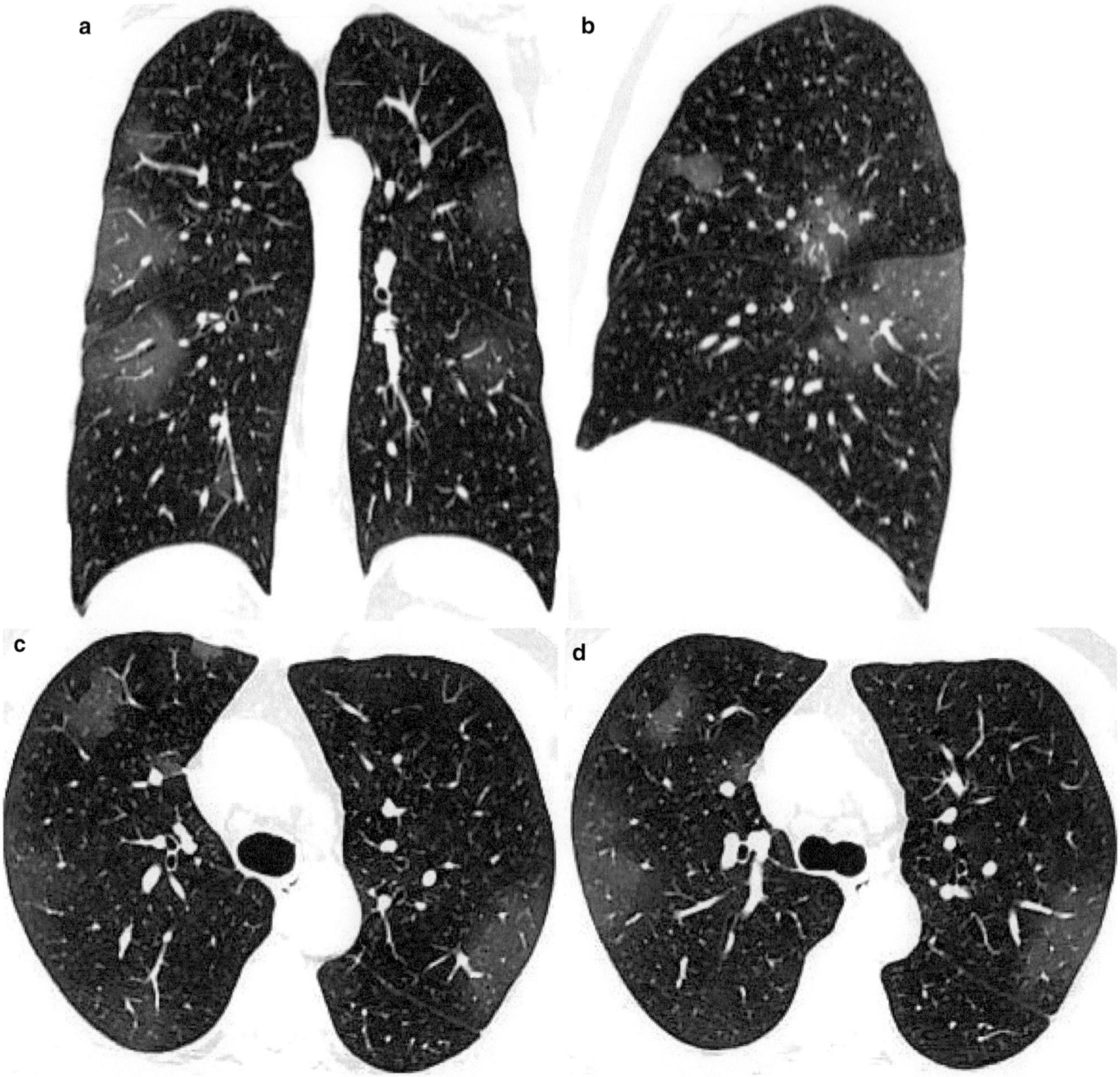

Fig. 7.6 CT images showed multiple patchy ground-glass opacities in bilateral lungs with enlarged vessels in the lesions (**j**)

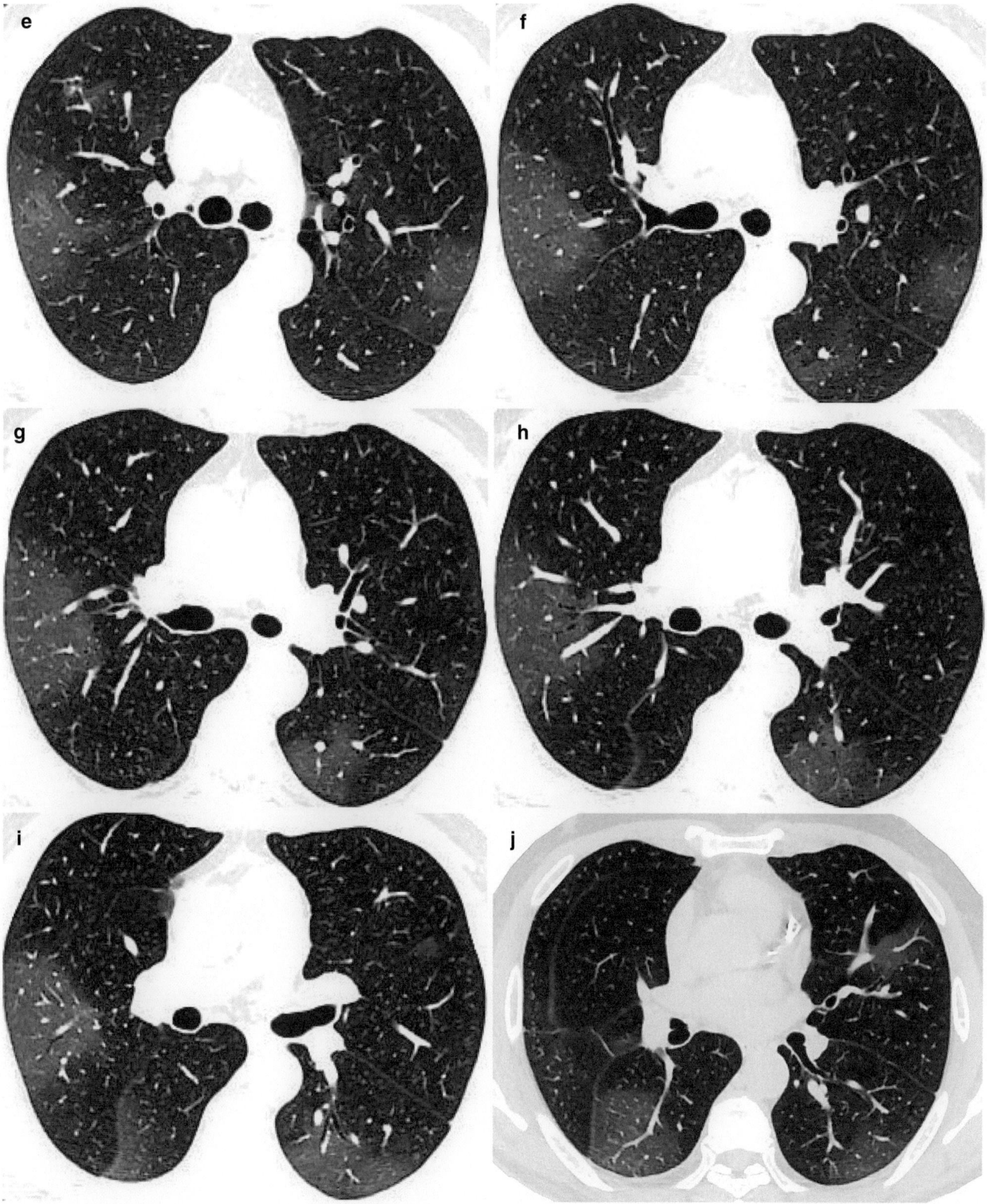

Fig. 7.6 (continued)

7.8 **Case 7** (Fig. 7.7a–j)

A 70-year-old male patient with a history of exposure to epidemic areas presented with cough and fever. He was admitted to the hospital on January 28, 2020. At the time of admission, the body temperature was 37.8 °C, the respiratory rate was 18 breaths per minute, total white blood cell count was 7.05×10^9 L, C-reactive protein was 92.82 mg/L, neutrophil count was 6.21×10^9 L,

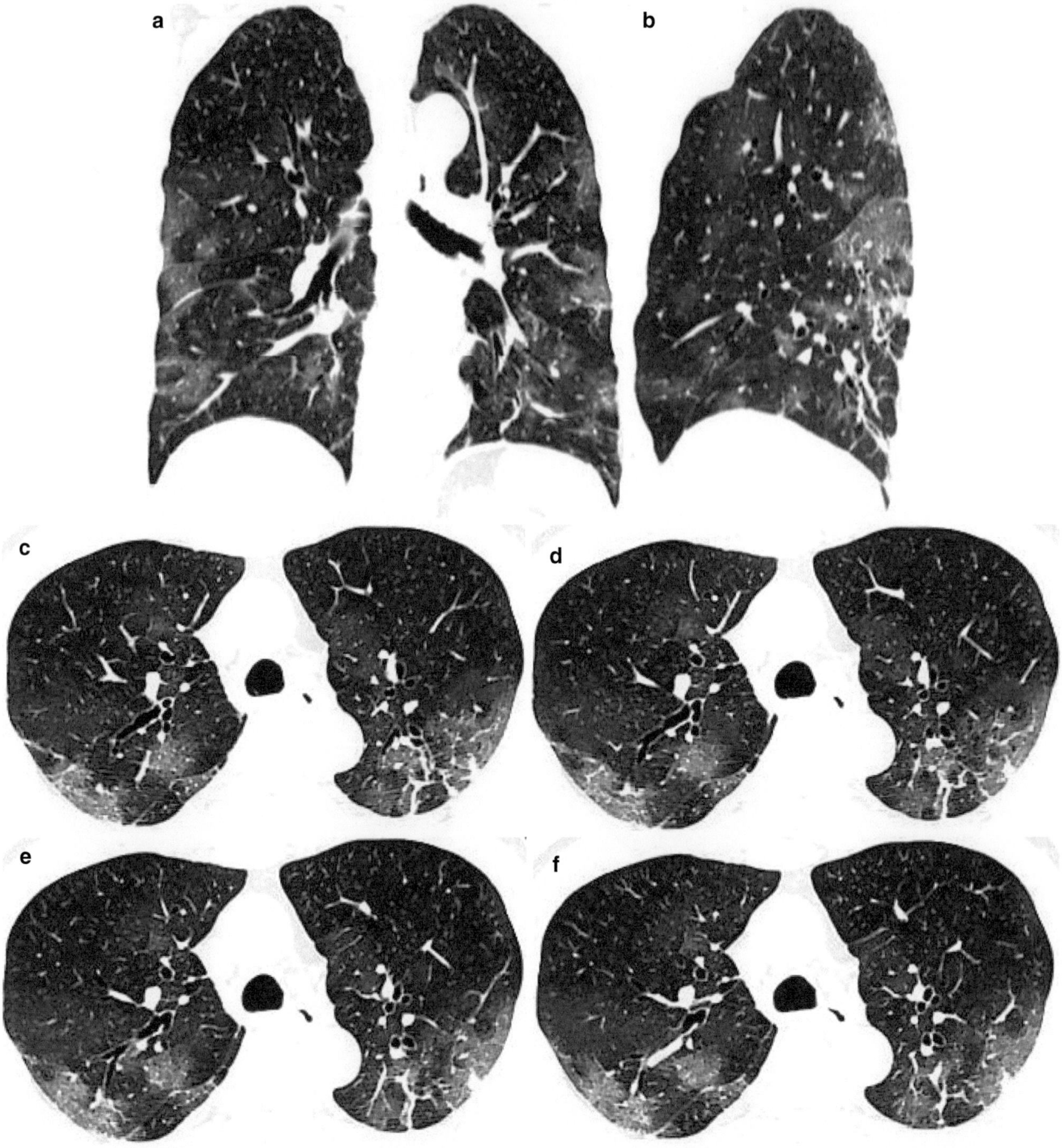

Fig. 7.7 CT images showed multiple patchy ground-glass opacities and linear opacities with interlobular septal thickening in bilateral lungs (**j**)

lymphocyte count was 0.56×10^9 L, platelet count was 175×10^9 L, and oxygen saturation was 92.5%. The viral RNA in throat swab was negative in his first examination. In his second examination, he was finally confirmed by Guangzhou CDC. On January 30, 2020, chest CT images showed multiple ground-glass opacities in bilateral lungs.

CT images showed multiple patchy ground-glass opacities and linear opacities with interlobular septal thickening in bilateral lungs (Fig. 7.7j).

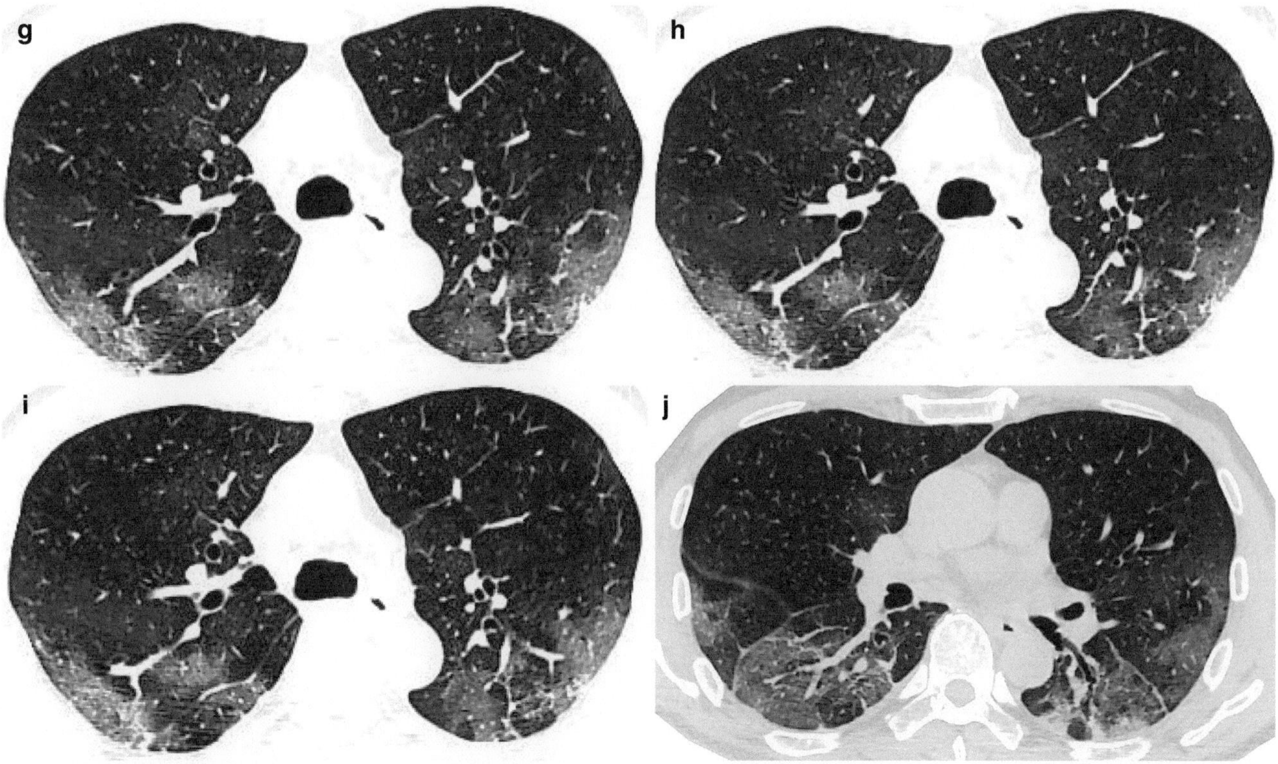

Fig. 7.7 (continued)

7.9 **Case 8** (Fig. 7.8a–j)

A 62-year-old female patient with a history of exposure to epidemic areas presented with cough and fever without obvious inducement on February 1, 2020. She was admitted to the hospital on February 3, 2020. At admission, the body temperature was 39 °C, the respiratory rate was 20 breaths per minute, white blood cell count was 3.75×10^9 L, C-reactive protein was 18.67 mg/L, neutrophil count was 1.97×10^9 L, lymphocyte count was 1.11×10^9 L, platelet count was 149×10^9 L, and oxygen saturation was 99%. The viral RNA in throat swab was negative for two examinations. In her third examination, she was finally confirmed by Guangzhou CDC. On February 5, 2020, chest CT images showed multiple ground-glass opacities in bilateral lungs.

CT images showed multiple patchy ground-glass opacities with blurred margin and thickened interlobular septa in bilateral lungs (Fig. 7.8a–j).

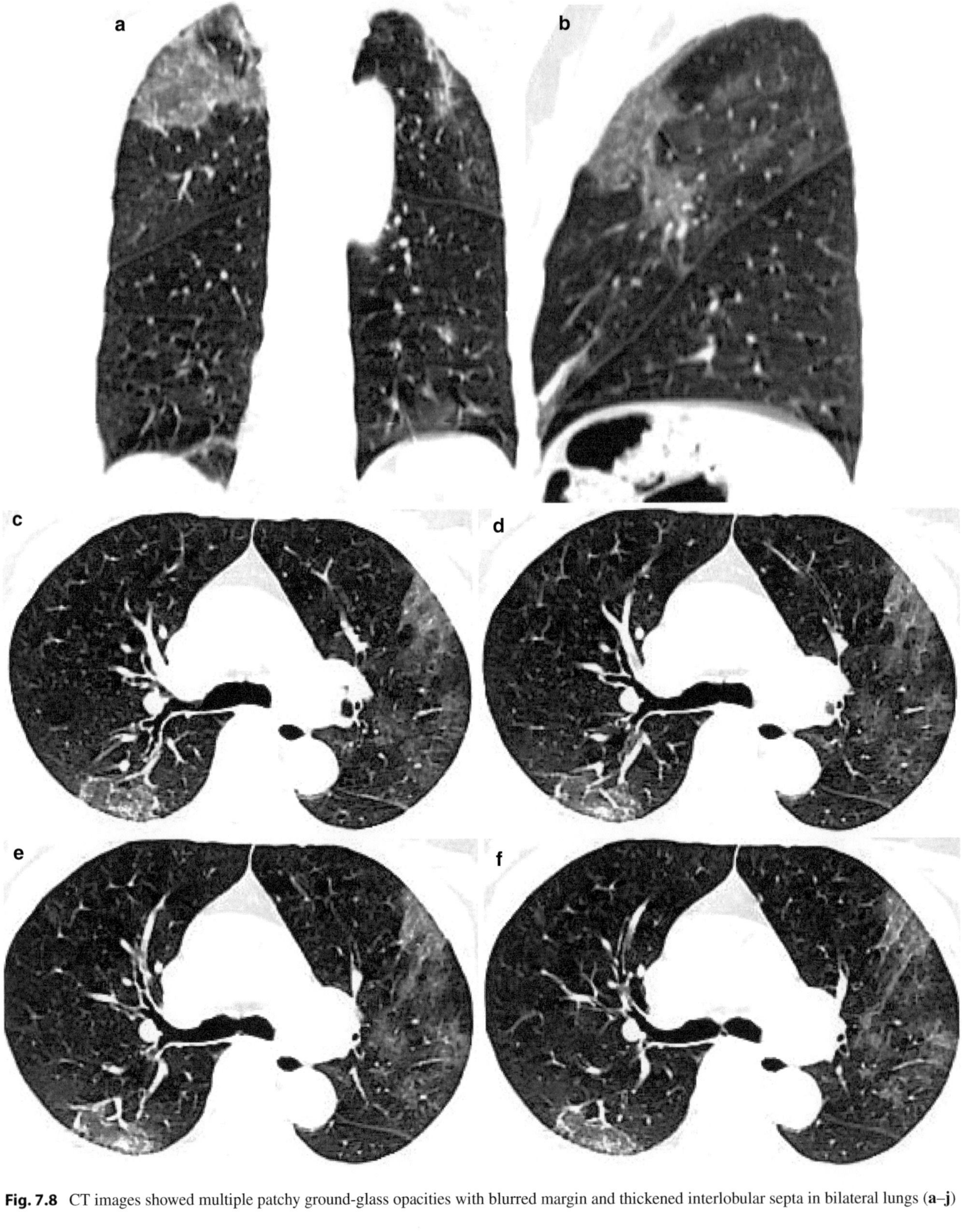

Fig. 7.8 CT images showed multiple patchy ground-glass opacities with blurred margin and thickened interlobular septa in bilateral lungs (**a**–**j**)

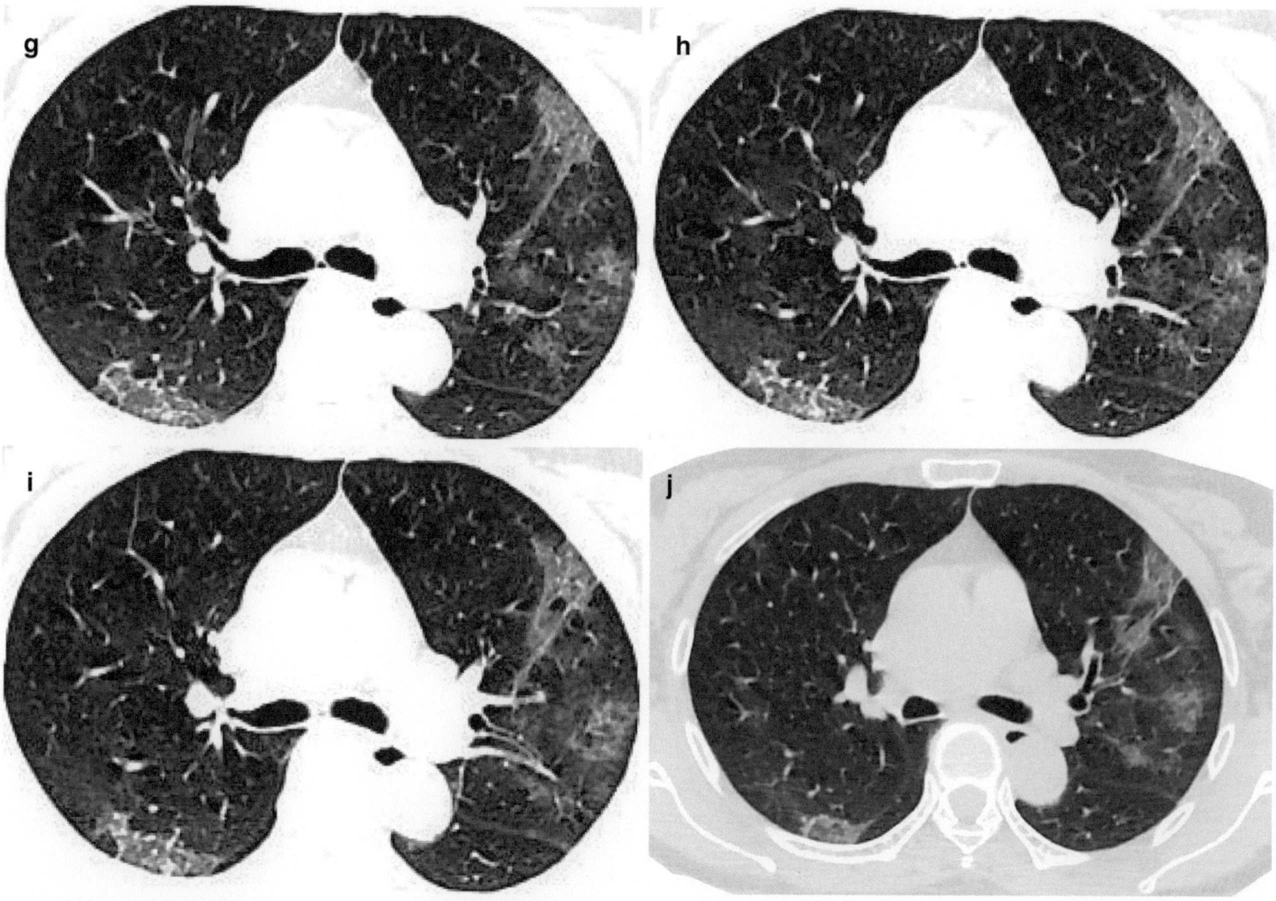

Fig. 7.8 (continued)

7.10 Case 9 (Fig. 7.9a–j)

A 43-year-old male patient with a history of exposure to epidemic areas presented with cough and fever without obvious inducement on January 22, 2020. He was admitted to the hospital on February 5, 2020. Admission temperature was 37.7 °C, the respiratory rate was 20 breaths per minute, peripheral white blood cell count was 4.2×10^9 L, C-reactive protein was 78.56 mg/L, neutrophil count was 2.50×10^9 L, lymphocyte count was 1.23×10^9 L, platelet count was 239×10^9 L, and oxygen saturation was 82.9%. The viral RNA in throat swab was negative for two examinations. In his third examination, he was finally confirmed by Guangzhou CDC. On February 5, 2020, chest CT images showed multiple ground-glass opacities and patchy consolidation in bilateral lungs.

CT images showed multiple patchy ground-glass opacities, consolidation, and thickening of the interlobular septa (Fig. 7.9a–j) in bilateral lungs. "Air bronchogram" can be seen in the upper lobe of the left lung (Fig. 7.9j).

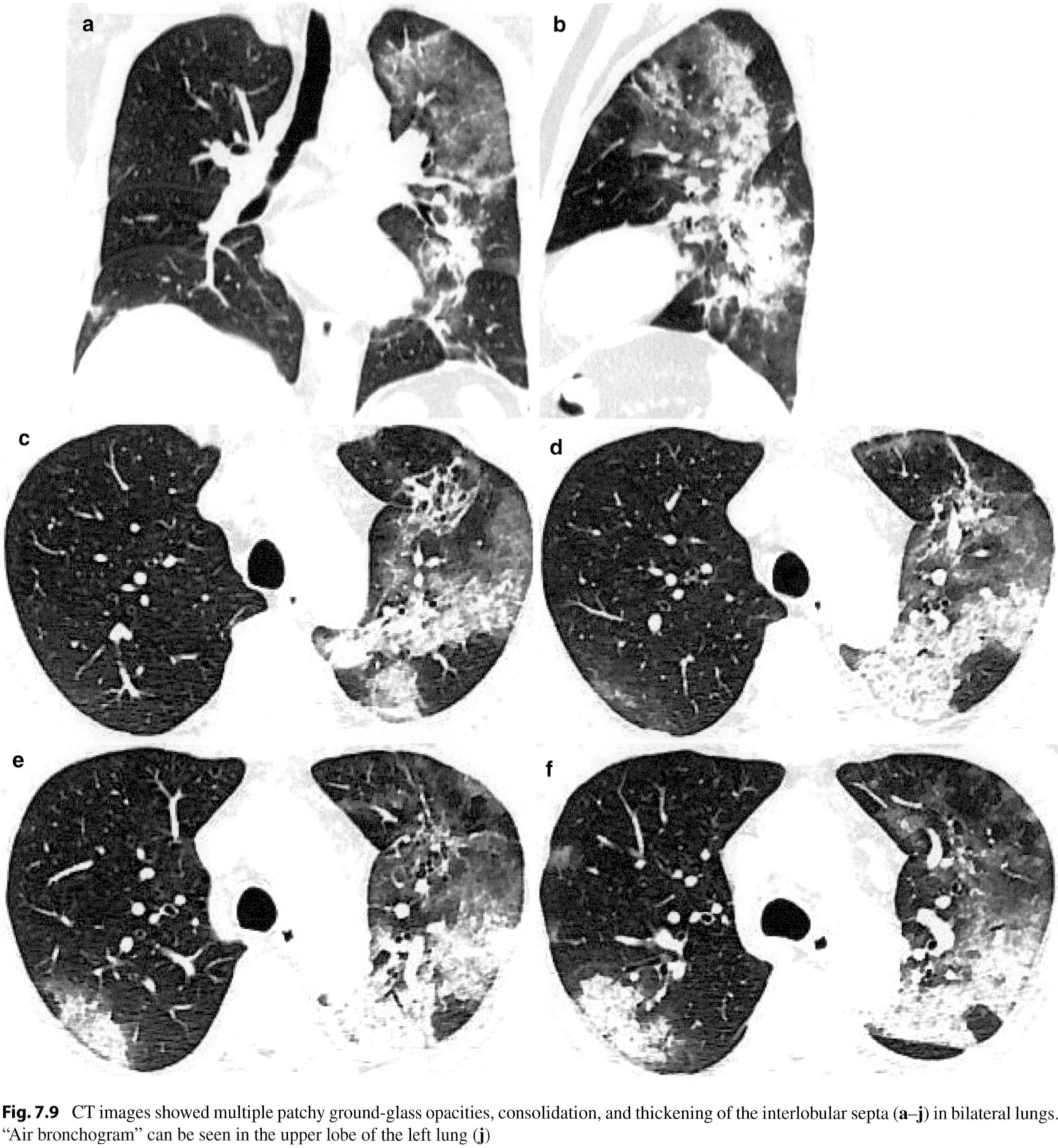

Fig. 7.9 CT images showed multiple patchy ground-glass opacities, consolidation, and thickening of the interlobular septa (**a**–**j**) in bilateral lungs. "Air bronchogram" can be seen in the upper lobe of the left lung (**j**)

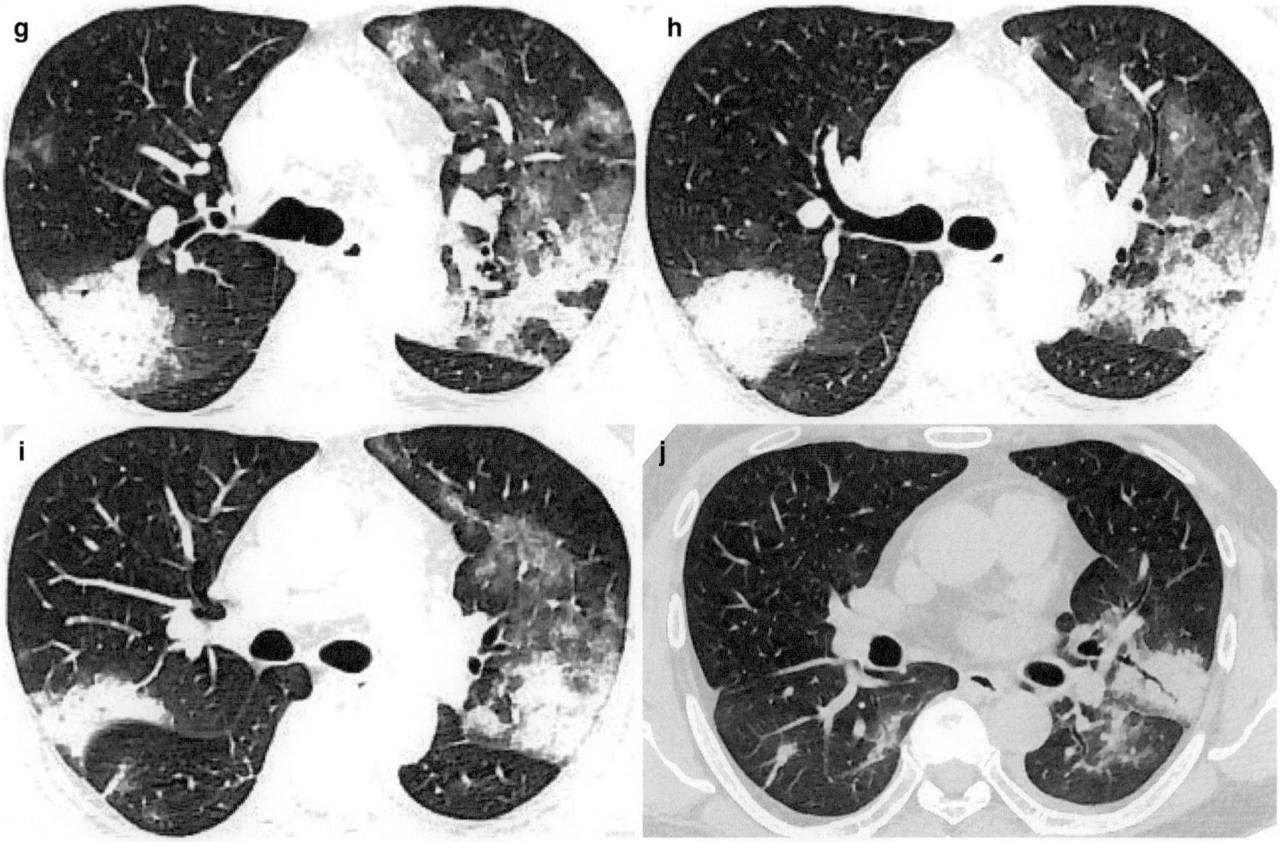

Fig. 7.9 (continued)

7.11 Case 10 (Fig. 7.10a–j)

A 23-year-old male patient with a history of close contact with a confirmed patient was admitted to the hospital on January 23, 2020. At the time of admission, the body temperature was 36.3 °C, the respiratory rate was 18 breaths per minute, total white blood cell count was 4.23×10^9 L, C-reactive protein was 18.4 mg/L, neutrophil count was 2.23×10^9 L, lymphocyte count was 1.53×10^9 L, platelet count was 187×10^9 L, and oxygen saturation was 98%. The viral RNA in throat swab was negative for four examinations. In his fifth examination, he was finally confirmed by Guangzhou CDC. On January 29, 2020, chest CT images showed multiple ground-glass opacities and multiple patchy consolidation in the right lower lobe.

CT images showed multiple patchy ground-glass opacities and focal consolidation in the lower lobe of the right lung (Fig. 7.10b, white arrow); "paving stone sign" (Fig. 7.10h) and "air bronchogram sign" (Fig. 7.10j) can be seen.

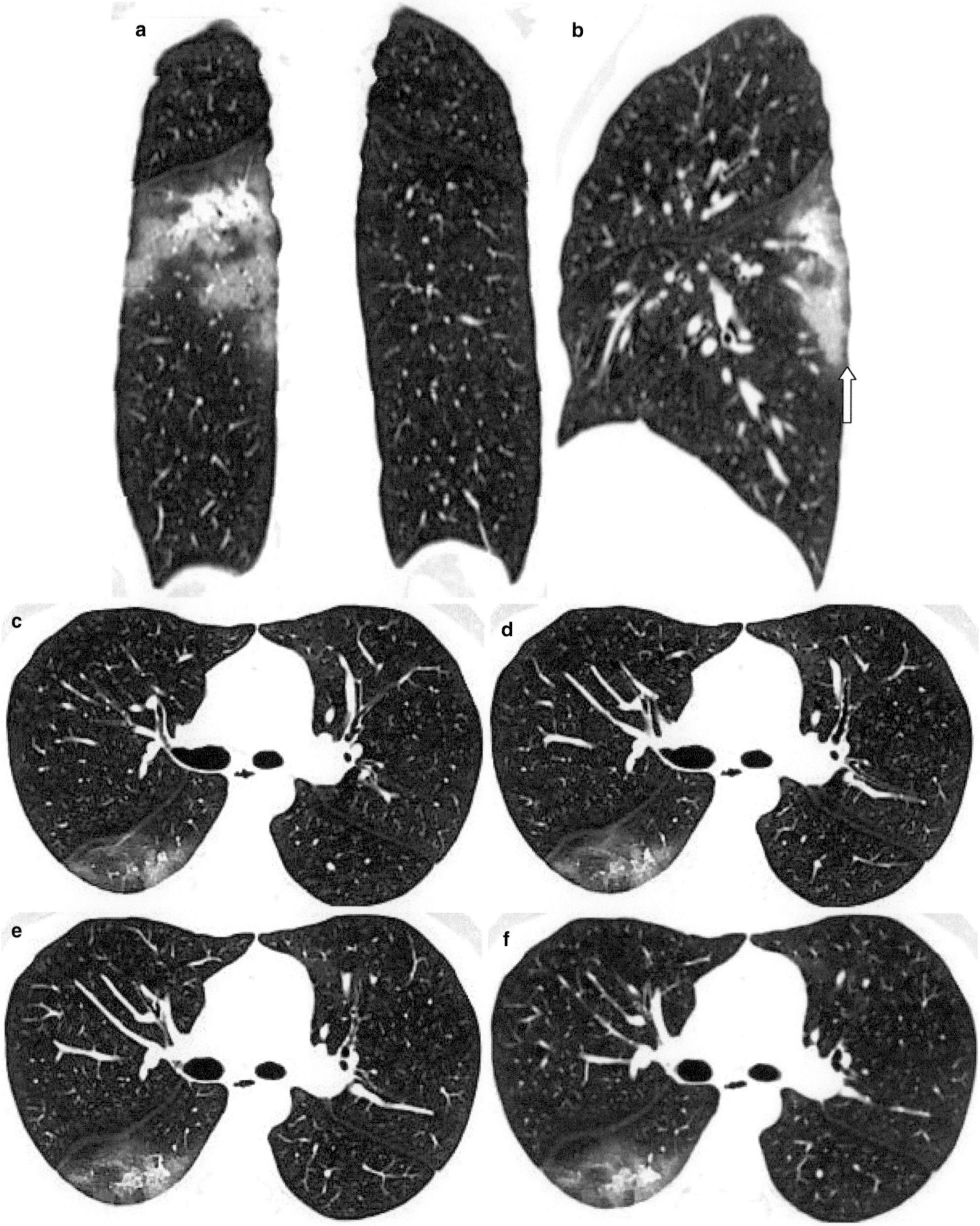

Fig. 7.10 CT images showed multiple patchy ground-glass opacities and focal consolidation in the lower lobe of the right lung (**b** white arrow); "paving stone sign" (**h**) and "air bronchogram sign" (**j**) can be seen

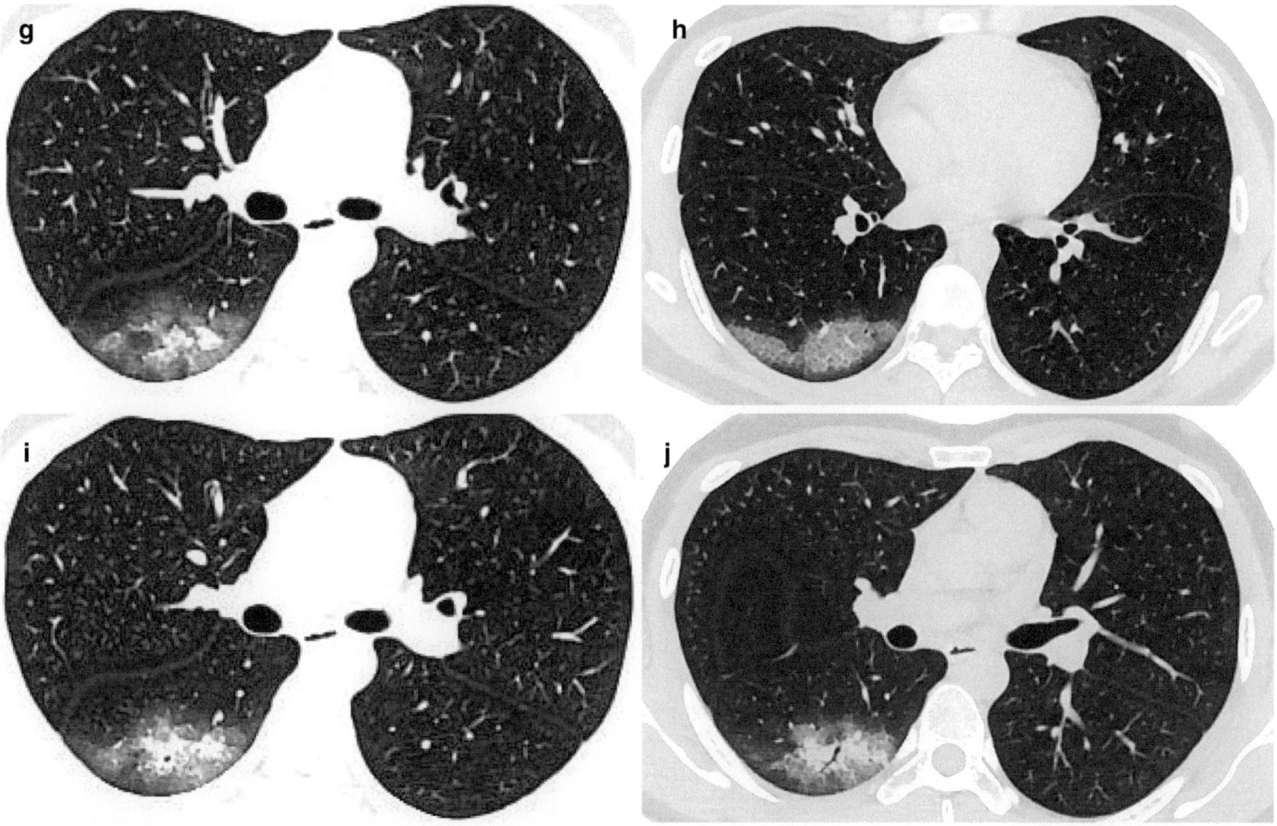

Fig. 7.10 (continued)

References

1. Li Q. The 2019-nCoV Outbreak joint Field Epidemiology Investigation team, Notes form the field: an outbreak of NCIP (2019-nCoV) infection in China-Wuhan, Hubei Province, 2019–2020. China CDC Weekly. 2020;2:79–80.
2. Dong N, Yang XM, Ye LW, et al. Genomic and protein structure modelling analysis depicts the origin and infectivity of 2019-nCoV, a new coronavirus which caused a pneumonia outbreak in Wuhan, China. bioRxiv 2020.01.20.913368; https://doi.org/10.1101/2020.01.20.913368.
3. Michael L, Vincent M. Functional assessment of cell entry and receptor usage for lineage B β-coronaviruses, including 2019-nCoV. bioRxiv 2020.01.22.915660; https://doi.org/10.1101/2020.01.22.915660.
4. Li Q, Guan WH, Wu P, et al. Early transmission dynamics in Wuhan, China, of novel coronavirus-infected pneumonia. N Engl J Med. https://doi.org/10.1056/NEJMoa2001316.
5. Chan JF, Yuan S, Kok KH, et al. A familial cluster of pneumonia associated with the 2019 novel coronavirus indicating person-to-person transmission: a study of a family cluster. Lancet. 2020 (Epub ahead of print).
6. Ju LE, Ri O, Christian L, et al. Pattern of early human-to-human transmission of Wuhan 2019-nCoV. Althaus. bioRxiv 2020.01.23.917351; https://doi.org/10.1101/2020.01.23.917351.
7. Paules CI, Marston HD, Fauci AS. Coronavirus infections–more than just the common cold. JAMA. 2020;323(8):707–8. https://doi.org/10.1001/jama.2020.0757.
8. Huang CL, Wang YM, Li XW, et al. Clinical features of patients infected with 2019 novel coronavirus in Wuhan China. Clinical features of patients infected with 2019 novel coronavirus in Wuhan, China. Lancet. 2020. ISSN0140-6736, https://doi.org/10.1016/S0140-6736(20)30183-5., http://www.sciencedirect.com/science/article/pii/S0140673620301835.
9. Chen NS, Zhou M, Dong X, et al. 2019 novel coronavirus pneumonia in Wuhan, China a descriptive study. Epidemiological and clinical characteristics of 99 cases of 2019 novel coronavirus pneumonia in Wuhan, China: a descriptive study. Lancet. 2020. ISSN0140-6736, https://doi.org/10.1016/S0140-6736(20)30211-7., http://www.sciencedirect.com/science/article/pii/S0140673620302117.
10. Wei JG, Zheng YN, Yu H, et al. Clinical characteristics of 2019 novel coronavirus infection in China. https://medrxiv.org/content/https://doi.org/10.1101/2020.02.06.20020974v1.

8 Follow-Up CT of Patients with First Negative CT But Positive PCR for COVID-19

Zhoukun Ling, Deyang Huang, and Chunliang Lei

8.1 Introduction

A recent outbreak of coronavirus disease 2019 (COVID-19) has become a public health emergency of international concern [1]. As of April 7, 2020, the coronavirus named as severe acute respiratory syndrome coronavirus 2 SARS-CoV-2 has infected more than 1,210,956 individuals, and caused 67,594 fatal cases [2].

In a familial cluster of COVID-19 pneumonia [3], a 10-year-old child had no clinical symptoms, but showed ground-glass lung opacification on CT, was viral RNA positive in subsequent laboratory test. This study supports that lung damage by viral infection is not necessary to result in obvious the clinical symptoms.

We observed 295 patients with laboratory-identified SARS-CoV-2 infection by RT-PCR between January 23, 2020 and February 18, 2020 in Guangzhou Eighth People's Hospital. Among them, 49 (17%) patients presented negative chest CT images at initial presentation; however, they had positive findings in the following CT scans after 3–14 days of onset. Most patients had no clinical symptoms or mild symptoms. According to the report of Lirong Zou et al., the asymptomatic and symptomatic patients showed similar viral loads [4]. Above findings suggest that suspected patients are also the potential sources of infection, thus individual isolation plays an important role in curbing the spread of COVID-19.

For those viral infected patients with the initial negative chest CT scan, some patients advance to the stage with notable new lung lesions during the following chest CT reexamination, while some patients keep persistently negative CT images until they met discharge criteria.

Because of the complex clinical situation among COVID-19 patients, chest CT examinations should be performed multiple times if possible and necessary for diagnosis and monitoring purposes.

8.2 **Case 1** (Fig. 8.1a–l)

A 66-year-old male was admitted without any symptoms. He had exposed in the epidemic area. Fever and chest tightness occurred on day-1 of admission, and the highest temperature in the course of the disease was 38.6 °C. White blood cell count, lymphocyte count, and C-reactive protein were 5.41×10^9/L, 0.98×10^9/L, and <10 mg/L, respectively. The patient was laboratory confirmed by novel coronavirus nucleic acid throat swab test in Guangzhou CDC. Chest CT examination was performed on 1 day (Fig. 8.1a, b), 5 days (Fig. 8.1c, d), 8 days (Fig. 8.1e, f), and 10 days (Fig. 8.1g–l) after onset of symptoms, respectively.

On 1 day after onset of symptoms, chest CT images showed no obvious abnormalities in both lungs (Fig. 8.1a, b); On 5 days after onset of symptoms, chest CT images showed multiple patchy ground-glass opacities in both lungs, presenting "crazy paving sign" (Fig. 8.1c, d); On 8 days after onset of symptoms, chest CT images demonstrated enlarged lesions and increased density of the lesions, compared with previous images, indicating disease progression, and the "crazy paving sign" was seen (Fig. 8.1e, f white arrow); On 10 days after onset of symptoms, chest CT images demonstrated enlarged lesions and increased density of the lesions, compared with previous images, and both lungs showed "white lung" changes (Fig. 8.1g, h); the coronal and sagittal positions show diffuse distribution of the lung lesions (Fig. 8.1i–l), showing thickening of the interlobar pleura (Fig. 8.1l white arrow).

Z. Ling (✉) · D. Huang · C. Lei
Guangzhou Eighth People's Hospital, Guangzhou Medical University, Guangzhou, China

J. Liu et al. (eds.), *Atlas of Chest Imaging in COVID-19 Patients*, https://doi.org/10.1007/978-981-16-1082-0_8

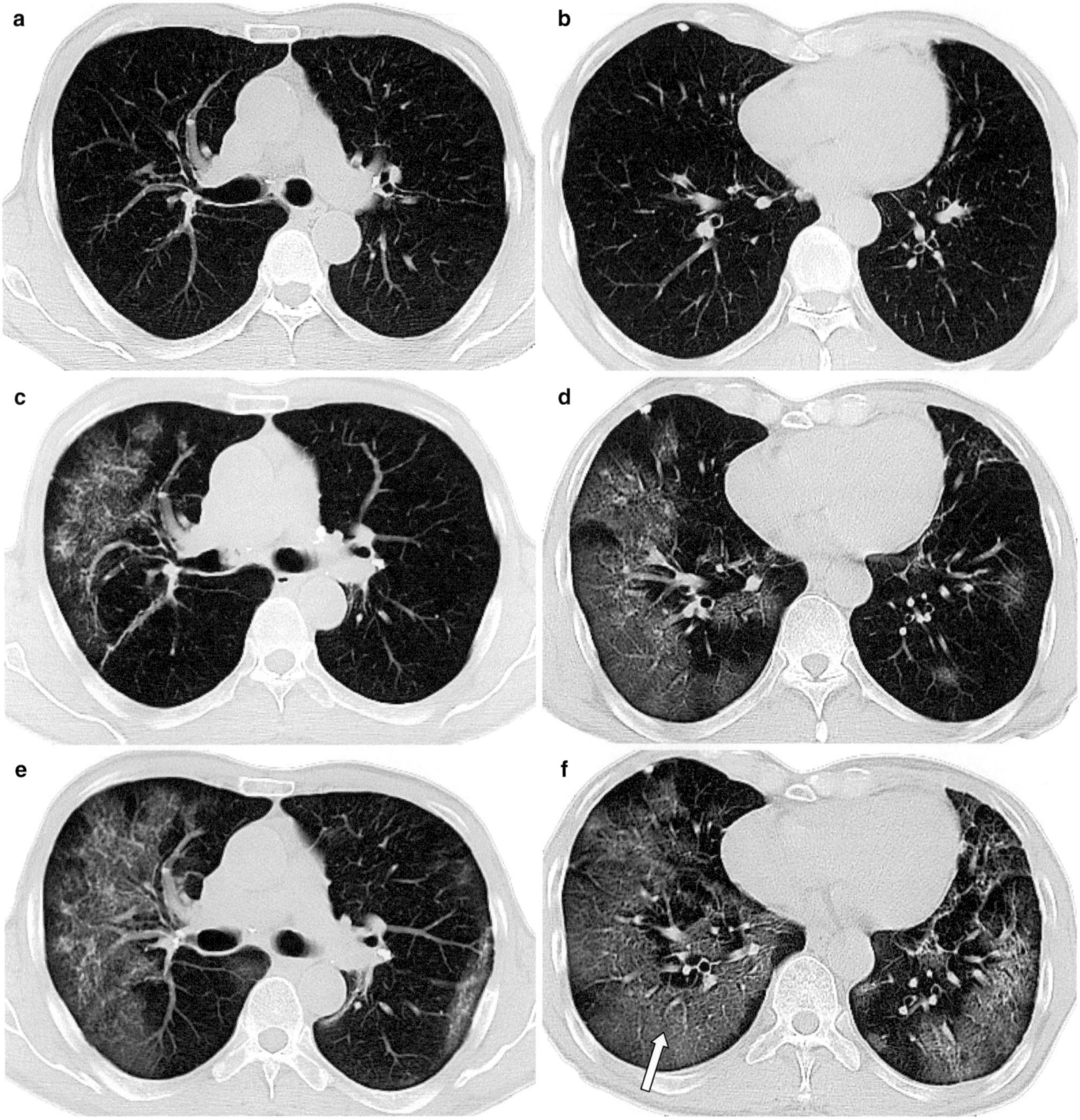

Fig. 8.1 On 1 day after onset of symptoms, chest CT images showed no obvious abnormalities in both lungs (**a**, **b**); On 5 days after onset of symptoms, chest CT images showed multiple patchy ground-glass opacities in both lungs, presenting "crazy paving sign" (**c**, **d**); On 8 days after onset of symptoms, chest CT images demonstrated enlarged lesions and increased density of the lesions, compared with previous images, indicating disease progression, and the "crazy paving sign" was seen (**e**, **f** white arrow); On 10 days after onset of symptoms, chest CT images demonstrated enlarged lesions and increased density of the lesions, compared with previous images, and both lungs showed "white lung" changes (**g**, **h**); the coronal and sagittal positions show diffuse distribution of the lung lesions (**i**–**l**), showing thickening of the interlobar pleura (**l** white arrow)

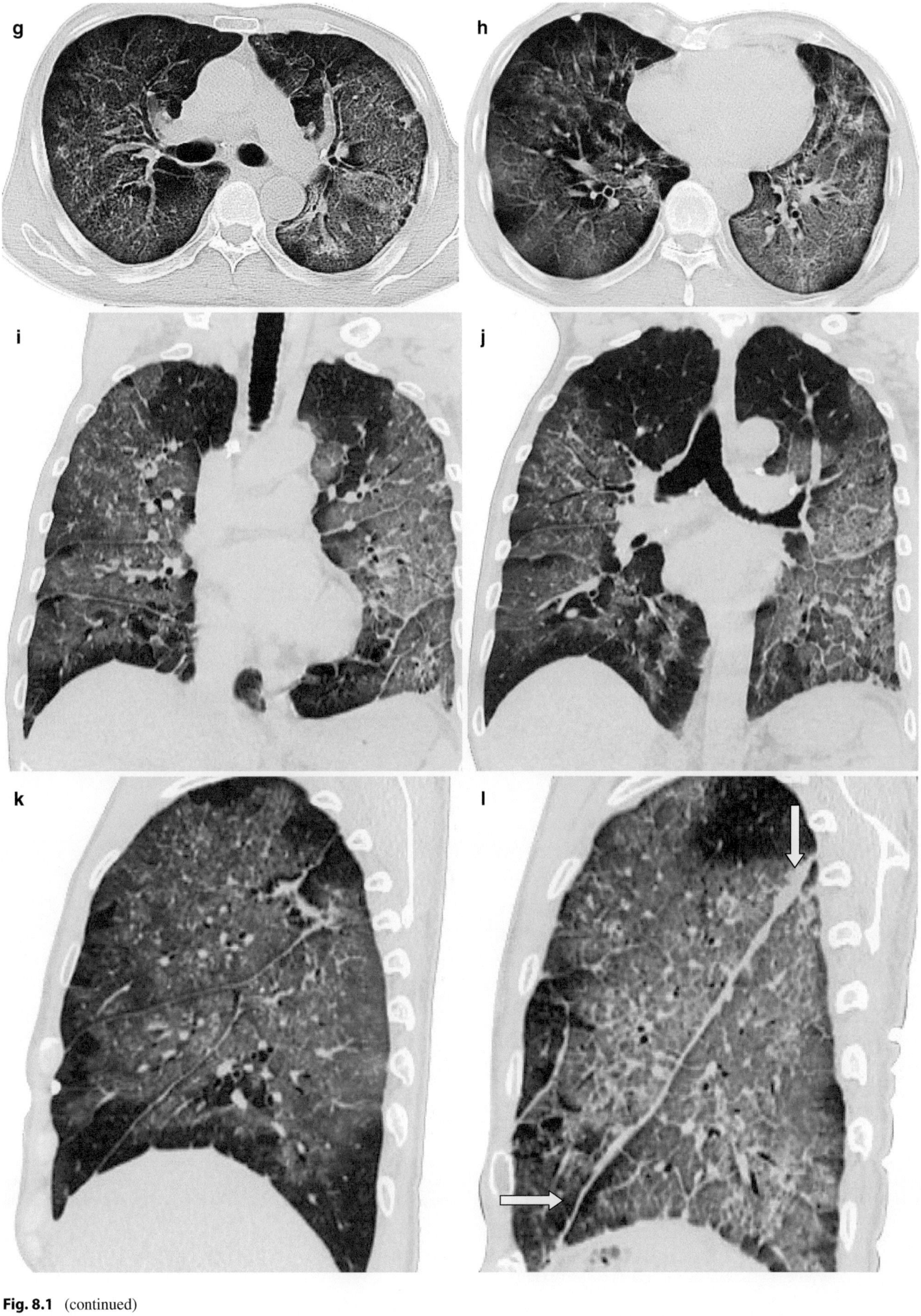

Fig. 8.1 (continued)

8.3 Case 2 (Fig. 8.2a–l)

A 41-year-old male was admitted with fever for 3 days, accompanied by chills and cough. He had exposed in the epidemic area. The body temperature at admission was 37.5 °C. White blood cell count, lymphocyte count, and C-reactive protein were 5.17×10^9/L, 1.31×10^9/L, and <10 mg/L, respectively. The patient was laboratory confirmed by novel coronavirus nucleic acid throat swab test in Guangzhou CDC. Chest CT examination was performed on 4 days (Fig. 8.2a, b), 10 days (Fig. 8.2c, d), 14 days (Fig. 8.2e, f, i, k), and 18 days (Fig. 8.2g, h, j, l) after onset of symptoms, respectively.

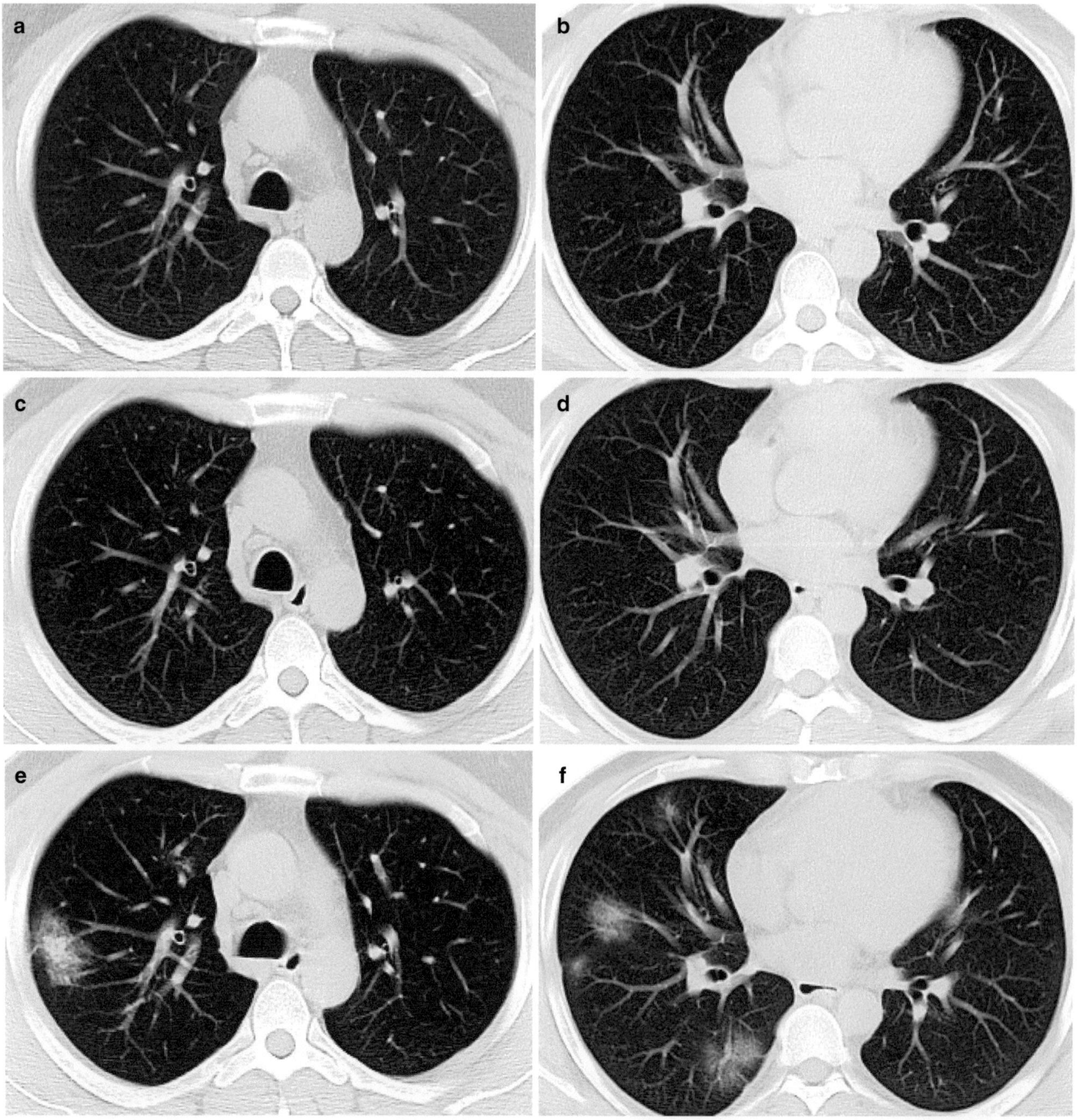

Fig. 8.2 On the 4th day after onset, the first chest CT on 4 days after onset of symptoms, chest CT images showed no obvious abnormality in both lungs (**a**, **b**). On 10 days after onset of symptoms, chest CT images showed patchy ground-glass opacities in the upper lobe of the right lung (**c**), and no obvious abnormality was observed in the lower lobe of both lungs (**d**). On 14 days after onset of symptoms, chest CT images showed multiple patchy ground-glass opacities in both lungs (**e**, **f**). On 18 days after onset of symptoms, chest CT images demonstrated enlarged lesions and increased density of the lesions, compared with previous images, indicating disease progression, and the "crazy paving sign" and subpleural curvilinear line were seen (**g** white arrow and **h**). The coronal and sagittal images showed patchy ground-glass opacities of both lungs (**i**–**l**)

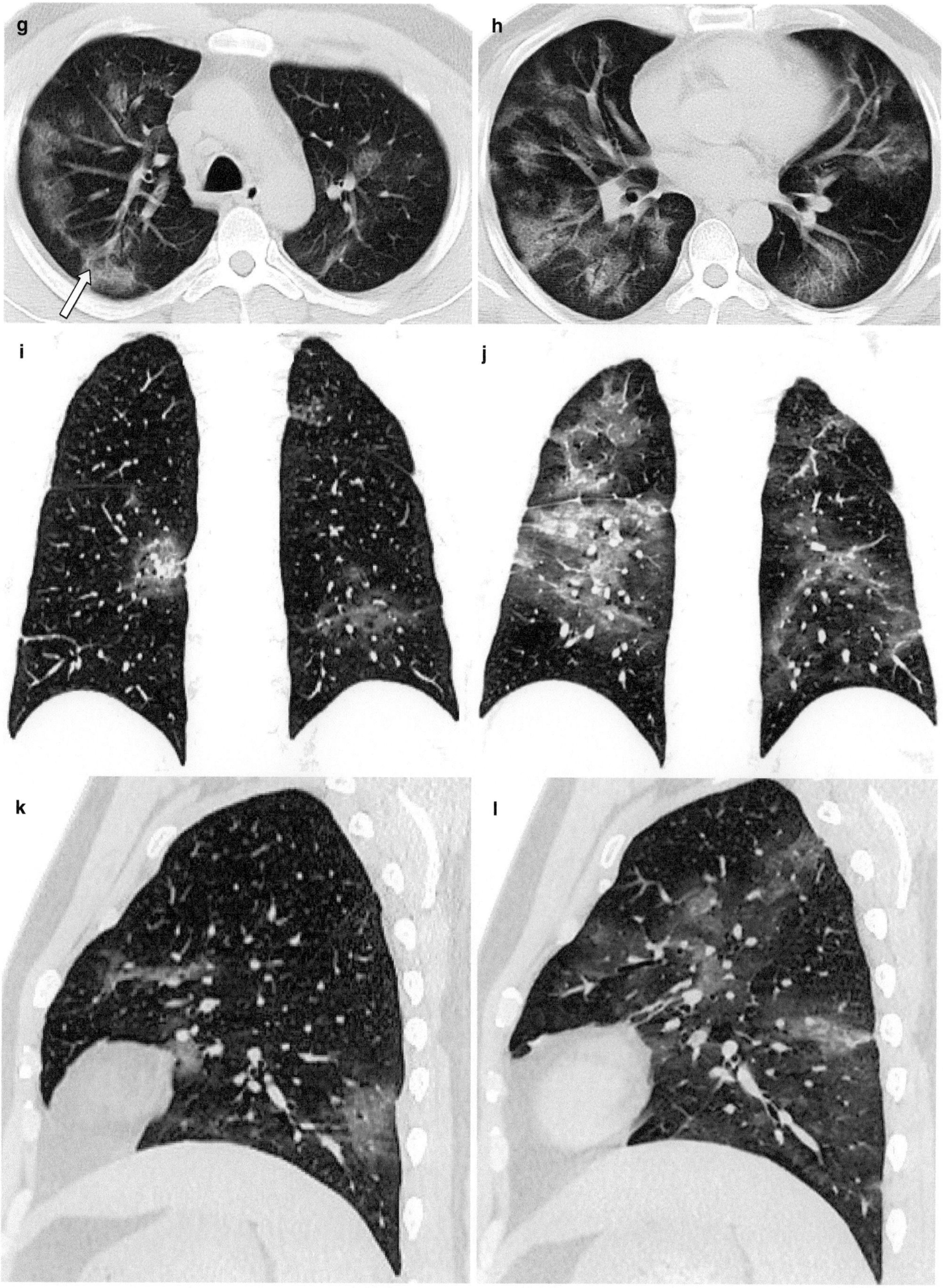

Fig. 8.2 (continued)

On the 4th day after onset, the first chest CT on 4 days after onset of symptoms, chest CT images showed no obvious abnormality in both lungs (Fig. 8.2a, b). On 10 days after onset of symptoms, chest CT images showed patchy ground-glass opacities in the upper lobe of the right lung (Fig. 8.2c), and no obvious abnormality was observed in the lower lobe of both lungs (Fig. 8.2d). On 14 days after onset of symptoms, chest CT images showed multiple patchy ground-glass opacities in both lungs (Fig. 8.2e, f). On 18 days after onset of symptoms, chest CT images demonstrated enlarged lesions and increased density of the lesions, compared with previous images, indicating disease progression, and the "crazy paving sign" and subpleural curvilinear line were seen (Fig. 8.2g white arrow and Fig. 8.2h). The coronal and sagittal images showed patchy ground-glass opacities of both lungs (Fig. 8.2i–l).

8.4 Case 3 (Fig. 8.3a–l)

A 44-year-old male was admitted with fever for 3 days, accompanied by chills and cough. He had exposed in the epidemic area. The body temperature at admission was 37.4 °C. White blood cell count, lymphocyte count, and C-reactive protein were 11.02×10^9/L, 3.02×10^9/L, and <10 mg/L, respectively. The patient was laboratory confirmed by novel coronavirus nucleic acid throat swab test in Guangzhou CDC. Chest CT examination was performed on 5 days (Fig. 8.3a, b), 10 days (Fig. 8.3c, d), 14 days (Fig. 8.3e, f), and 17 days (Fig. 8.3g–l) after onset of symptoms, respectively.

On 5 days after onset of symptoms, chest CT images showed no obvious abnormality in both lungs (Fig. 8.3a, b). On 10 days after onset of symptoms, chest CT images showed patchy ground-glass opacities in both lungs (Fig. 8.3c, d). On 14 days after onset of symptoms, chest CT images demonstrated enlarged lesions and increased density of the lesions, compared with previous images, indicating disease progression (Fig. 8.3e, f). On 17 days after onset of symptoms, chest CT images showed decreased lesions in bilateral lungs, and subpleural arc band shadow in the lower lobe of both lungs. The lesions gradually disappeared/vanished (Fig. 8.3g, h). Coronal and sagittal images showed patchy ground-glass opacities in both lungs (Fig. 8.3i–l), and "reverse halo sign" was seen locally (Fig. 8.3j, l white arrow).

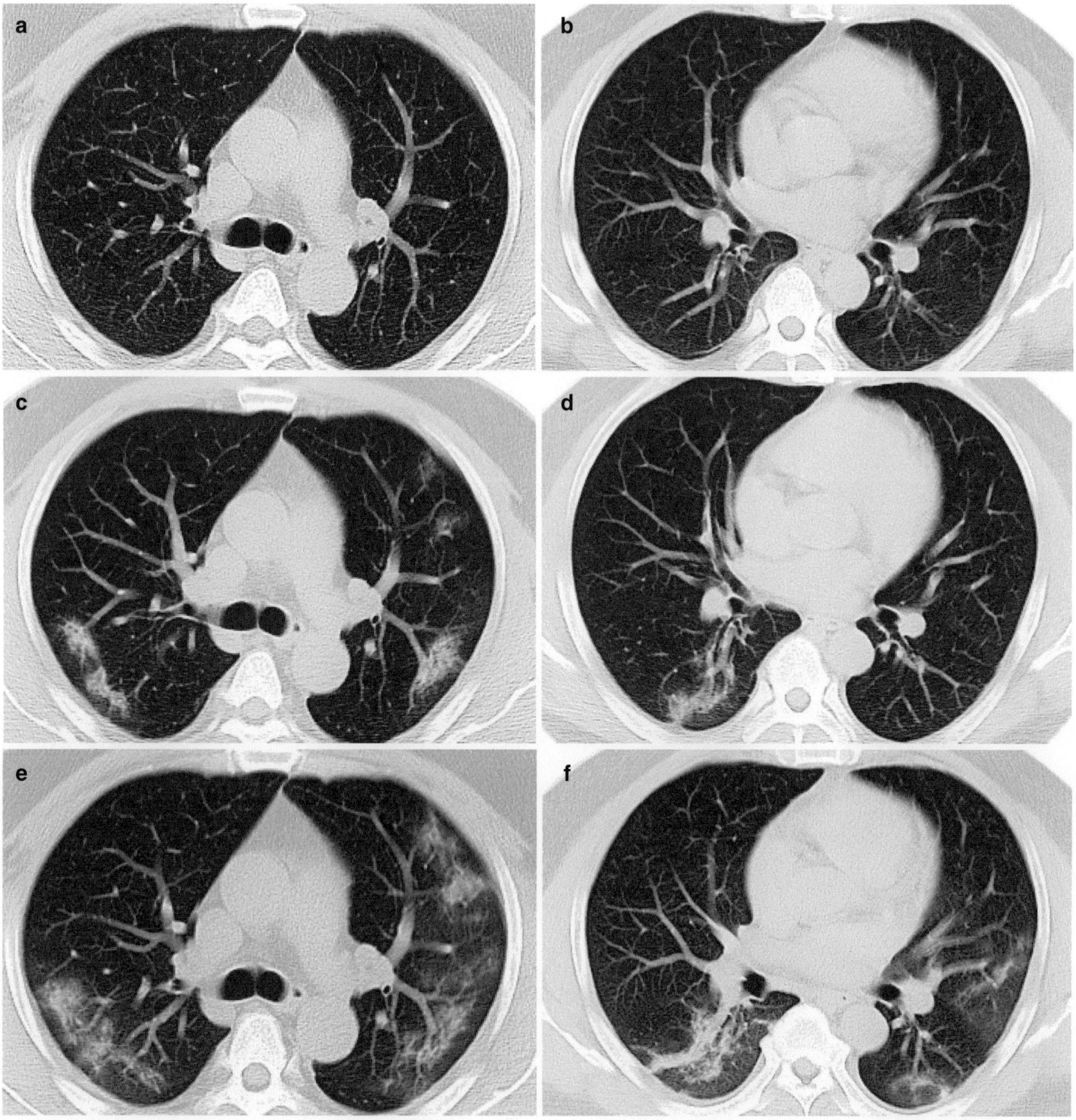

Fig. 8.3 On 5 days after onset of symptoms, chest CT images showed no obvious abnormality in both lungs (**a**, **b**). On 10 days after onset of symptoms, chest CT images showed patchy ground-glass opacities in both lungs (**c**, **d**). On 14 days after onset of symptoms, chest CT images demonstrated enlarged lesions and increased density of the lesions, compared with previous images, indicating disease progression (**e**, **f**). On 17 days after onset of symptoms, chest CT images showed decreased lesions in bilateral lungs, and subpleural arc band shadow in the lower lobe of both lungs. The lesions gradually disappeared/vanished (**g**, **h**). Coronal and sagittal images showed patchy ground-glass opacities in both lungs (**i**–**l**), and "reverse halo sign" was seen locally (**j**, **l** white arrow)

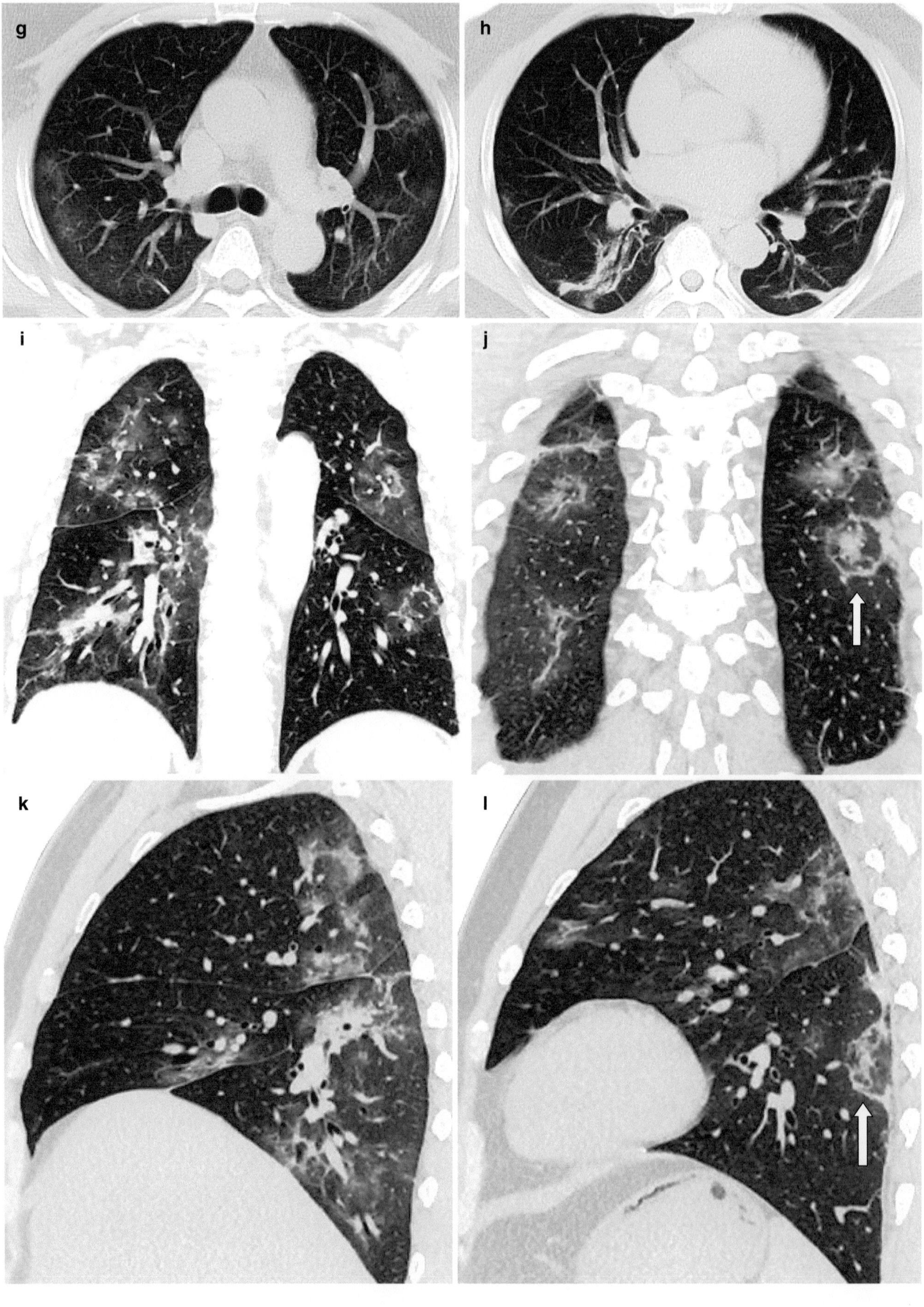

Fig. 8.3 (continued)

8.5 Case 4 (Fig. 8.4a–l)

A 41-year-old male was admitted with fever for 3 days, accompanied by pharyngeal dryness and cough. He had exposed in the epidemic area. The body temperature at admission was 37.3 °C. White blood cell count, lymphocyte count, and C-reactive protein were 3.74×10^9/L, 1.49×10^9/L, and <10 mg/L, respectively. The patient was laboratory confirmed by novel coronavirus nucleic acid throat swab test in Guangzhou CDC. Chest CT examination was performed on 4 days (Fig. 8.4a, b), 8 days (Fig. 8.4c, d, i, j), 11 days (Fig. 8.4e, f, k), and 16 days (Fig. 8.4g, h, l), respectively.

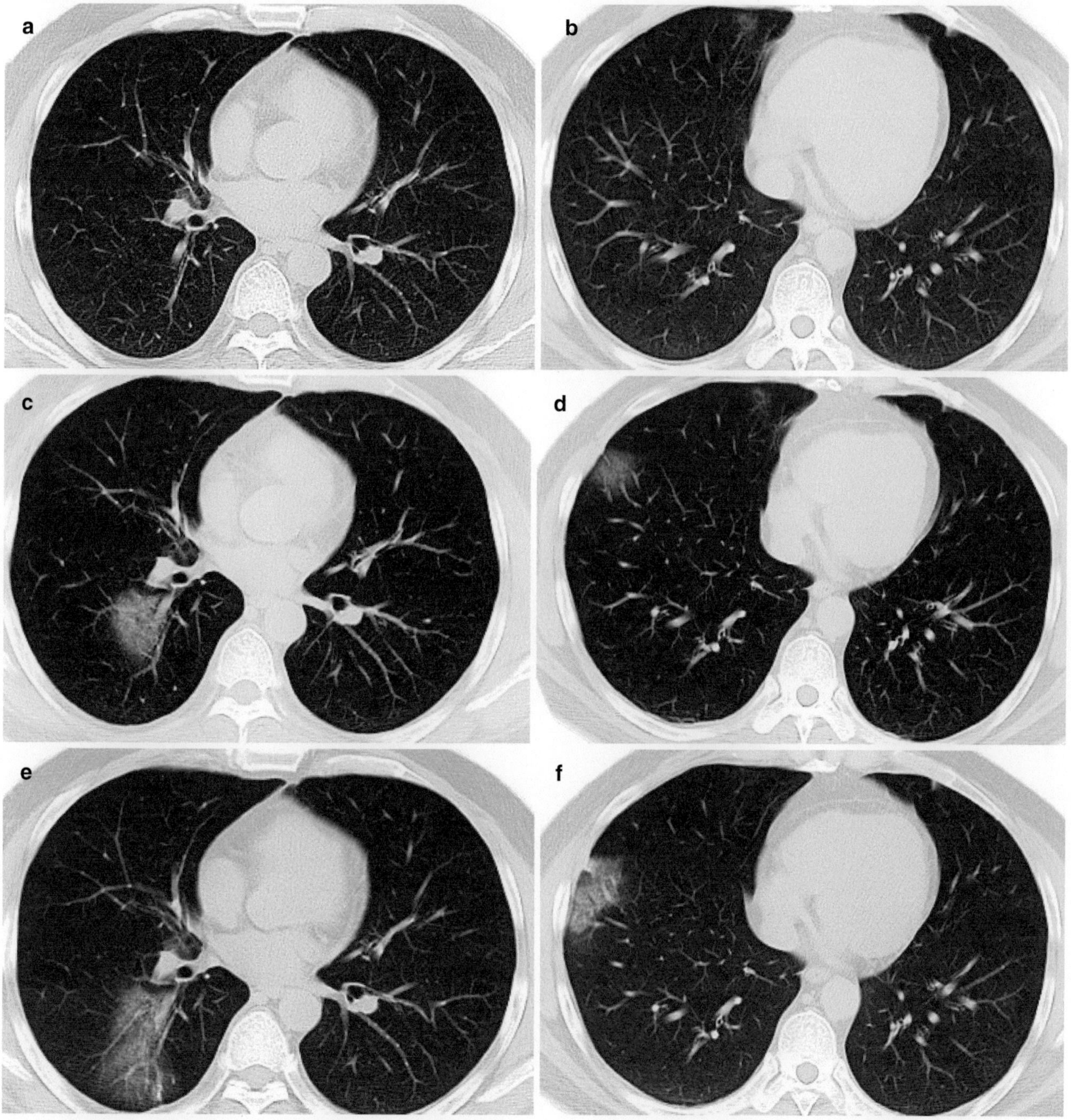

Fig. 8.4 On 4 days after onset of symptoms, chest CT images showed no obvious abnormality in both lungs (**a**, **b**). On 8 days after onset of symptoms, chest CT images showed patchy ground-glass opacities in the lower lobe of the right lung (**c**, **d**). On 11 days after onset of symptoms, chest CT images demonstrated enlarged lesions and increased density of the lesions, compared with previous images, indicating disease progression (**e**, **f**). On 16 days after onset of symptoms, chest CT images showed that the scope of the lesion in the lower lobe of the right lung was smaller than before (**g**, **h**). Coronal and sagittal images showed patchy ground-glass opacities in the lower lobe of the right lung (**i**–**l**), and "reverse halo sign" in the dorsal segment of the lower lobe of the right lung (**k** white arrow)

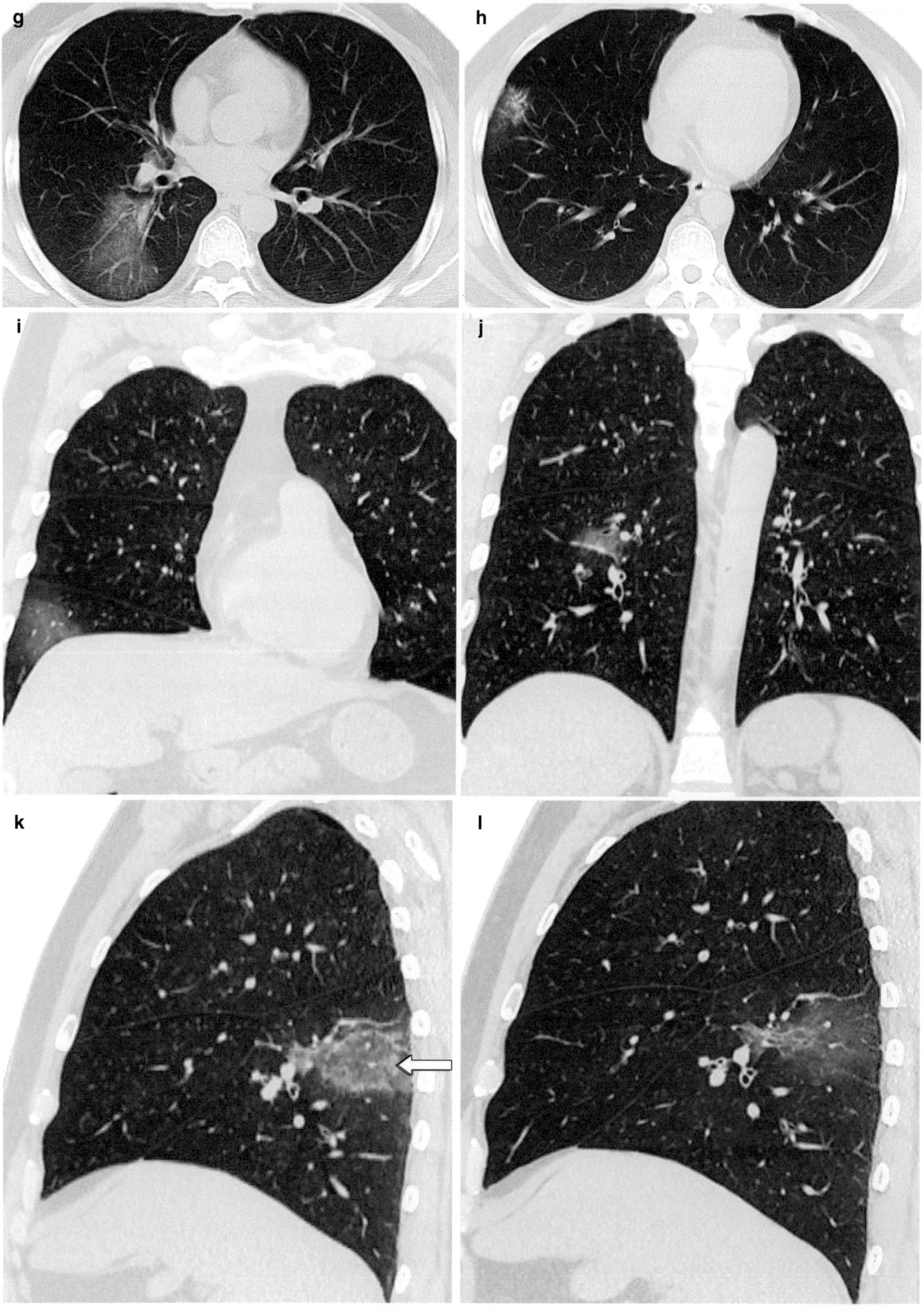

Fig. 8.4 (continued)

On 4 days after onset of symptoms, chest CT images showed no obvious abnormality in both lungs (Fig. 8.4a, b). On 8 days after onset of symptoms, chest CT images showed patchy ground-glass opacities in the lower lobe of the right lung (Fig. 8.4c, d). On 11 days after onset of symptoms, chest CT images demonstrated enlarged lesions and increased density of the lesions, compared with previous images, indicating disease progression (Fig. 8.4e, f). On 16 days after onset of symptoms, chest CT images showed that the scope of the lesion in the lower lobe of the right lung was smaller than before (Fig. 8.4g, h). Coronal and sagittal images showed patchy ground-glass opacities in the lower lobe of the right lung (Fig. 8.4i–l), and "reverse halo sign" in the dorsal segment of the lower lobe of the right lung (Fig. 8.4k white arrow).

8.6 **Case 5** (Fig. 8.5a–j)

A 50-year-old male was admitted with pharyngeal discomfort for 1 day. He had exposed to confirmed cases with novel coronavirus pneumonia. The body temperature at admission was 36.3 °C. White blood cell count, lymphocyte count, and C-reactive protein were 5.85×10^9/L, 0.86×10^9/L, and <10 mg/L, respectively. The patient was laboratory confirmed by novel coronavirus nucleic acid throat swab test in Guangzhou CDC. Chest CT examination was performed on 3 days (Fig. 8.5a), 6 days (Fig. 8.5b), 10 days (Fig. 8.5c, g, i), 13 days (Fig. 8.5d, h), 16 days (Fig. 8.5e), and 24 days (Fig. 8.5f, j) after onset of symptoms, respectively.

On 3 days after onset of symptoms, chest CT images showed no obvious abnormalities in both lungs (Fig. 8.5a). On 6 days after onset of symptoms, chest CT images showed patchy ground-glass opacities in the lower lobe of the left lung (Fig. 8.5b). On 10 days after onset of symptoms, chest CT images showed new lesions in the right lung, increased density of lesions in the lower lobe of the left lung, and pleural subline (Fig. 8.5c). On 13 days after onset of symptoms, chest CT images showed that the lesion in the lower lobe of both lungs was slightly more absorbed than before, with strip-shaped shadows (Fig. 8.5d). On 16 days after onset of symptoms, chest CT images showed no significant changes in the bilateral lung lesions (Fig. 8.5e). On 24 days after onset of symptoms, chest CT images showed that the lesions in bilateral lungs were more absorbed than before, with strip-shaped shadows (Fig. 8.5f). Coronal and sagittal images showed multiple patchy ground-glass opacities and strip-shaped shadows in both lungs (Fig. 8.5g, h). Multiple strip-shaped shadows were seen under the pleura in the lower lobe of the right lung (Fig. 8.5i). The range of lesions in the right lung was smaller than before, and the pleural subline was seen (Fig. 8.5j white arrow).

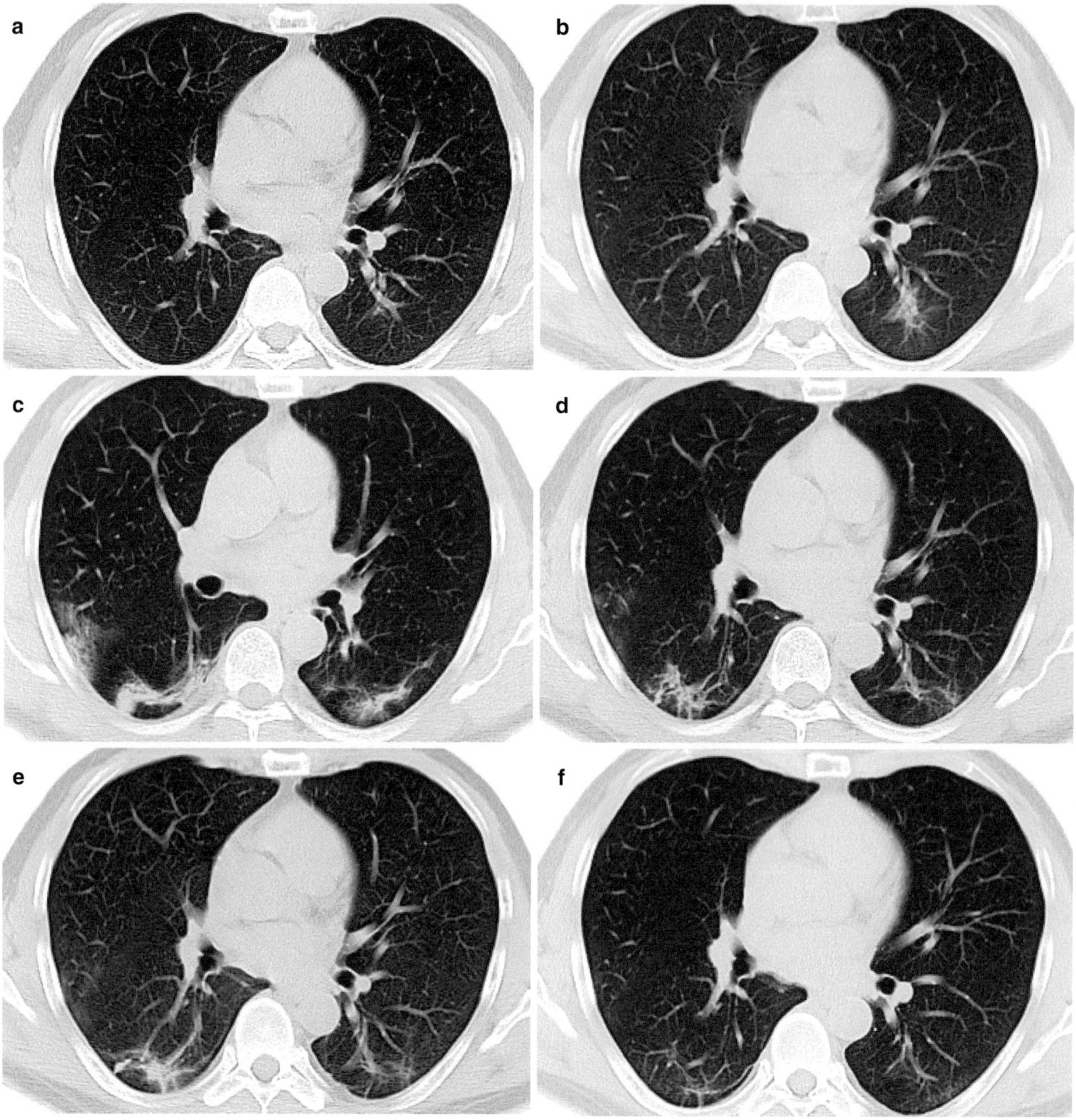

Fig. 8.5 On 3 days after onset of symptoms, chest CT images showed no obvious abnormalities in both lungs (**a**). On 6 days after onset of symptoms, chest CT images showed patchy ground-glass opacities in the lower lobe of the left lung (**b**). On 10 days after onset of symptoms, chest CT images showed new lesions in the right lung, increased density of lesions in the lower lobe of the left lung, and pleural subline (**c**). On 13 days after onset of symptoms, chest CT images showed that the lesion in the lower lobe of both lungs was slightly more absorbed than before, with strip-shaped shadows (**d**). On 16 days after onset of symptoms, chest CT images showed no significant changes in the bilateral lung lesions (**e**). On 24 days after onset of symptoms, chest CT images showed that the lesions in bilateral lungs were more absorbed than before, with strip-shaped shadows (**f**). Coronal and sagittal images showed multiple patchy ground-glass opacities and strip-shaped shadows in both lungs (**g**, **h**). Multiple strip-shaped shadows were seen under the pleura in the lower lobe of the right lung (**i**). The range of lesions in the right lung was smaller than before, and the pleural subline was seen (**j** white arrow)

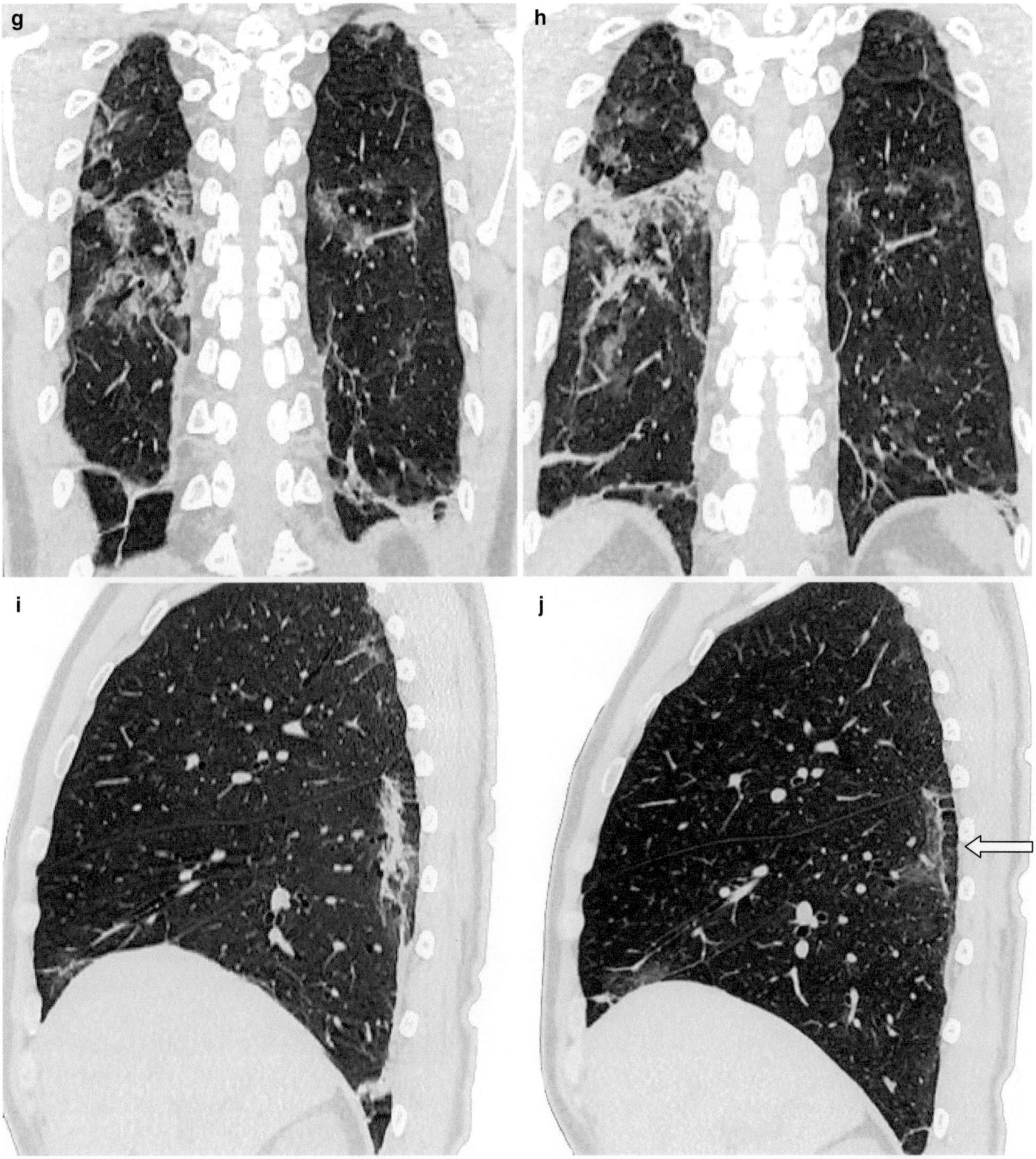

Fig. 8.5 (continued)

8.7 Case 6 (Fig. 8.6a–l)

A 47-year-old male was admitted with fever for 4 days, accompanied by pharyngalgia and cough. He had exposed to confirmed cases with novel coronavirus pneumonia. The body temperature at admission was 37.6 °C. White blood cell count, lymphocyte count, and C-reactive protein were 5.65×10^9/L, 2.79×10^9/L, and <10 mg/L, respectively. The patient was laboratory confirmed by novel coronavirus nucleic acid throat swab test in Guangzhou CDC. Chest CT examination was performed on 7 days (Fig. 8.6a, b), 11 days (Fig. 8.6c, d), days 16 (Fig. 8.6e, f, i, k), and days 21 (Fig. 8.6g, h, j, l) after onset of symptoms, respectively.

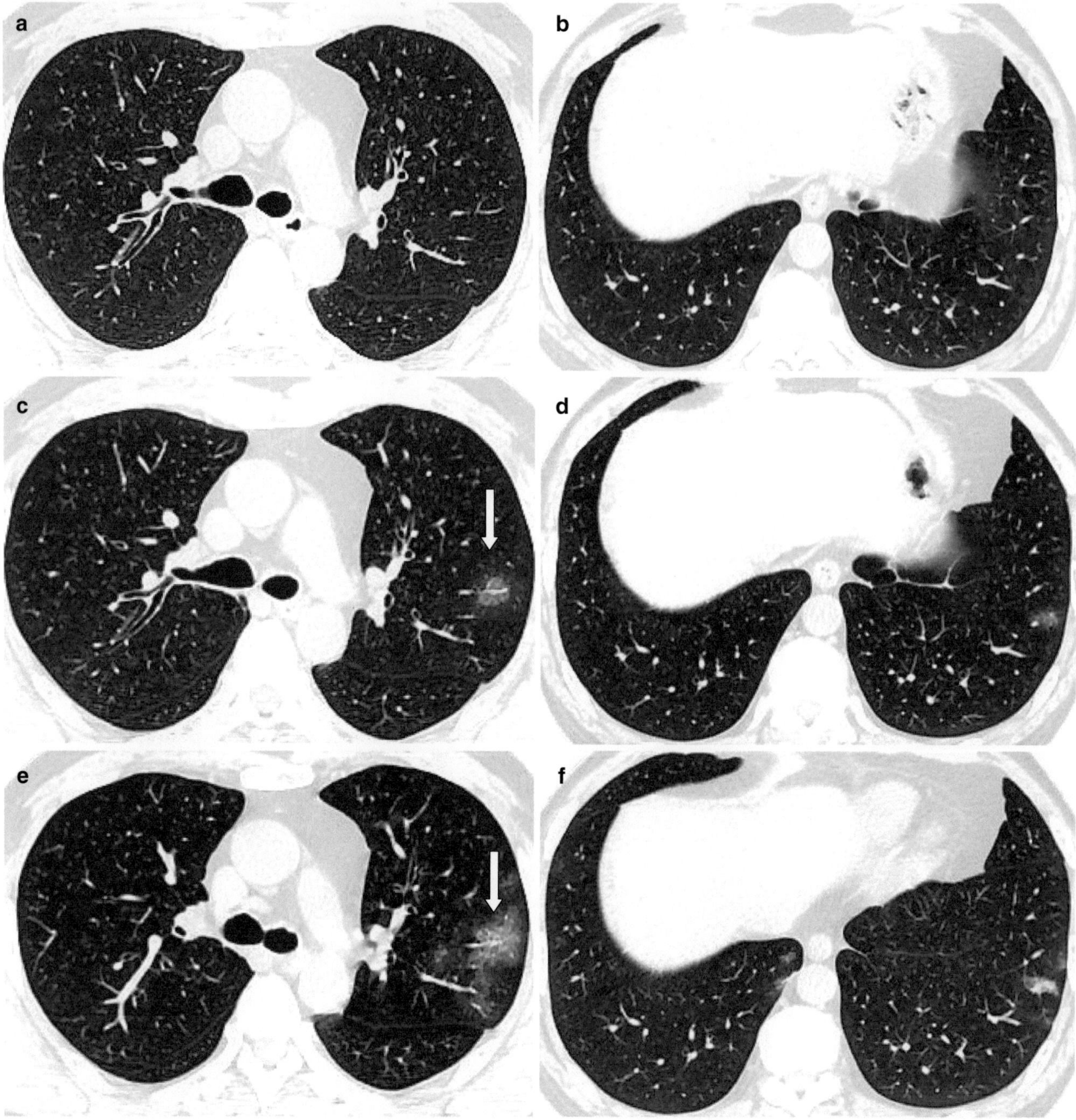

Fig. 8.6 On 7 days after onset of symptoms, chest CT images showed no obvious abnormality in both lungs (**a**, **b**). On 11 days after onset of symptoms, chest CT images showed nodular/patchy ground-glass opacities in the upper and lower lobes of the left lung (**c**, **d**), and thickened vascular shadows in the lesions in the upper lobe of the left lung (**c**, **e**). On 16 days after onset of symptoms, chest CT images showed more lesions than before (**e**, **f**). On 21 days after onset of symptoms, chest CT images demonstrated enlarged lesions and increased density of the lesions, compared with previous images, indicating disease progression (**g**, **h**). Coronal and sagittal images showed patchy ground-glass opacities in the upper lobe of the left lung (**i**–**l**), and "crazy paving sign" in the posterior segment of the upper lobe tip of the left lung (**l** empty arrow)

On 7 days after onset of symptoms, chest CT images showed no obvious abnormality in both lungs (Fig. 8.6a, b). On 11 days after onset of symptoms, chest CT images showed nodular/patchy ground-glass opacities in the upper and lower lobes of the left lung (Fig. 8.6c, d), and thickened vascular shadows in the lesions in the upper lobe of the left lung (Fig. 8.6c, e). On 16 days after onset of symptoms, chest CT images showed more lesions than before (Fig. 8.6e, f). On 21 days after onset of symptoms, chest CT images demonstrated enlarged lesions and increased density of the lesions, compared with previous images, indicating disease progression (Fig. 8.6g, h). Coronal and sagittal images

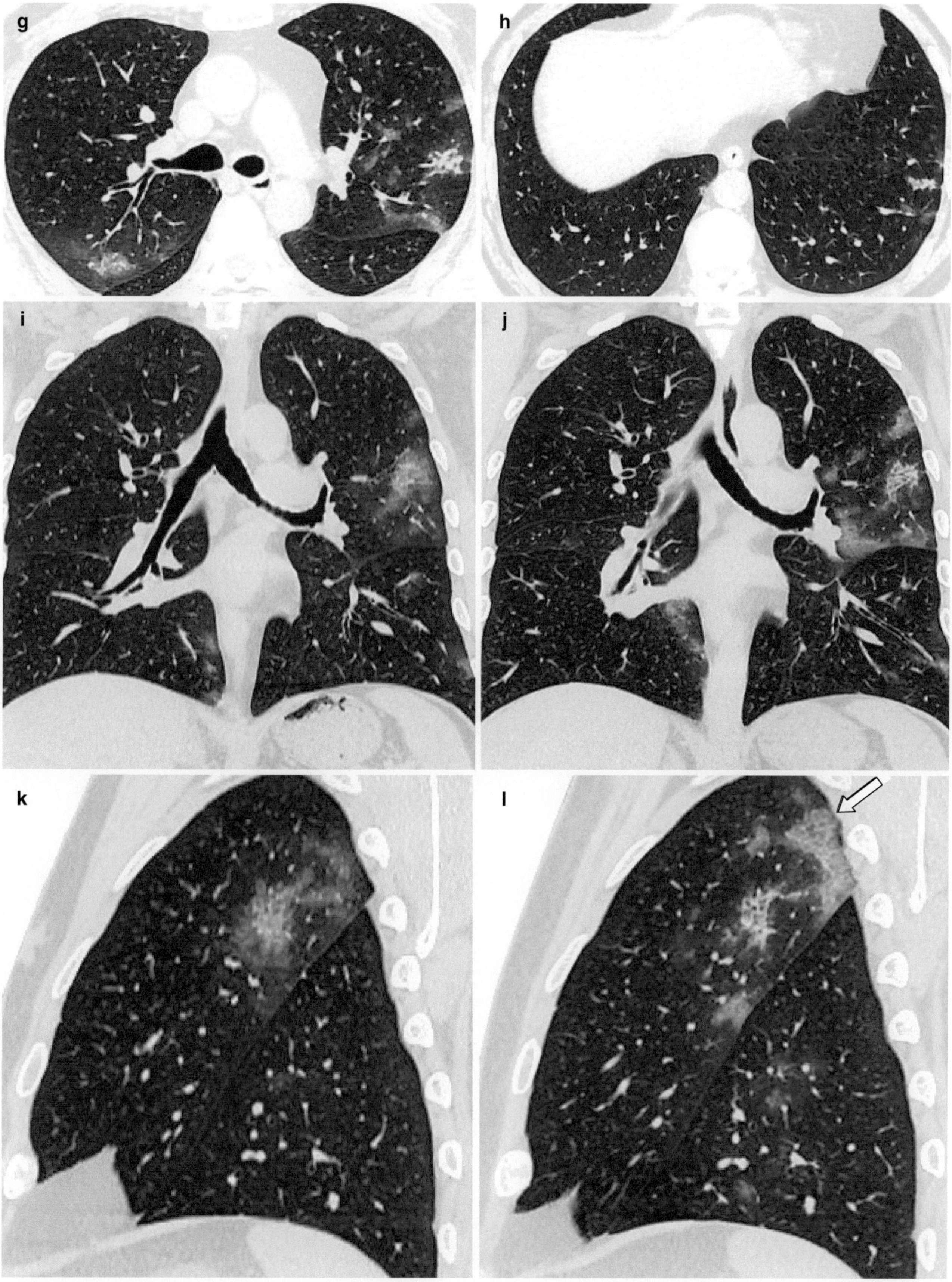

Fig. 8.6 (continued)

showed patchy ground-glass opacities in the upper lobe of the left lung (Fig. 8.6i–l), and "crazy paving sign" in the posterior segment of the upper lobe tip of the left lung (Fig. 8.6l empty arrow).

8.8 Case 7 (Fig. 8.7a–l)

A 45-year-old male was admitted with fever for 4 days, accompanied by cough and sputum for 3 days. He had exposed to confirmed cases with novel coronavirus pneumonia. The body temperature at admission was 37.3 °C. White blood cell count, lymphocyte count, and C-reactive protein were 4.59×10^9/L, 2.10×10^9/L, and <10 mg/L, respectively. The patient was laboratory confirmed by novel coronavirus nucleic acid throat swab test in Guangzhou CDC. Chest CT examination was performed on 5 days (Fig. 8.7a, b), 9 days (Fig. 8.7c, d, i), 12 days (Fig. 8.7e, f, k), and 22 days (Fig. 8.7g, h, j, l) after onset of symptoms, respectively.

On 5 days after onset of symptoms, chest CT images showed no obvious abnormalities in both lungs (Fig. 8.7a, b). On 9 days after onset of symptoms, chest CT images showed patchy ground-glass opacities in the lower lobe of the right lung (Fig. 8.7c, d). On 12 days after onset of symptoms, chest CT images showed that the density of lesions in the lower lobe of the right lung was higher than before (Fig. 8.7e, f). On 22 days after onset of symptoms, chest CT images showed that the scope and density of the lesion in the lower lobe of the right lung were smaller than before (Fig. 8.7g, h), and the lesion in the lower lobe of the right lung presented strip-shaped shadows after absorption (Fig. 8.7g empty arrow). Patchy ground-glass opacities were seen in the lower lobe of the right lung at coronal and sagittal positions (Fig. 8.7i–k).

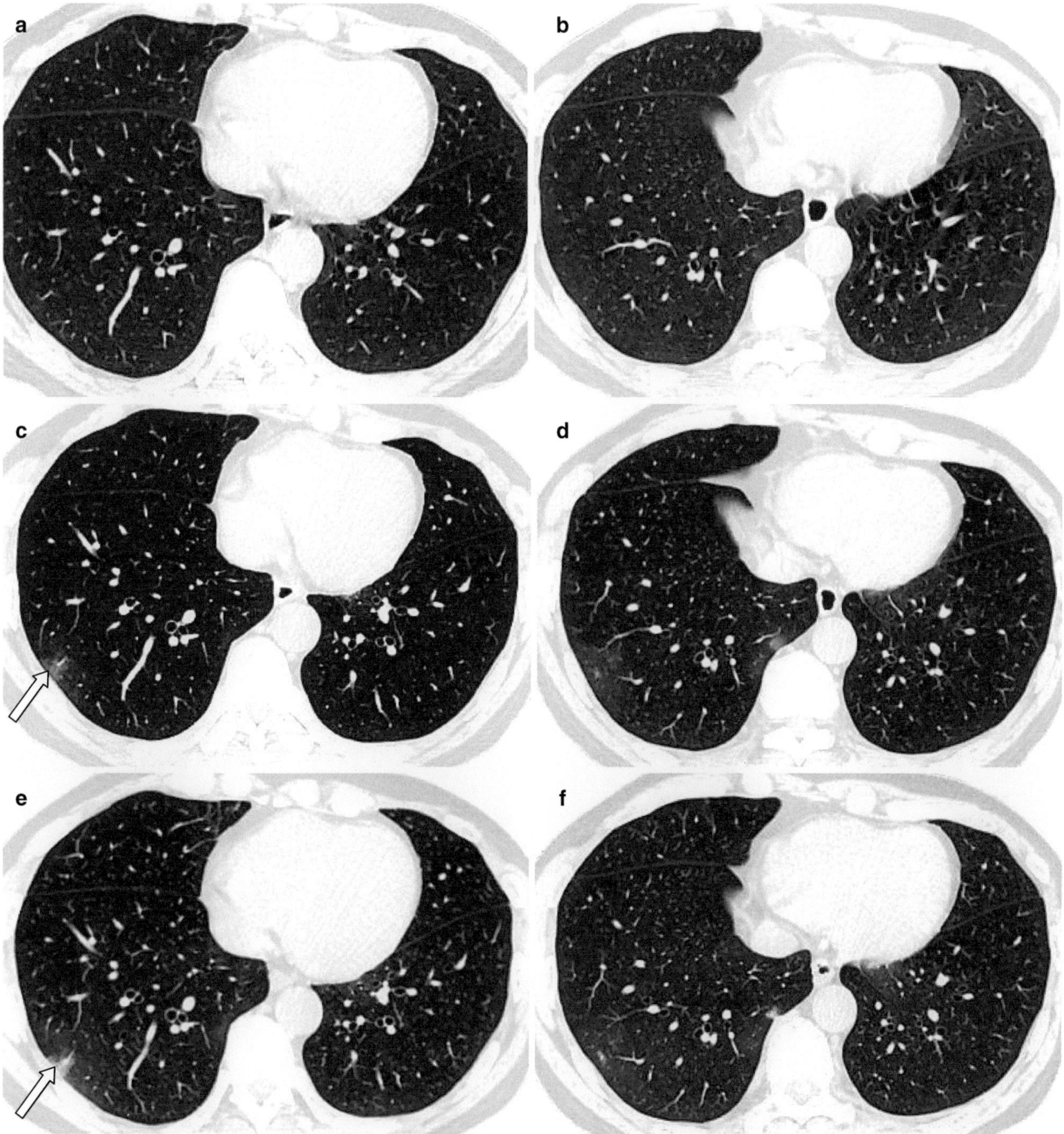

Fig. 8.7 On 5 days after onset of symptoms, chest CT images showed no obvious abnormalities in both lungs (**a**, **b**). On 9 days after onset of symptoms, chest CT images showed patchy ground-glass opacities in the lower lobe of the right lung (**c**, **d**). On 12 days after onset of symptoms, chest CT images showed that the density of lesions in the lower lobe of the right lung was higher than before (**e**, **f**). On 22 days after onset of symptoms, chest CT images showed that the scope and density of the lesion in the lower lobe of the right lung were smaller than before (**g**, **h**), and the lesion in the lower lobe of the right lung presented strip-shaped shadows after absorption (**g** empty arrow). Patchy ground-glass opacities were seen in the lower lobe of the right lung at coronal and sagittal positions (**i**–**k**)

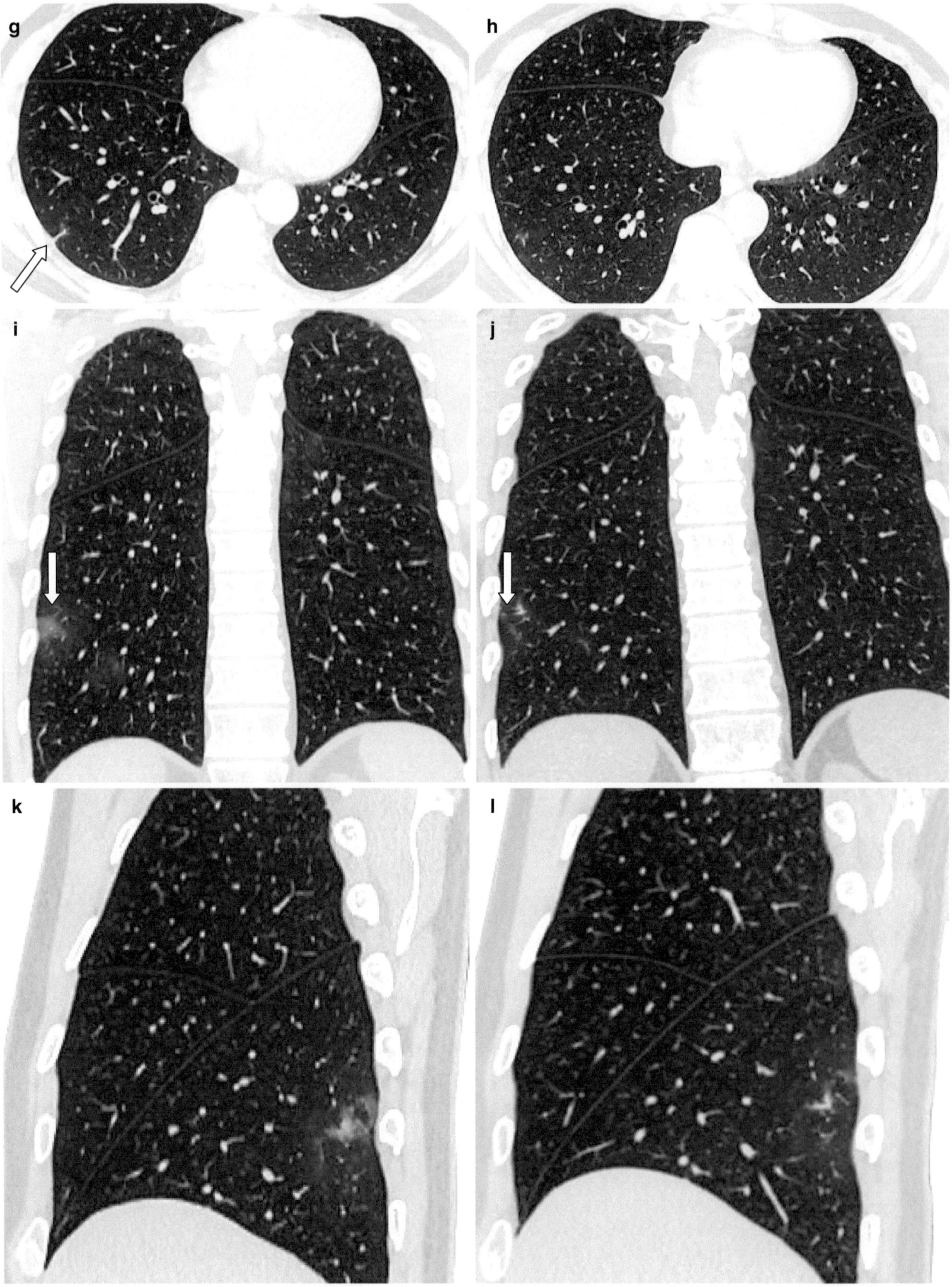

Fig. 8.7 (continued)

8.9 **Case 8** (Fig. 8.8a–j)

A 45-year-old male patient was admitted with fever and cough for 2 days. He had exposed in the epidemic area. The body temperature at admission was 38.0 °C. White blood cell count, lymphocyte count, and C-reactive protein were $5.35 \times 10^9/L$, $2.05 \times 10^9/L$, and <10 mg/L, respectively. The patient was laboratory confirmed by novel coronavirus nucleic acid throat swab test in Guangzhou CDC. Chest CT examination was performed on 3 days (Fig. 8.8a), 7 days (Fig. 8.8b, i), 10 days (Fig. 8.8c, g), 15 days (Fig. 8.8d) 19 days (Fig. 8.8e), and 21 days (Fig. 8.8f, h, j) after onset of symptoms, respectively.

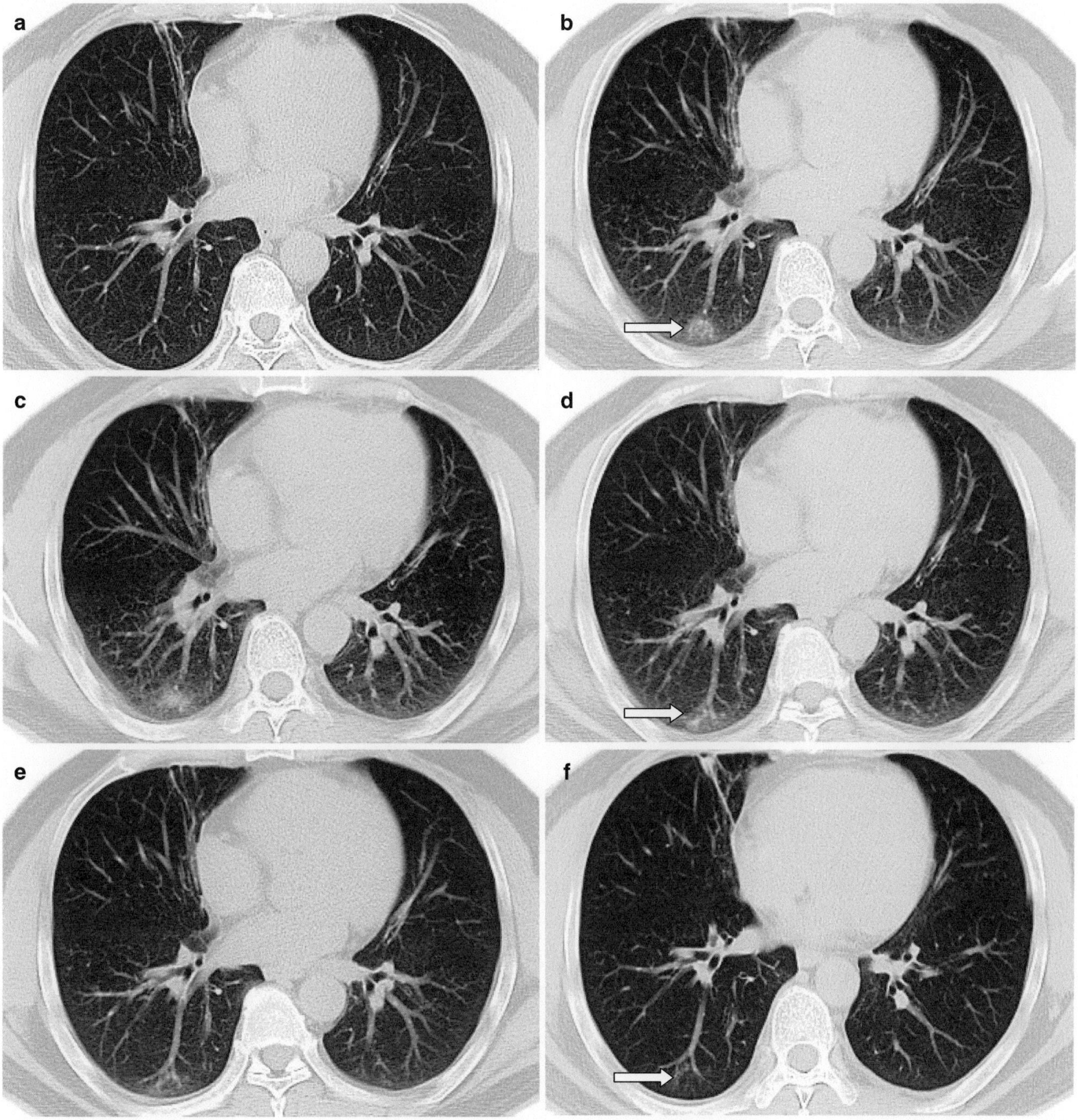

Fig. 8.8 On 3 days after onset of symptoms, chest CT images showed stripy shadows in the middle lobe of the right lung (**a**). On 7 days after onset of symptoms, chest CT images showed patchy ground-glass opacities in the lower lobe of the right lung (**b**). On 10 days after onset of symptoms, chest CT images showed an enlarged lesion in the lower lobe of the right lung (**c**). On 15 days and 19 days after onset of symptoms, chest CT images showed that the scope of the lesion in the lower lobe of the right lung was smaller than before, with strip-shaped shadows (**d**, **e**). On 21 days after onset of symptoms, chest CT images showed that the lesion in the lower lobe of the right lung disappeared (**f**). Scattered patchy ground-glass opacities were seen in the upper lobe of the right lung at coronal and sagittal positions (**g**–**j**)

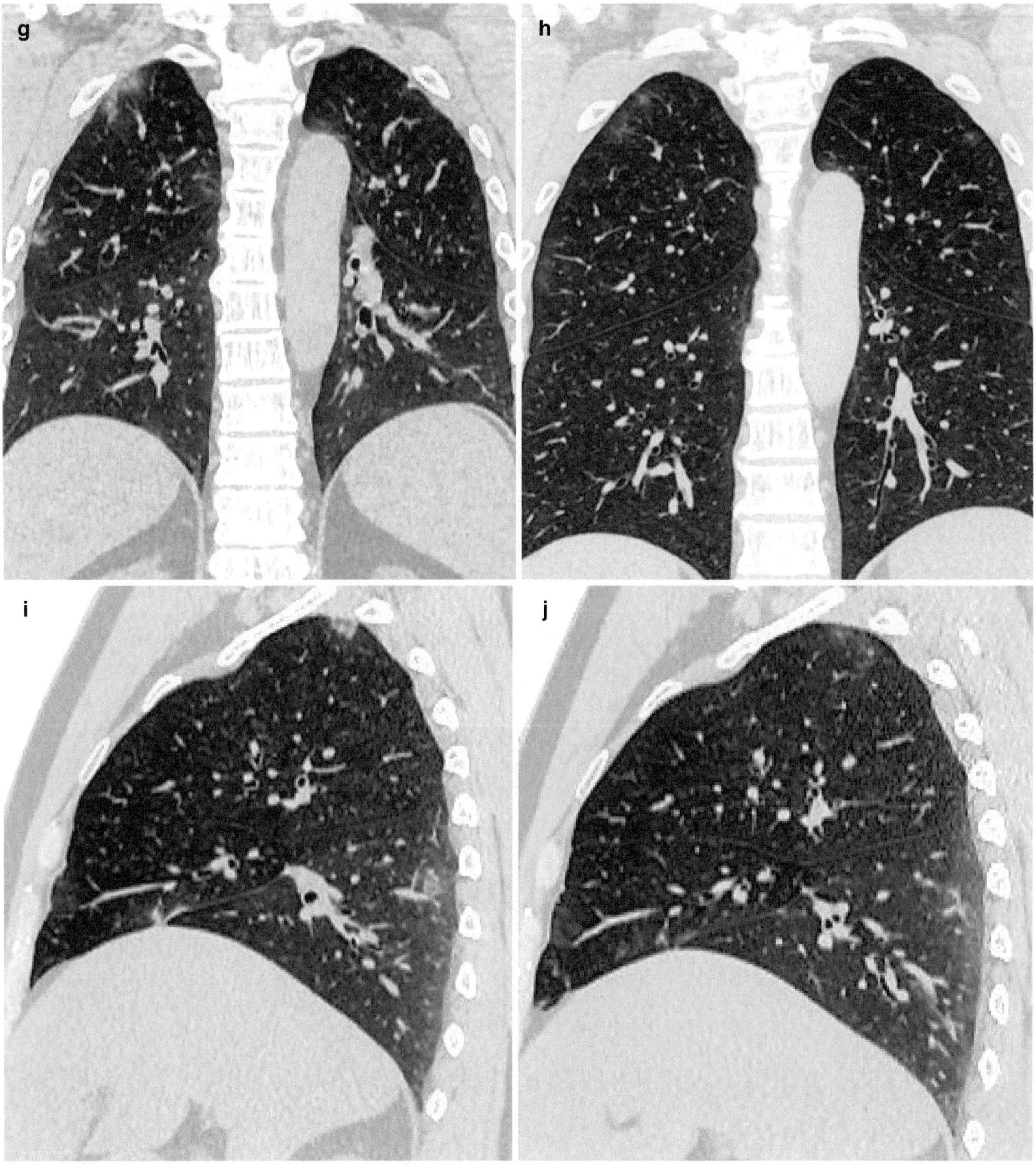

Fig. 8.8 (continued)

On 3 days after onset of symptoms, chest CT images showed stripy shadows in the middle lobe of the right lung (Fig. 8.8a). On 7 days after onset of symptoms, chest CT images showed patchy ground-glass opacities in the lower lobe of the right lung (Fig. 8.8b). On 10 days after onset of symptoms, chest CT images showed an enlarged lesion in the lower lobe of the right lung (Fig. 8.8c). On 15 days and 19 days after onset of symptoms, chest CT images showed that the scope of the lesion in the lower lobe of the right lung was smaller than before, with strip-shaped shadows (Fig. 8.8d, e). On 21 days after onset of symptoms, chest CT images showed that the lesion in the lower lobe of the right lung disappeared (Fig. 8.8f). Scattered patchy ground-glass opacities were seen in the upper lobe of the right lung at coronal and sagittal positions (Fig. 8.8g–j).

8.10 Case 9 (Fig. 8.9a–j)

A 43-year-old female was admitted with pharyngalgia for 1 day. She had exposed to confirmed cases with novel coronavirus pneumonia. White blood cell count, lymphocyte count, and C-reactive protein were 4.44×10^9/L, 0.86×10^9/L, and <10 mg/L, respectively. The patient was laboratory confirmed by novel coronavirus nucleic acid throat swab test in Guangzhou CDC. Chest CT examination was performed on 1 day (Fig. 8.9a), 5 days (Fig. 8.9b), 8 days (Fig. 8.9c), 11 days (Fig. 8.9d, g, i), 14 days (Fig. 8.9e, h, j), and 18 days (Fig. 8.9f) after onset of symptoms, respectively.

On 1 day after onset of symptoms, chest CT images showed no obvious abnormalities in both lungs (Fig. 8.9a). On 5 days

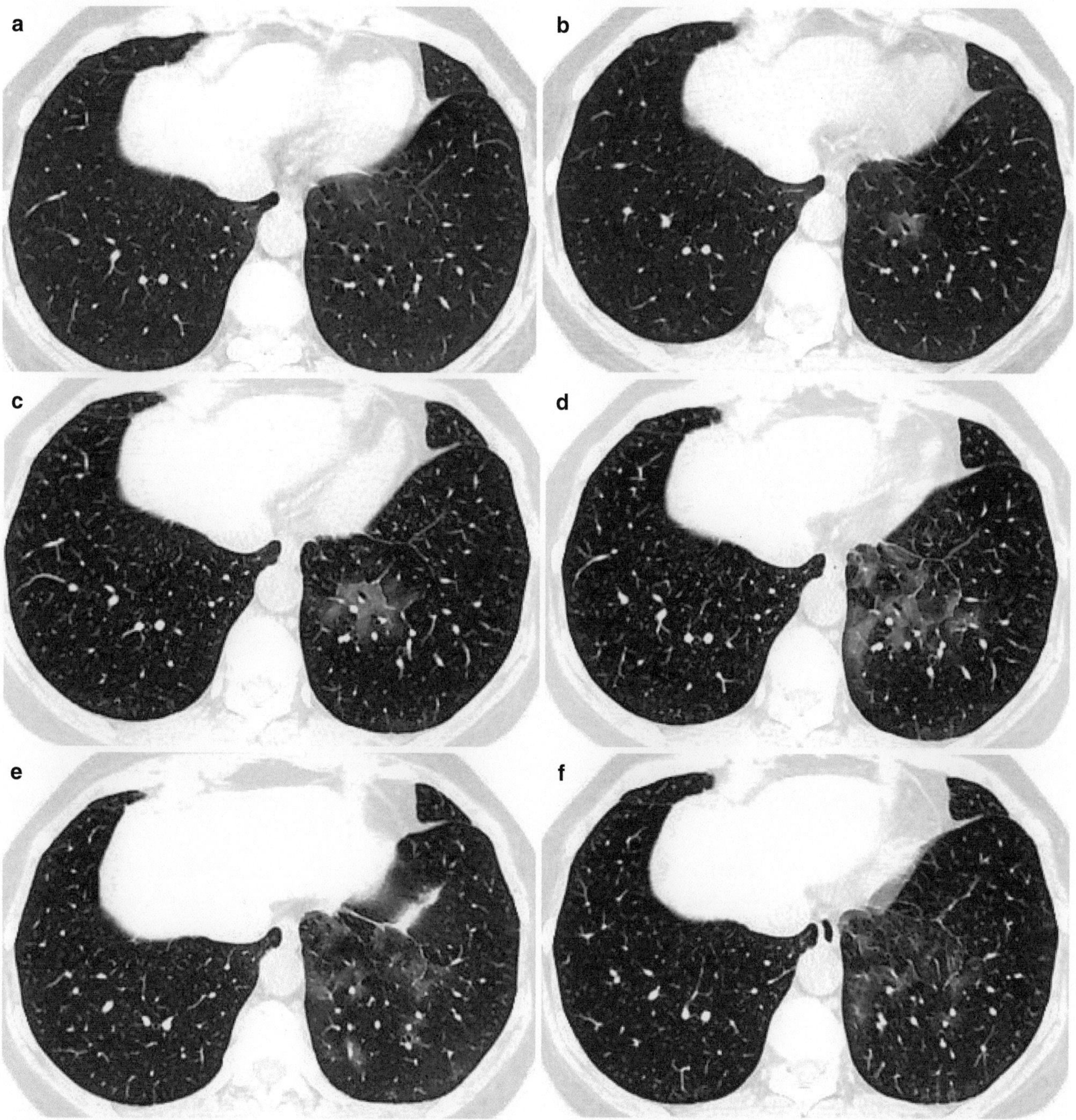

Fig. 8.9 On 1 day after onset of symptoms, chest CT images showed no obvious abnormalities in both lungs (**a**). On 5 days after onset of symptoms, chest CT images showed patchy ground-glass opacities in the lower lobe of the right lung (**b**). On 8 days and 11 days after onset of symptoms, chest CT images showed increased lesions in the lower lobe of the right lung (**c**, **d**). On 14 and 18 days after onset of symptoms, chest CT images showed that the lesion was smaller, and the density is lower than before (**e**, **f**). Patchy ground-glass opacities were seen in the lower lobe of the right lung at coronal and sagittal positions (**g**–**j**)

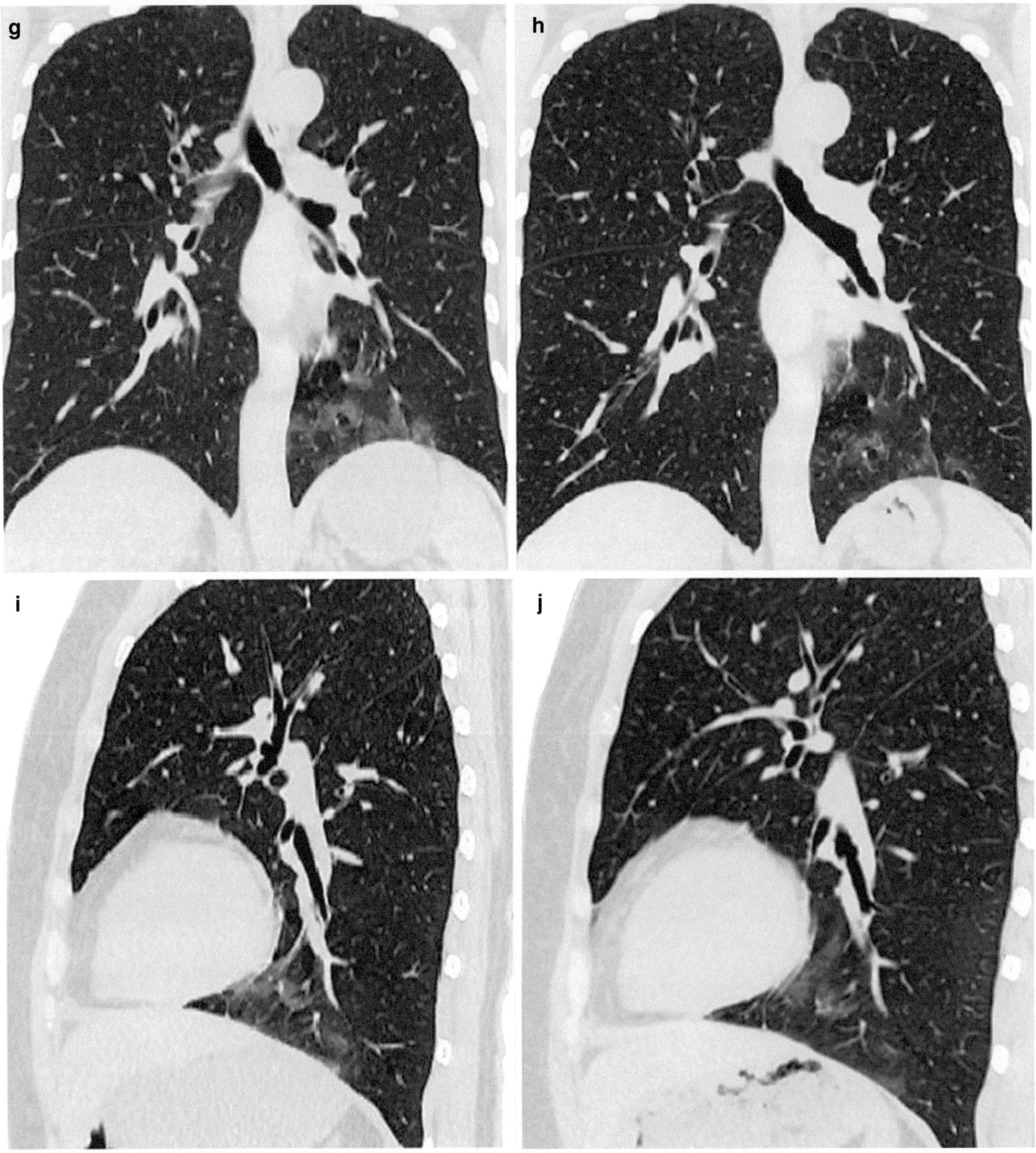

Fig. 8.9 (continued)

after onset of symptoms, chest CT images showed patchy ground-glass opacities in the lower lobe of the right lung (Fig. 8.9b). On 8 days and 11 days after onset of symptoms, chest CT images showed increased lesions in the lower lobe of the right lung (Fig. 8.9c, d). On 14 and 18 days after onset of symptoms, chest CT images showed that the lesion was smaller, and the density is lower than before (Fig. 8.9e, f). Patchy ground-glass opacities were seen in the lower lobe of the right lung at coronal and sagittal positions (Fig. 8.9g–j).

8.11 Case 10 (Fig. 8.10a–j)

A 45-year-old female was admitted with fever for 2 days, accompanied by cough. She had exposed to confirmed cases with novel coronavirus pneumonia. The body temperature at admission was 37.5 °C. White blood cell count, lymphocyte count, and C-reactive protein were 7.11 × 10^9/L, 0.61 × 10^9/L, and <10 mg/L, respectively. The patient was laboratory confirmed by novel coronavirus nucleic acid

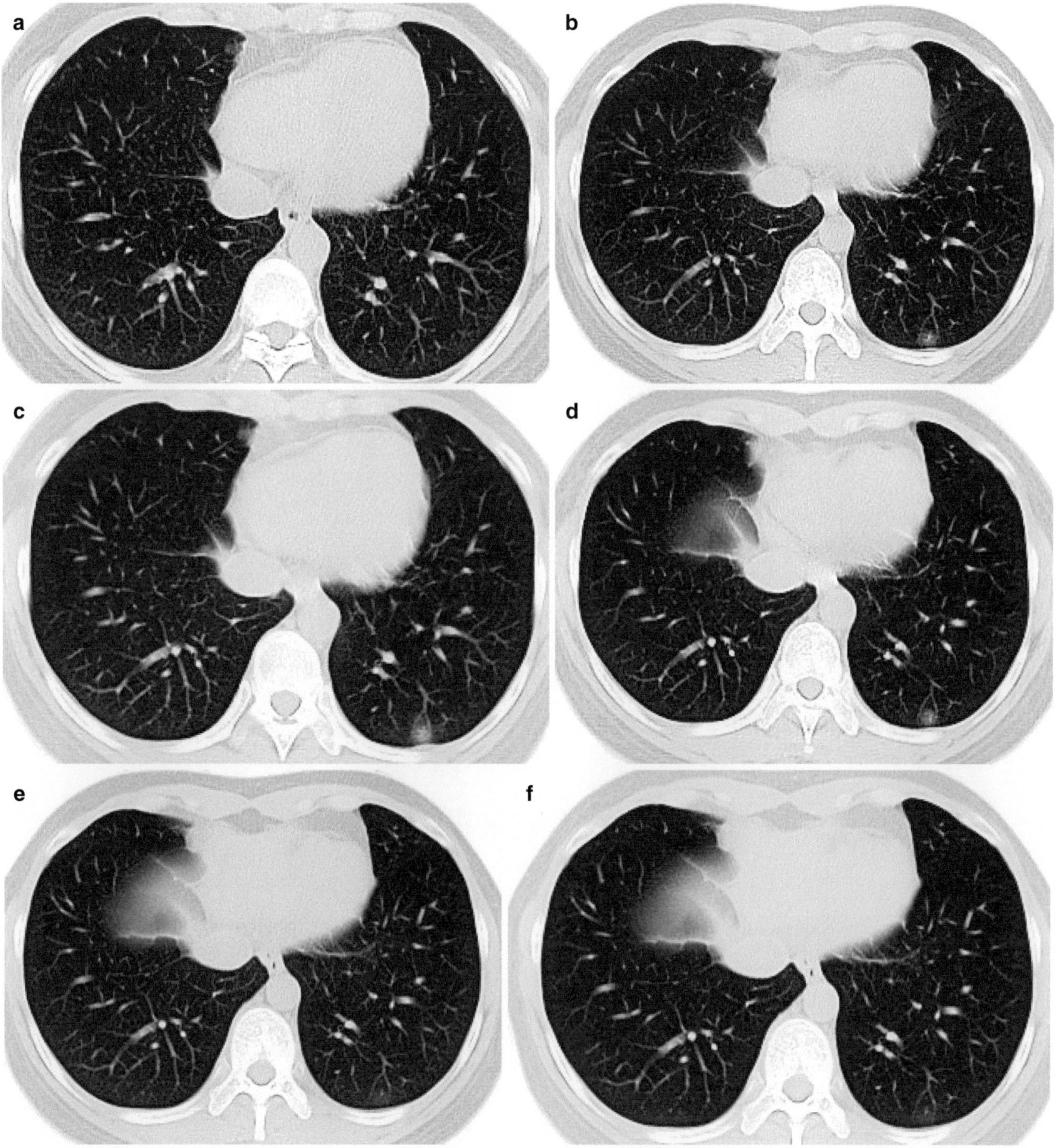

Fig. 8.10 On 3 days after onset of symptoms, chest CT images showed no obvious abnormalities in both lungs (**a**). On 6 days after onset of symptoms, chest CT images showed new nodular ground-glass opacities in the lower lobe of the right lung, and the thickening of the central structure of the lobule was observed (**b**). On 10 days and 13 days after onset of symptoms, chest CT images showed a slightly larger range of lesions in the lower lobe of the right lung (**c**, **d**). On 18 days after onset of symptoms, chest CT images showed a slight decrease in the density of the lesion in the lower lobe of the right lung (**e**). On 23 days after onset of symptoms, chest CT images showed the lesion in the lower lobe of the right lung disappeared (**f**). At the coronal and sagittal position, a small nodular ground hyaline density shadow was seen in the lower lobe of the right lung, and the central node of the lobule was thickened (**g**, **i** empty arrow), and the lesion disappeared after treatment (**h**, **j** white arrow)

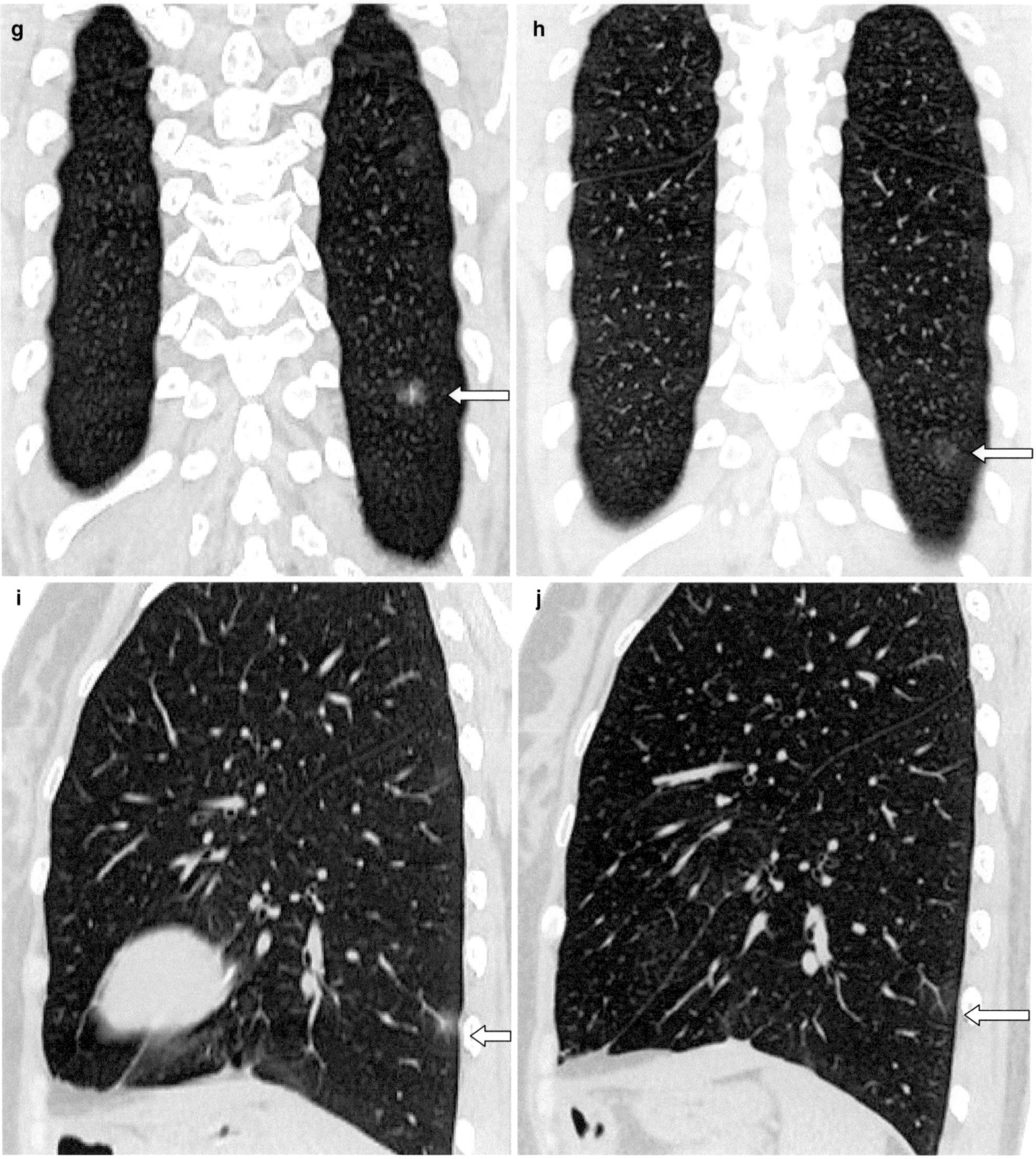

Fig. 8.10 (continued)

throat swab test in Guangzhou CDC. Chest CT examination was performed on 3 days (Fig. 8.10a), 6 days (Fig. 8.10b, g, i), 10 days (Fig. 8.10c), 13 days (Fig. 8.10d), 18 days (Fig. 8.10e), and 23 days (Fig. 8.10f, h, j) after onset of symptoms, respectively.

On 3 days after onset of symptoms, chest CT images showed no obvious abnormalities in both lungs (Fig. 8.10a). On 6 days after onset of symptoms, chest CT images showed new nodular ground-glass opacities in the lower lobe of the right lung, and the thickening of the central structure of the lobule was observed (Fig. 8.10b). On 10 days and 13 days after onset of symptoms, chest CT images showed a slightly larger range of lesions in the lower lobe of the right lung (Fig. 8.10c, d). On 18 days after onset of symptoms, chest CT images showed a slight decrease in the density of the lesion in the lower lobe of the right lung (Fig. 8.10e). On 23 days after onset of symptoms, chest CT images showed the lesion in the lower lobe of the right lung disappeared (Fig. 8.10f). At the coronal and sagittal position, a small nodular ground hyaline density shadow was seen in the lower lobe of the right lung, and the central node of the lobule was thickened (Fig. 8.10g, i empty arrow), and the lesion disappeared after treatment (Fig. 8.10h, j white arrow).

References

1. Zhu N, Zhang D, Wang W, et al. A novel coronavirus from patients with pneumonia in China, 2019. N Engl J Med. 2020;382(8):727–33. https://doi.org/10.1056/NEJMoa2001017.
2. World Health Organization (WHO). Coronavirus disease 2019 (COVID-19) situation report-78. https://www.who.int/docs/default-source/coronaviruse/situation-reports/20200407-sitrep-78-covid-19.pdf?sfvrsn=bc43e1b_2
3. Chan JF, Yuan S, Kok KH, et al. A familial cluster of pneumonia associated with the 2019 novel coronavirus indicating person-to-person transmission: a study of a family cluster. Lancet. 2020;395(10223):514–23. https://doi.org/10.1016/S0140-6736(20)30154-9.
4. Zou L, Ruan F, Huang M, et al. SARS-CoV-2 viral load in upper respiratory specimens of infected patients. N Engl J Med. 2020;382(12):1177–9. https://doi.org/10.1056/NEJMc2001737.

Imaging Analysis of Family Clustering COVID-19

9

Rui Jiang, Xiaoneng Mo, and Yueping Li

9.1 Introduction

According to the four items in the sixth edition of the "New Coronavirus Infection Pneumonia Diagnosis and Treatment Program" diagnostic criteria, if any two of the clinical manifestations are met, suspected infection can be diagnosed.

1. A history of travel or residence in disease-relative area [1] and its surrounding areas, or other communities with reported cases, within 14 days before the onset of illness;
2. Have a history of contact with a new coronavirus infection (positive nucleic acid test) within 14 days before onset;
3. Have contacted patients with fever or respiratory symptoms from Wuhan and its surrounding areas, or from communities with case reports within 14 days before onset of illness;
4. Clustering.

Cluster disease refers to the occurrence of the same disease in one family, one unit, and there is an epidemiological association between them. Familial aggregative morbidity is one of the most common forms. Due to individual differences in age, gender, health conditions, each cluster member will have a different incubation period before disease onset, clinical manifestations. Therefore, one familial member is confirmed, the rest members with a close contact history should have chest CT examination and viral RNA test as early as possible. There is no obvious specificity in the CT manifestation of family agglomerative coronavirus pneumonia, which can be manifested as multiple grinding glass densities with lung solidification, thickening of leaflet spacing and fibrosis of lung tissue in the peripheral zone of both lungs.

R. Jiang (✉) · X. Mo · Y. Li
Guangzhou Eighth People's Hospital, Guangzhou Medical University, Guangzhou, China

As of February 11, 20 provinces outside of Hubei had reported 1183 clusters of cases, 88% of which contained 2–4 confirmed cases [2]. More notably, 64% of the clusters recorded to date were within families. Family clustering [3] is characterized by rapid nucleic acid testing when members of the family have a history of contact with infected areas and early onset of fever-related symptoms, which facilitates timely identification of COVID-19 patients [4]. During the epidemic, Guangzhou CDC worked quickly to grasp the onset of symptoms in family members of infected patients, so some patients were isolated and treated early before symptoms appeared.

9.2 Family 1

Families in this group: the mother first developed symptoms and the remaining three successively; the mother was of the critical type with a poor prognosis; the daughter-in-law was the mild type, the father and son were of the moderate type with a good prognosis.

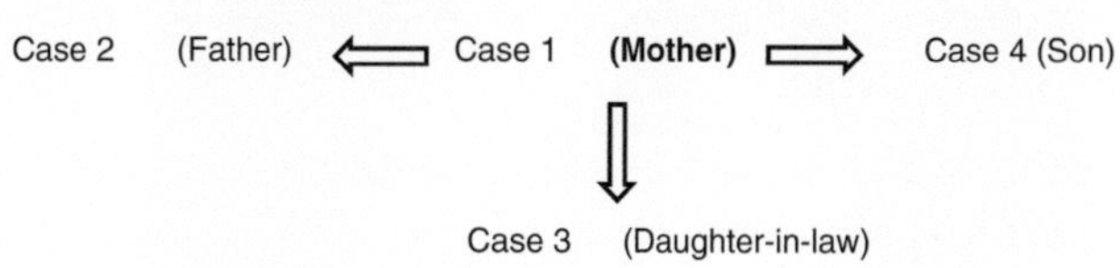

9.2.1 Case 1

A 72-year-old female patient with a disease-related exposure history. Cough occurred 12 days ago. Fever occurred 5 days ago and diarrhoea occurred 1 day ago. Admission body temperature was 39 °C, with a maximum temperature of 39.6 °C during the course of the illness. White blood cell count was17.8 × 10^9/L, lymphocyte count was 0.4 × 10^9/L, and C-reactive protein was 72.88 mg/L. (Critical: oxygen satura-

J. Liu et al. (eds.), *Atlas of Chest Imaging in COVID-19 Patients*, https://doi.org/10.1007/978-981-16-1082-0_9

tion was 80–92%, D-2 aggregates was 3340 μg/L, lactate dehydrogenase was 425 U/L). The patient underwent chest CT scanned at day 13 and day 17 after onset of symptoms, and was confirmed by CDC in Guangzhou.

CT scan showed multiple ground-glass opacities in bilateral lungs on day 13 of onset (Fig. 9.1a, c, e). On day 17, CT showed an exacerbation of the bilateral lung lesions with a "paving stone sign" and an increase in the number of bars (Fig. 9.1b, d, f). A significant increase in the number and extent of bilateral lung lesions was seen on day 13 versus day 17 CT (Fig. 9.1e, f).

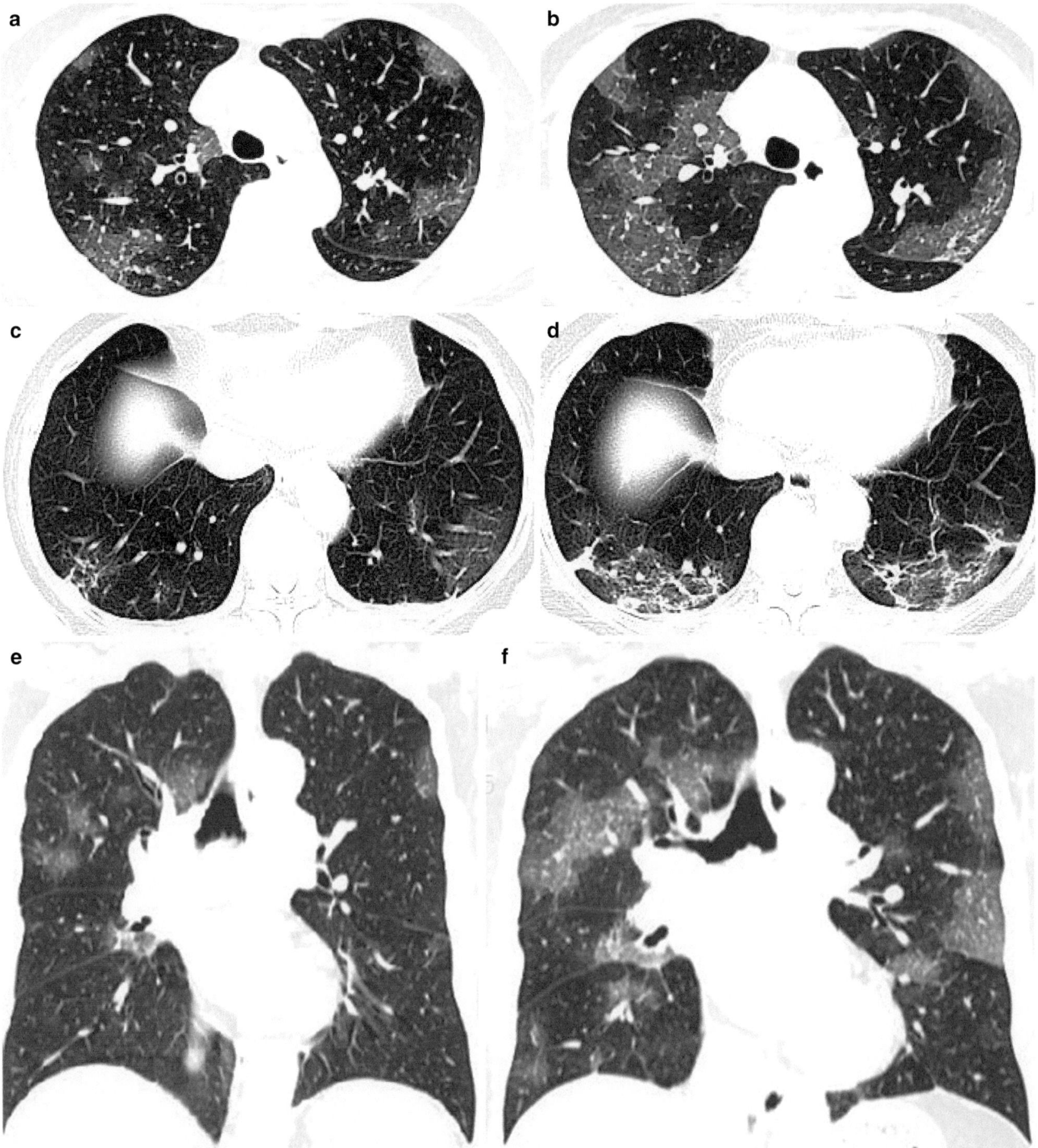

Fig. 9.1 CT scan showed multiple ground-glass opacities in bilateral lungs on day 13 of onset (**a**, **c**, **e**). On day 17, CT showed an exacerbation of the bilateral lung lesions with a "paving stone sign" and an increase in the number of bars (**b**, **d**, **f**). A significant increase in the number and extent of bilateral lung lesions was seen on day 13 versus day 17 CT (**e**, **f**)

9.2.2 Case 2

A 73-year-old male patient with a history of family clustering. Cough and fever occurred 2 days ago. Admission body temperature was 38.4 °C. White blood cell count was 3.59×10^9/L, lymphocyte count was 1.12×10^9/L, C-reactive protein was <10 mg/L. (Normal: oxygen saturation was 94%, D-2 aggregates was 1520 μg/L). The patient was confirmed by CDC in Guangzhou.

CT of the chest on day 3 showed multiple ground-glass opacities in bilateral lungs (Fig. 9.2a, b); CT of the chest on day 6 showed multiple stripe shadows in the bilateral lobes

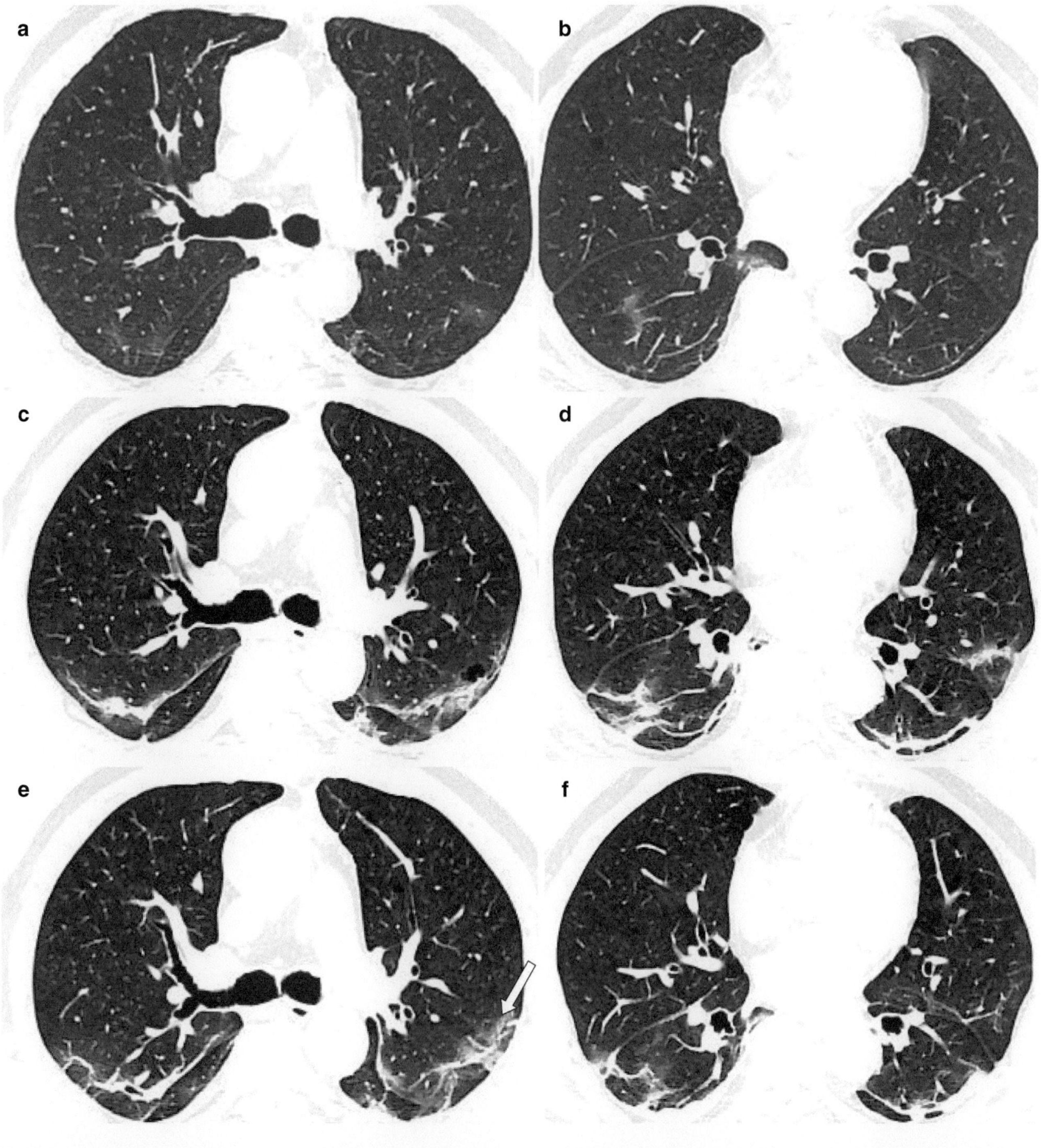

Fig. 9.2 CT of the chest on day 3 showed multiple ground-glass opacities in bilateral lungs (**a**, **b**); CT of the chest on day 6 showed multiple stripe shadows in the bilateral lobes (**c**, **d**). Day 9 CT showed increased bilateral pulmonary stripe shadows, (**e**, **f**) with subpleural line formation visible (**e** white arrow). On day 22, CT showed a significant decrease in bilateral (**f**) lung lesions (**g**, **h**). Coronal position (day 9 vs. day 22 CT), significant reduction and partial disappearance of lesions (**i**, **j**)

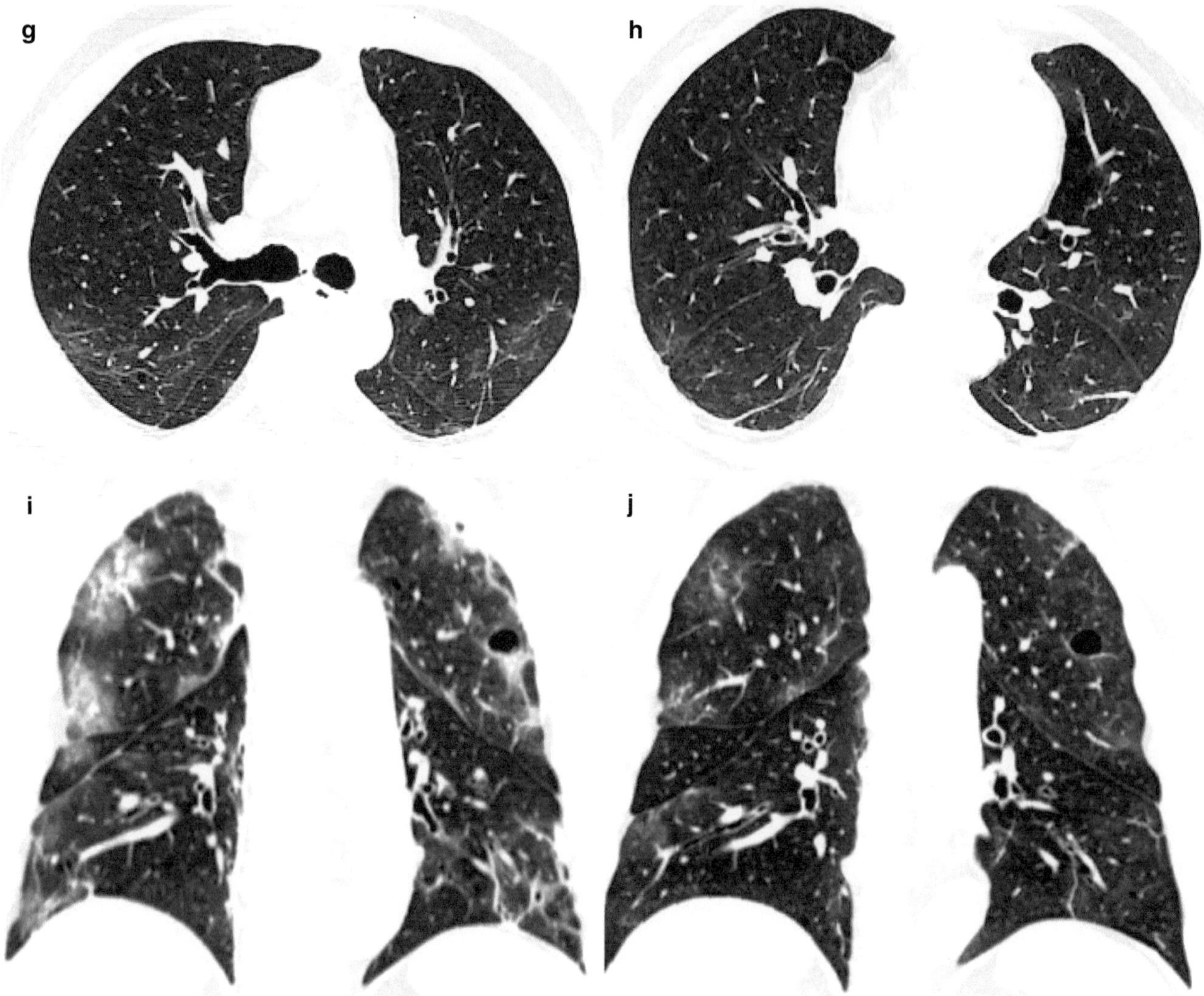

Fig. 9.2 (continued)

(Fig. 9.2c, d). Day 9 CT showed increased bilateral pulmonary stripe shadows with subpleural line formation visible (Fig. 9.2e, f white arrow). On day 22, CT showed a significant decrease in bilateral lung lesions (Fig. 9.2g, h). Coronal position (day 9 vs. day 22 CT), significant reduction and partial disappearance of lesions (Fig. 9.2i, j).

9.2.3 Case 3

A 35-year-old female patient with a history of family clustering. Admitted to hospital due to "pharyngeal discomfort for 3 days". The body temperature was 37 °C at the time of admission and there was no fever during the hospitalization.

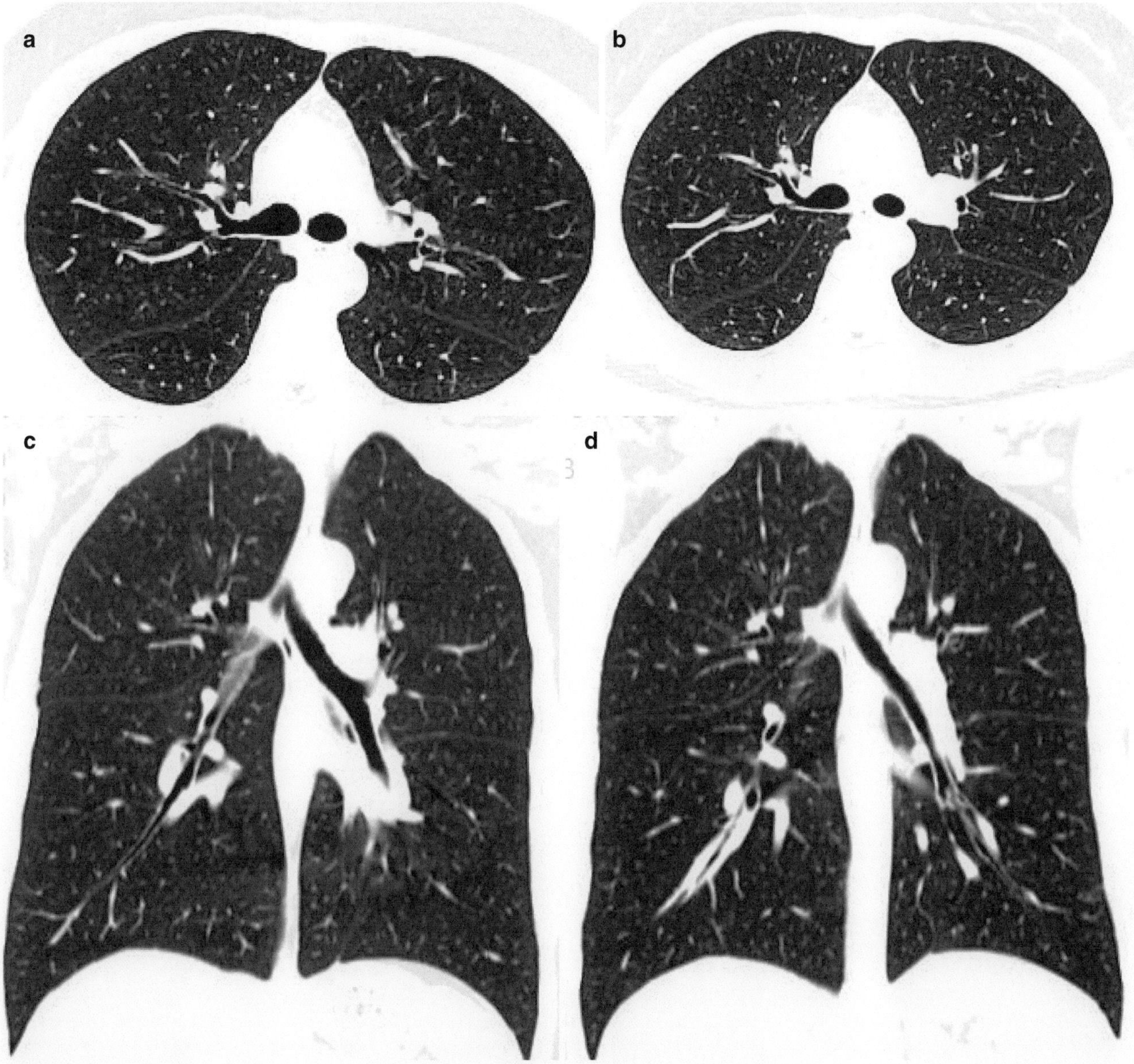

Fig. 9.3 Chest CT was not positive on days 5 and 13 (**a**–**d**)

White blood cell count was 5.64 × 10^9/L, lymphocyte count was 2.07 × 10^9/L, C-reactive protein was <10 g/L. The patient was confirmed by CDC in Guangzhou.

Chest CT was not positive on days 5 and 13 (Fig. 9.3a–d).

9.2.4 Case 4

A 43-year-old male patient with a history of family clustering. Admitted to hospital due to fever for 1 day and decreased sense of smell for 2 days. Admission body temperature was 38.5 °C. White blood cell count was 4.30 × 10^9/L, lymphocyte count were1.76 × 10^9/L, C-reactive protein was <10 mg/L. (Common type: blood oxygen saturation was 97.9%). The patient was confirmed by CDC in Guangzhou.

CT of the chest on day 7 of the onset showed scattered patchy ground-glass opacity in bilateral lungs (Fig. 9.4a). CT on day 10 showed an increased range of intrapulmonary plaques in both lungs (Fig. 9.4b). Day 13 CT showed an increased density of bilateral lung plaques compared to the anterior (Fig. 9.4c).

Day 17 CT showed a partial reduction in the extent of the lesion (Fig. 9.4d).

Day 21 CT showed a further reduction in the extent of bilateral lung lesions (Fig. 9.4e). Day 25 CT shows partial lesions that are more or less resorbed than before (Fig. 9.4f). The coronal position is shown (day 17 vs. day 25 CT) and the lesion is clearly resorbed (Fig. 9.4g, h white arrow).

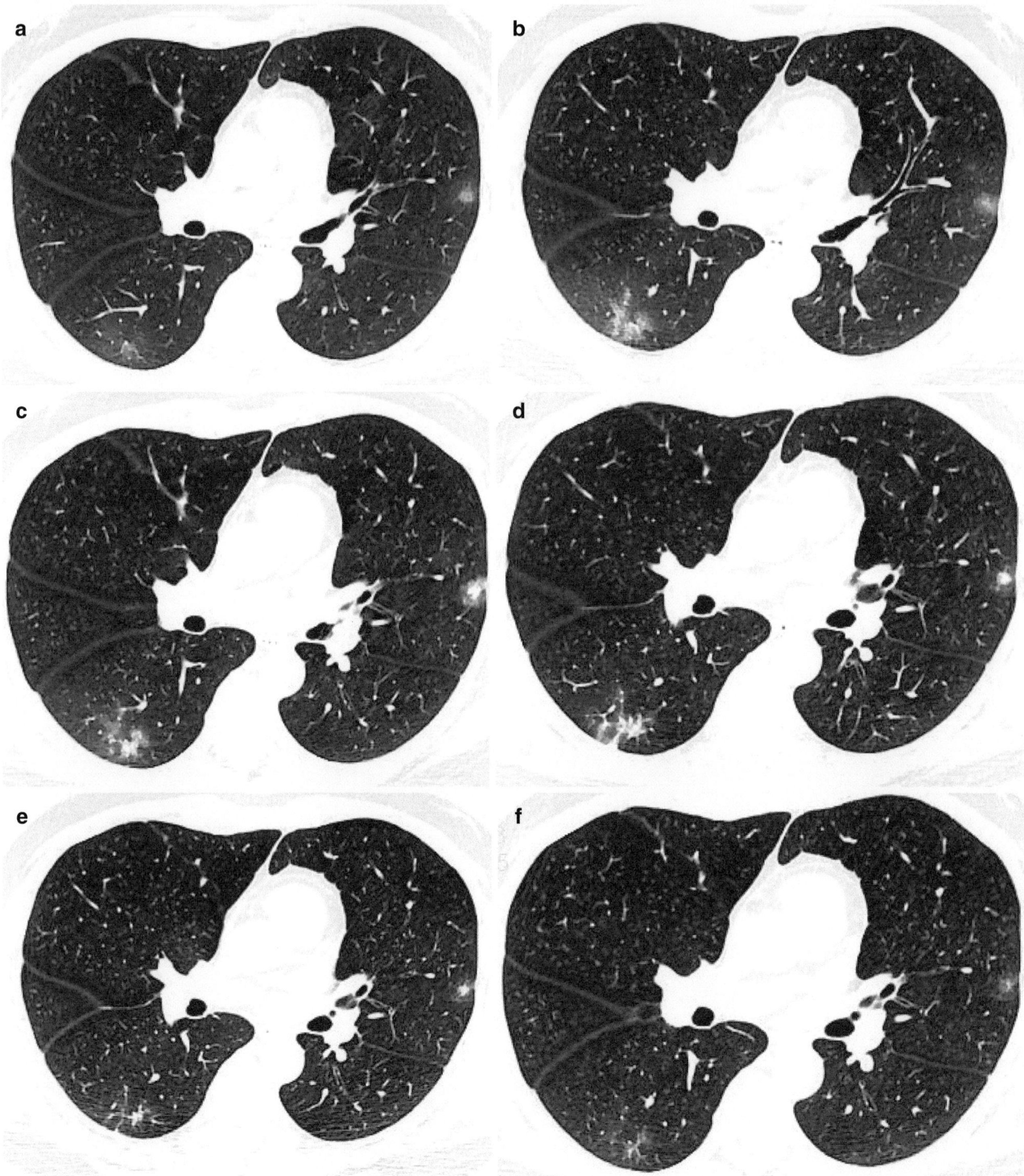

Fig. 9.4 CT of the chest on day 7 of the onset showed scattered patchy ground-glass opacity in bilateral lungs (**a**). CT on day 10 showed an increased range of intrapulmonary plaques in both lungs (**b**). Day 13 CT showed an increased density of bilateral lung plaques compared to the anterior (**c**). Day 17 CT showed a partial reduction in the extent of the lesion (**d**). Day 21 CT showed a further reduction in the extent of bilateral lung lesions (**e**). Day 25 CT shows partial lesions that are more or less resorbed than before (**f**). The coronal position is shown (day 17 vs. day 25 CT) and the lesion is clearly resorbed (**g**, **h** white arrow)

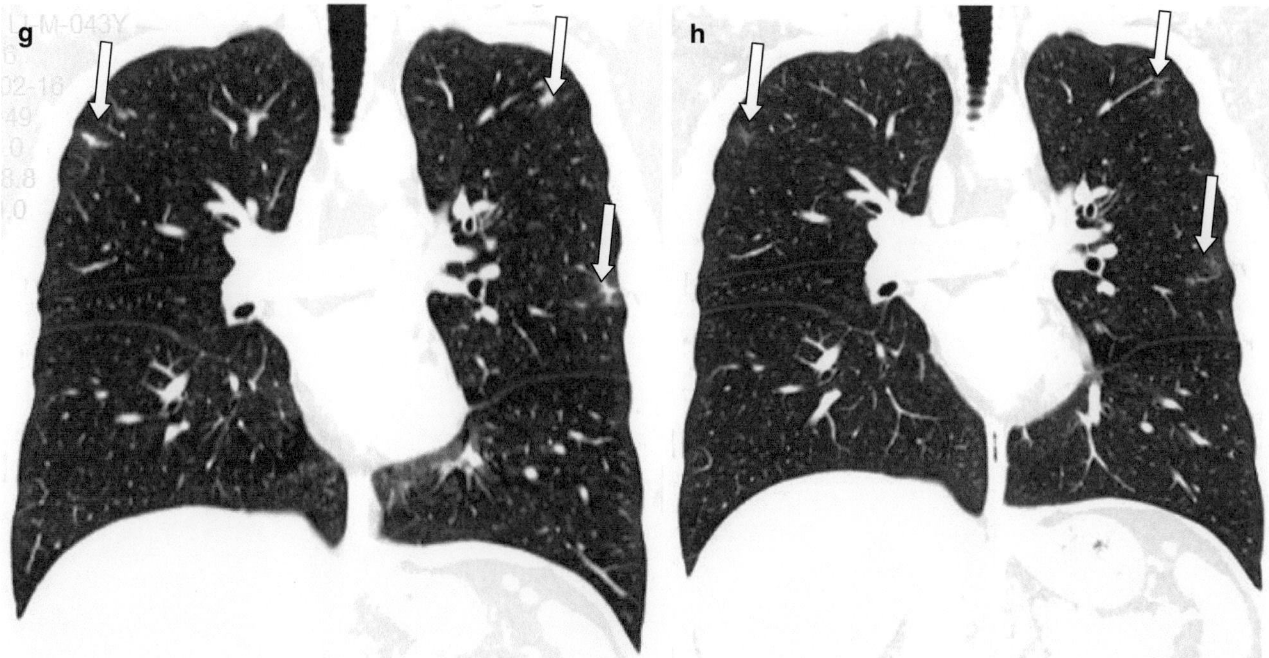

Fig. 9.4 (continued)

9.3 Family 2

Families in this group: Daughters with first symptoms and parents with successive illnesses; daughters with mild symptoms and parents with moderate symptoms with a good prognosis.

Case 6 **(Mother)** ⟸ Case 5 (Daughter) ⟹ Case 7 (Father)

9.3.1 Case 5

A 19-year-old female patient with a disease-related exposure history. Admitted to hospital due to fever for 3 days. Maximum body temperature was 39.6 °C during the course of the disease. White blood cell count was 2.74×10^9/L, lymphocyte count was 1.28×10^9/L, C-reactive protein was <10 mg/L. The patient was confirmed by CDC in Guangzhou.

Chest CT was not positive on days 5 and 18 (Fig. 9.5a–d).

9.3.2 Case 6

A 43-year-old female patient with a history of family clustering. Admitted to hospital due to "Novel coronavirus nucleic acid positive found 1 day". The body temperature was 36.3 °C at the time of admission and there was no fever during the hospitalization. White blood cell count was 4.44×10^9/L, lymphocyte count was 0.86×10^9/L, C-reactive protein was <10 mg/L. The patient was confirmed by CDC in Guangzhou.

Chest CT on day 2 of admission was not significantly positive (Fig. 9.6a).

Day 5 CT scan shows ground-glass opacity in the left lower lobe (Fig. 9.6b). Day 11 CT showed an increased extent of lesions in the lower left lobe of the lung (Fig. 9.6c). Day 18 CT showed significant resorption of the left lower lobe of the lung (Fig. 9.6d). On day 11 compared with day 18, the lesion range was reduced (Fig. 9.6e, f white arrows).

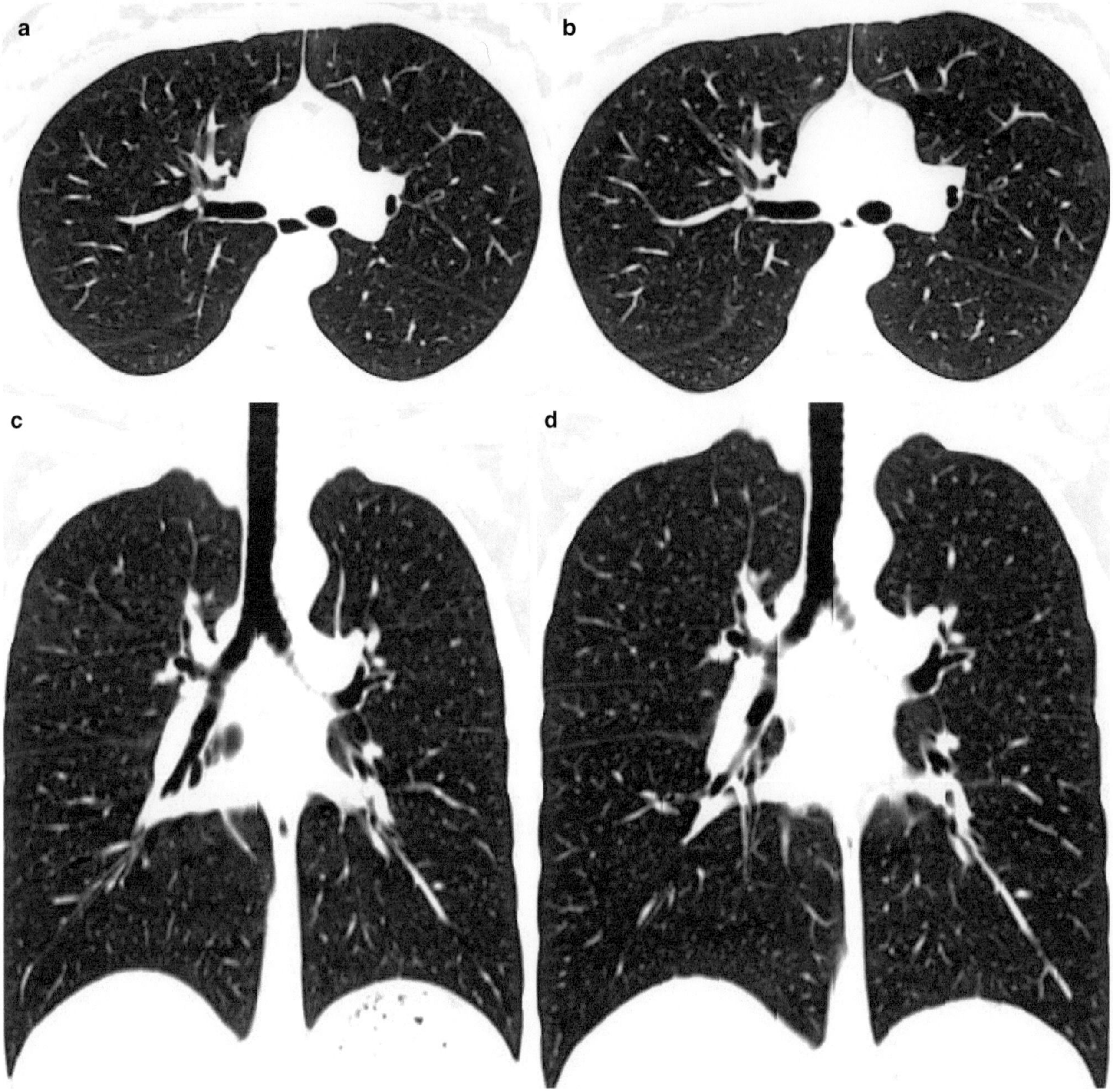

Fig. 9.5 Chest CT was not positive on days 5 and 18 (**a–d**)

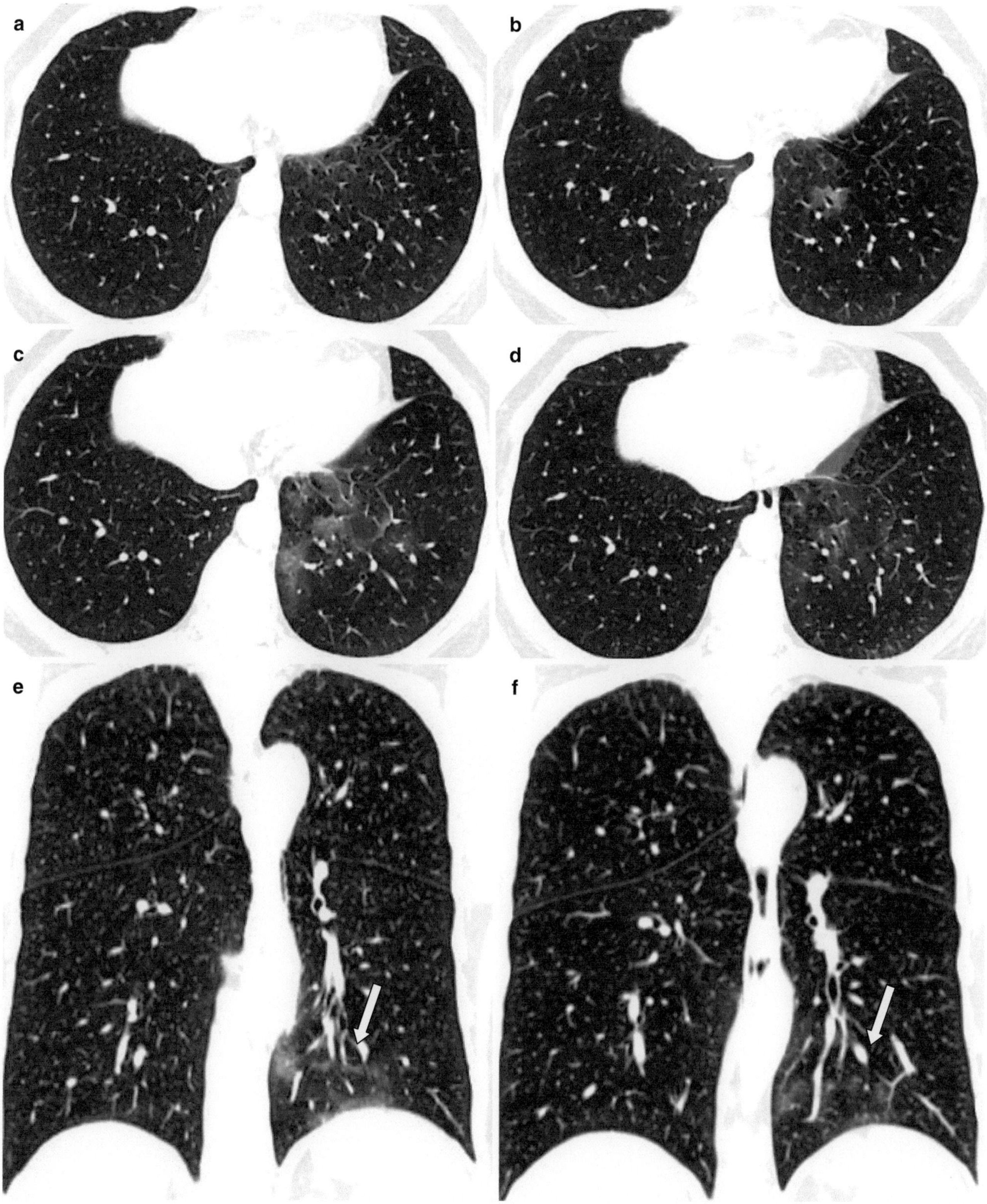

Fig. 9.6 Chest CT on day 2 of admission was not significantly positive (**a**). Day 5 CT scan shows ground-glass opacity in the left lower lobe (**b**). Day 11 CT showed an increased extent of lesions in the lower left lobe of the lung (**c**). Day 18 CT showed significant resorption of the left lower lobe of the lung (**d**). On day 11 compared with day 18, the lesion range was reduced (**e**, **f** white arrows)

9.3.3 Case 7

A 48-year-old female patient with a history of family clustering. Admitted to hospital due to "Fever for 4 days with cough and sputum for 3 days". The body temperature was 37.8 °C at the time of admission and there was no fever during the hospitalization. White blood cell count was 4.59×10^9/L, lymphocyte count was 2.10×10^9/L, C-reactive protein was <10 mg/L. The patient was confirmed by CDC in Guangzhou.

CT on day 5 of the onset showed a ground-glass nodules in the right lower lobe, with unclear boundary (Fig. 9.7a empty arrow). On day 9, CT showed an increase in plaque grinding ground-glass nodules in the lower lobe of the right lung with a thickened central lobe structure and an increased lesion extent (Fig. 9.7b1, b2 empty arrows). Day 21 CT showed a decrease in right lobe lesions (Fig. 9.7c).

Day 9 vs. day 21 CT, with reduced lesion extent and increased density (Fig. 9.7d, e white arrows).

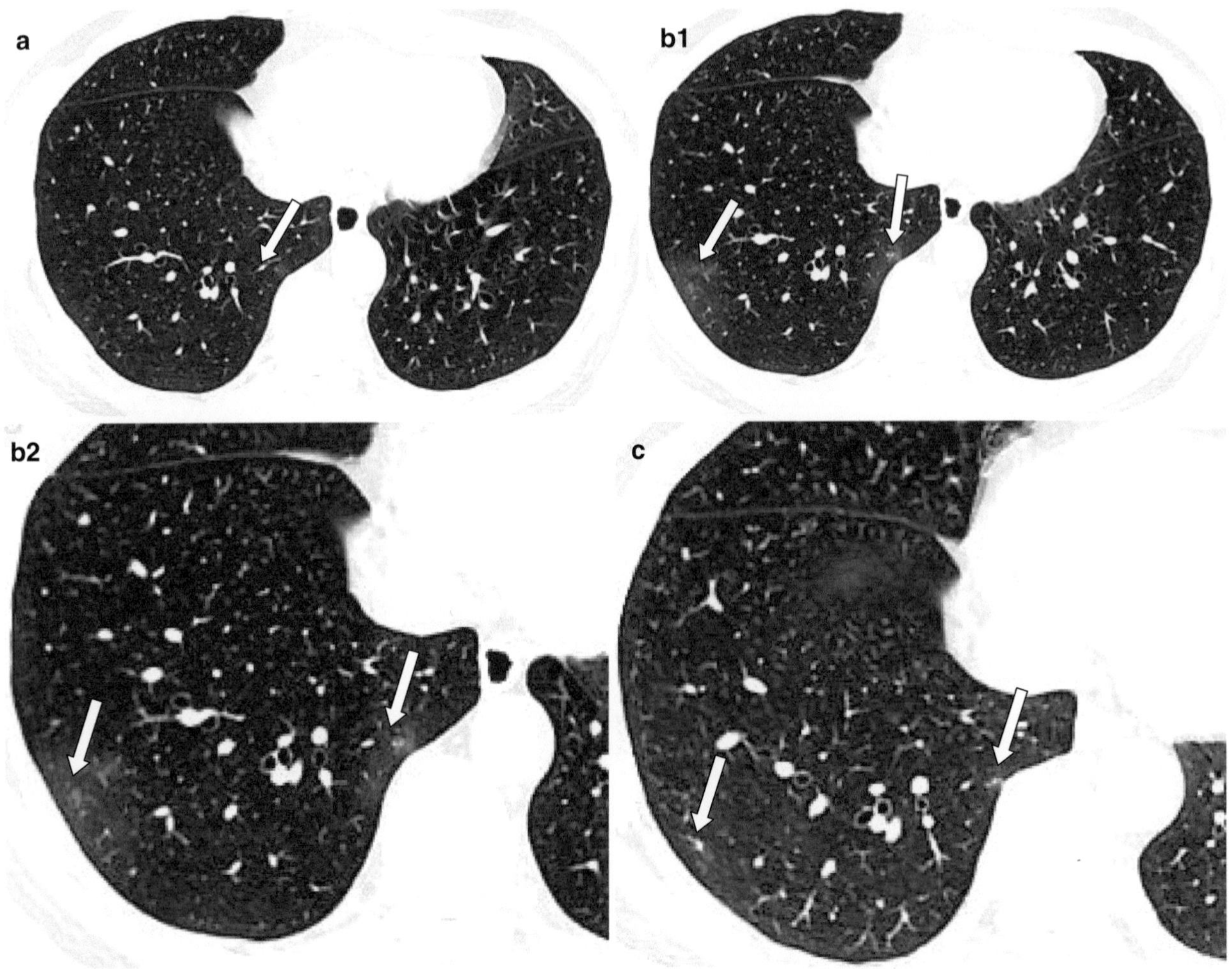

Fig. 9.7 CT on day 5 of the onset showed a ground-glass nodules in the right lower lobe, with unclear boundary (**a** empty arrow). On day 9, CT showed an increase in plaque grinding ground-glass nodules in the lower lobe of the right lung with a thickened central lobe structure and an increased lesion extent (**b1**, **b2** empty arrows). Day 21 CT showed a decrease in right lobe lesions (**c**). Day 9 vs. day 21 CT, with reduced lesion extent and increased density (**d**, **e** white arrows)

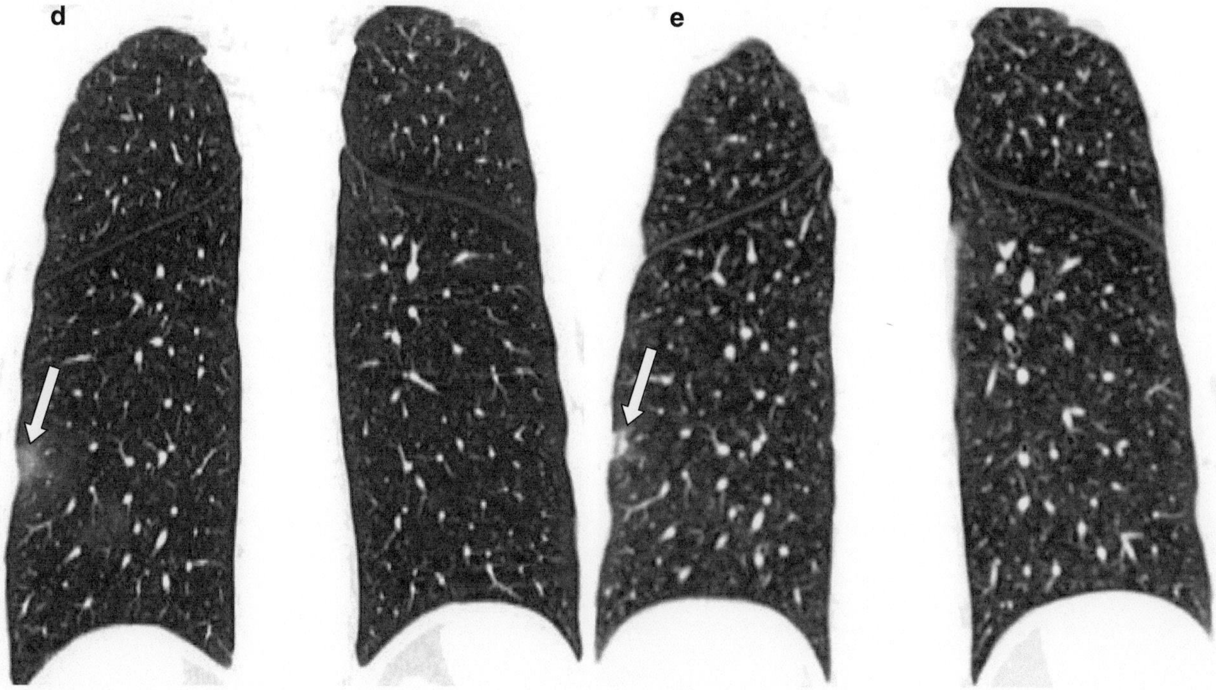

Fig. 9.7 (continued)

9.4 Family 3

Families in this group: the older brother first developed symptoms and his mother and brother successively; all three were seriously ill and had a poor prognosis.

Case 10 **(Mother)** ⟸ Case 8 (**T**he older brother) ⟹ Case 9 (Brother)

9.4.1 Case 8

A 64-year-old male patient with a disease-related exposure history. Admitted to the hospital with "fever, shortness of breath for 9 days after activity, exacerbated for 3 days". The body temperature on admission was 37.2 °C and there was no fever during the hospital stay. White blood cell count was 10.03×10^9/L, lymphocyte count was 0.55×10^9/L, C-reactive protein was 124.1 mg/L. (Critical type: blood oxygen saturation was <90%, plasma D-dimer was >10 mg/L, lactate dehydrogenase was 649 U/L) The patient was confirmed by CDC in Guangzhou.

A diffuse patchy, slightly dense, "white lung-like" manifestation was seen in both lungs on the 10th day of illness on a paraplegic chest piece (Fig. 9.8a).

On day 11, the bilateral lung lesions were smaller in extent and less dense than before (Fig. 9.8b).

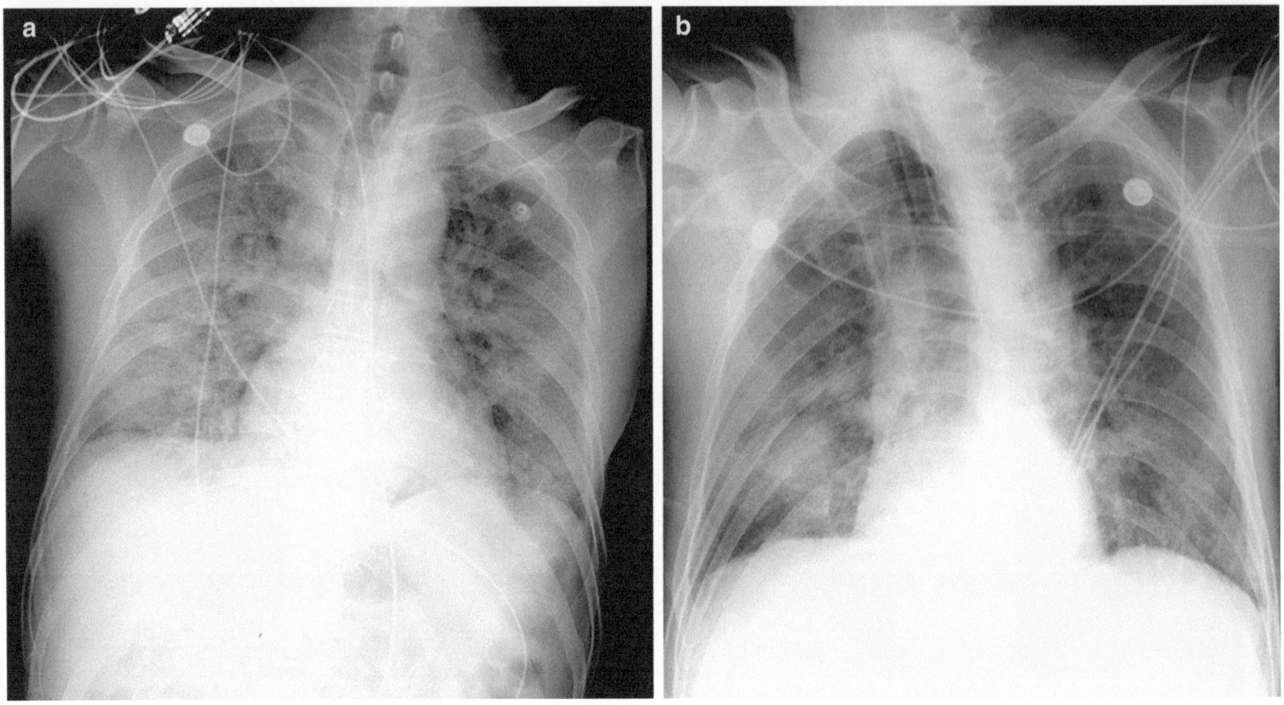

Fig. 9.8 A diffuse patchy, slightly dense, "white lung-like" manifestation was seen in both lungs on the 10th day of illness on a paraplegic chest piece (**a**). On day 11, the bilateral lung lesions were smaller in extent and less dense than before (**b**)

9.4.2 Case 9

A 58-year-old male patient was admitted to the hospital for "9 days of contact with a suspected case of novel coronavirus pneumonia" with a body temperature of 38 °C on admission and a maximum temperature of 38.4 °C during the course of the illness. White blood cell count was 6.69×10^9/L, lymphocyte count was 2.14×10^9/L, C-reactive protein was 25.1 mg/L. (Critical: oxygen saturation was 86–90%). The patient was confirmed by CDC in Guangzhou.

CT of the chest on day 3 of hospital admission showed scattered bilateral lung dense in the form of a patchy milliglass (Fig. 9.9a). On day 6, CT showed multiple patches and bars in both lungs, with a larger area and more lesions (Fig. 9.9b).

On day 9, CT showed a significant increase in lesions with thickening of the lobule interval and intrafollicular interval (Fig. 9.9c, d). On day 3 compared with day 9 CT, there was a significant increase in lesions, an increase in extent, and a decrease in partial lung volume (Fig. 9.9e, f).

9.4.3 Case 10

A 84-year-old female patient admitted to hospital with "cough and chest tightness for 2 days" with a family history of gathering. The temperature on admission was 36.4 °C, with a maximum temperature of 38 °C during the course of the illness. White blood cell count was 4.75×10^9/L, lymphocyte count was 1.54×10^9/L, C-reactive protein was 70.2 mg/L. (Critical type: blood oxygen saturation was <90%, plasma D-dimer was 1.1 mg/L) The patient was confirmed by CDC in Guangzhou.

CT of the chest on day 3 of the onset showed scattered, patchy, ground-glass opacity of both lungs (Fig. 9.10a, a1). CT on day 6 showed an increased range of bilateral lung lesions (Fig. 9.10b, b1). Diffuse densities of both lungs on the paraplegic chest piece on day 11 with a "white lung" presentation (Fig. 9.10c).

The range and density of bilateral lung lesions on days 19, 21, and 26 of the onset were smaller and less dense than before (Fig. 9.10d–f).

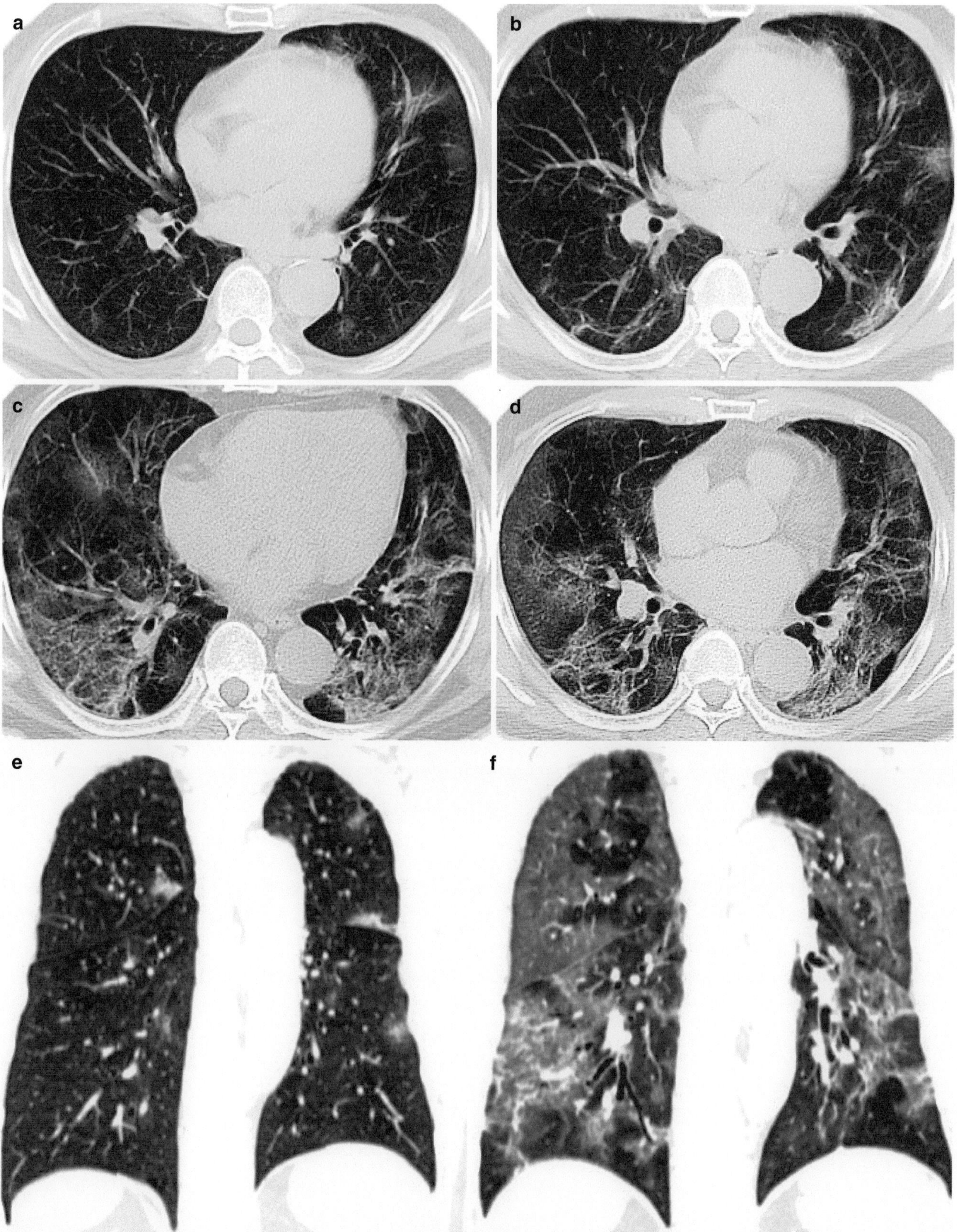

Fig. 9.9 CT of the chest on day 3 of hospital admission showed scattered bilateral lung dense in the form of a patchy milliglass (**a**). On day 6, CT showed multiple patches and bars in both lungs, with a larger area and more lesions (**b**). On day 9, CT showed a significant increase in lesions with thickening of the lobule interval and intrafollicular interval (**c**, **d**). On day 3 compared with day 9 CT, there was a significant increase in lesions, an increase in extent, and a decrease in partial lung volume (**e**, **f**)

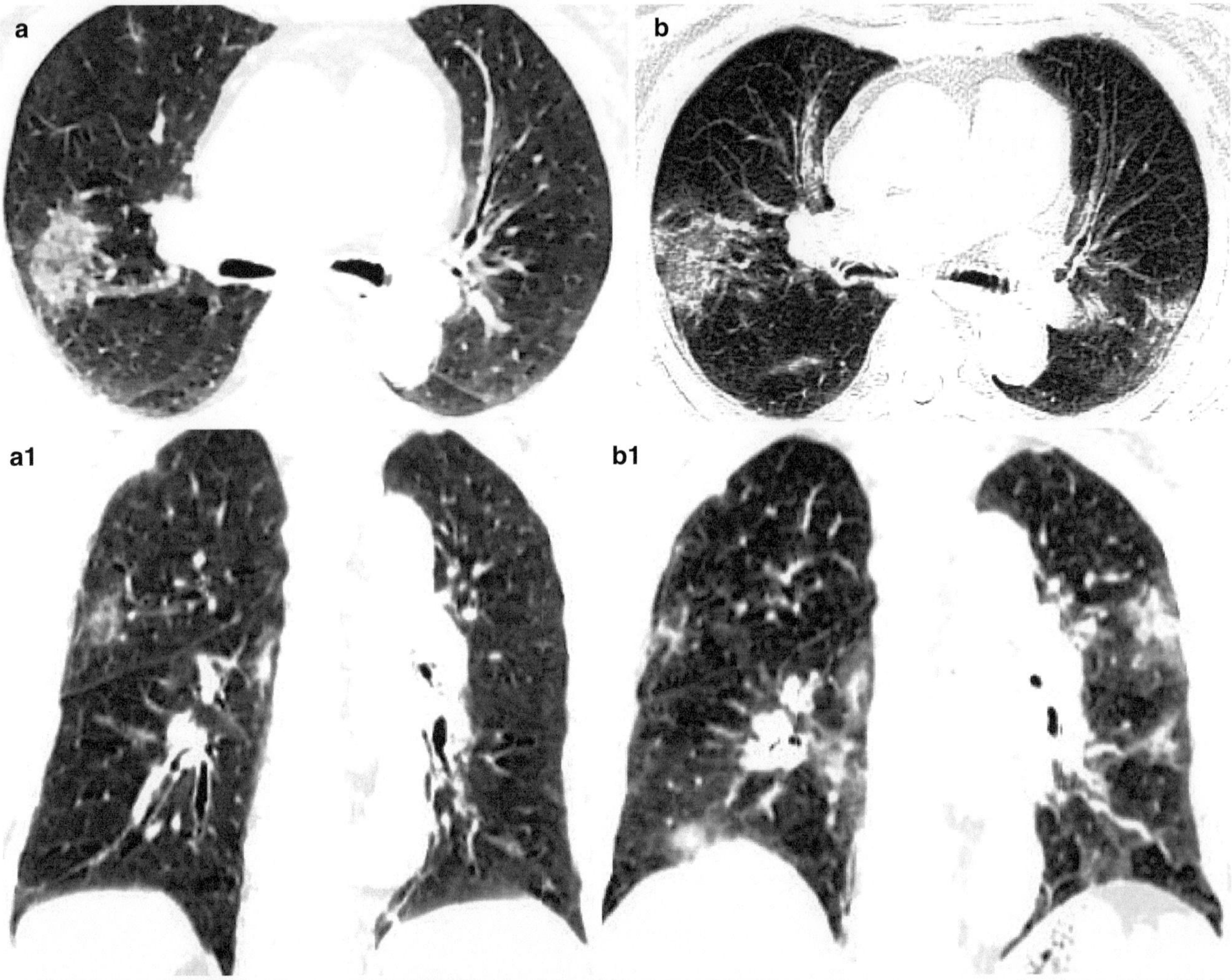

Fig. 9.10 CT of the chest on day 3 of the onset showed scattered, patchy, ground-glass opacity of both lungs (**a**, **a1**). CT on day 6 showed an increased range of bilateral lung lesions (**b**, **b1**). Diffuse densities of both lungs on the paraplegic chest piece on day 11 with a "white lung" presentation (**c**). The range and density of bilateral lung lesions on days 19, 21, and 26 of the onset were smaller and less dense than before (**d**–**f**)

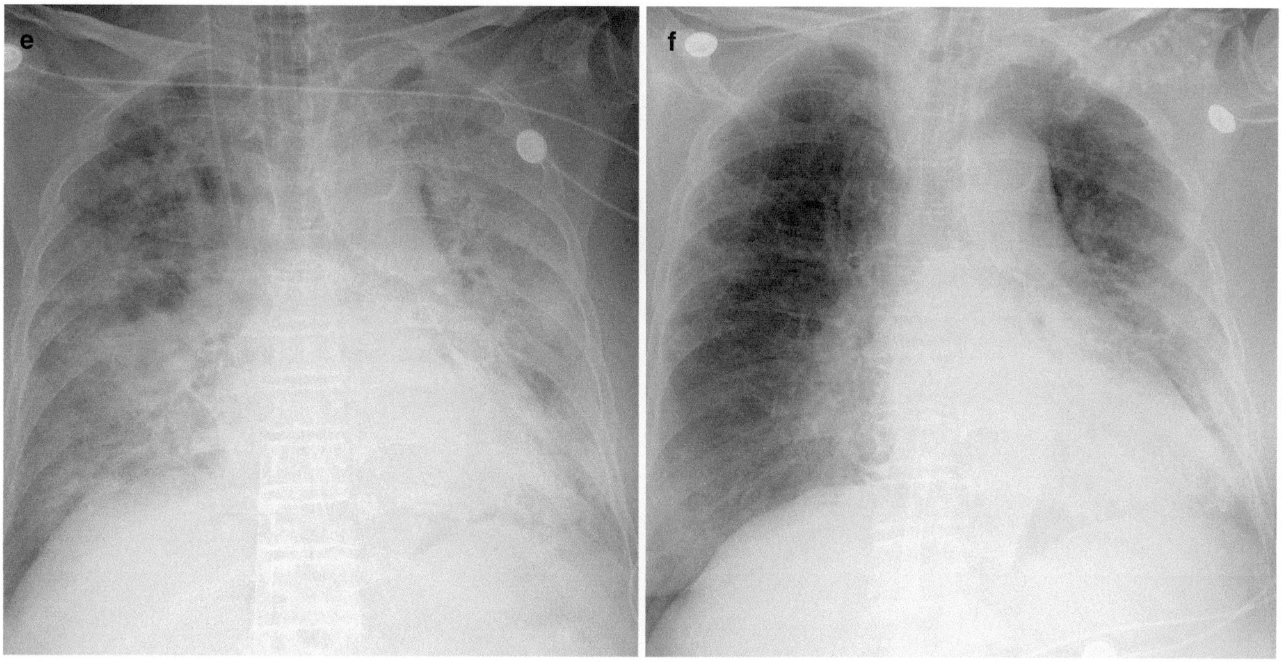

Fig. 9.10 (continued)

References

1. Wang X, Zhou Q, He Y, et al. Nosocomial outbreak of COVID-19 pneumonia in Wuhan, China. Eur Respir J. 2020;55(6):2000544. https://doi.org/10.1183/13993003.00544-2020. Print 2020 Jun. PMID: 32366488
2. Wu Z, McGoogan JM. Characteristics of and important lessons from the coronavirus disease 2019 (COVID-19) outbreak in China. Summary of a report of 72 314 cases from the Chinese center for disease control and prevention. JAMA. 2020;323(13):1239–42. https://doi.org/10.1001/jama.2020.2648. PMID: 32091533
3. Zhuang YL, et al. Analysis on the cluster epidemic of coronavirus disease 2019 in Guangdong Province. Zhonghua Yu Fang Yi Xue Za Zhi. 2020;54(7):720–5. https://doi.org/10.3760/cma.j.cn112150-20200326-00446.
4. Guan Q, Liu M, Zhuang YJ, Yuan Y. Epidemiological investigation of a family clustering of COVID-19. Zhonghua Liu Xing Bing Xue Za Zhi. 2020;41(5):629–33. https://doi.org/10.3760/cma.j.cn112338-20200223-00152.

Residual CT Features in Recovery Stage of COVID-19 Pneumonia

10

Yanhong Yang, Lieguang Zhang, Haiyan Shi, and Sufang Tian

10.1 Introduction

CT scan is not only used to initially assess the degree of lung involvement, but also to determine complications, guide treatment plans, and monitor the progression and changes of pneumonia, especially patients with functional respiratory disorder and/or hypoxemia after recovery from COVID-19 [1–5].

There are many published researches focused on the dynamic changes of chest CT, Liu N. et al. showed that the occurrence rate of ground-glass opacity, crazy paving pattern, pleural thickening in severe and critical group is higher [6]. Meanwhile, some researchers found that more than half of patients still had abnormal imaging findings on chest CT such as linear opacities, especially in severe or critical patients [7, 8].

According to the follow-up data of COVID-19 patients treated in Guangzhou Eighth People's Hospital, we found that ground-glass opacities and linear opacities could be seen in some patients although they had recovered and discharged from hospital, and others showed negative results on chest CT.

10.2 Case 1 (Fig. 10.1a–f)

A 65-year-old male was admitted with fever for 11 days, accompanied by diarrhea for 5 days and short-breathed for 3 days. He had no exposure to infected patient or epidemic area. The body temperature at admission was 39.2 °C. White blood cell count, neutrophil count, lymphocyte count, and the C-reactive protein were 6.74×10^9/L, 5.82×10^9/L, 0.67×10^9/L, and 68.0 mg/L, respectively. The patient was laboratory confirmed by novel coronavirus nucleic acid throat swab test in Guangzhou CDC. Chest CT examination was performed on 213 days after onset of symptoms (Fig. 10.1a–f).

On 213 days after onset of symptoms, chest CT images (Fig. 10.1a–f) showed patchy ground-glass opacities with thickening of the interlobular septa and linear opacities in bilateral lung.

Y. Yang (✉) · L. Zhang · H. Shi
Guangzhou Eighth People's Hospital, Guangzhou Medical University, Guangzhou, China

S. Tian
Zhongnan Hospital of Wuhan University, Wuhan, China

J. Liu et al. (eds.), *Atlas of Chest Imaging in COVID-19 Patients*, https://doi.org/10.1007/978-981-16-1082-0_10

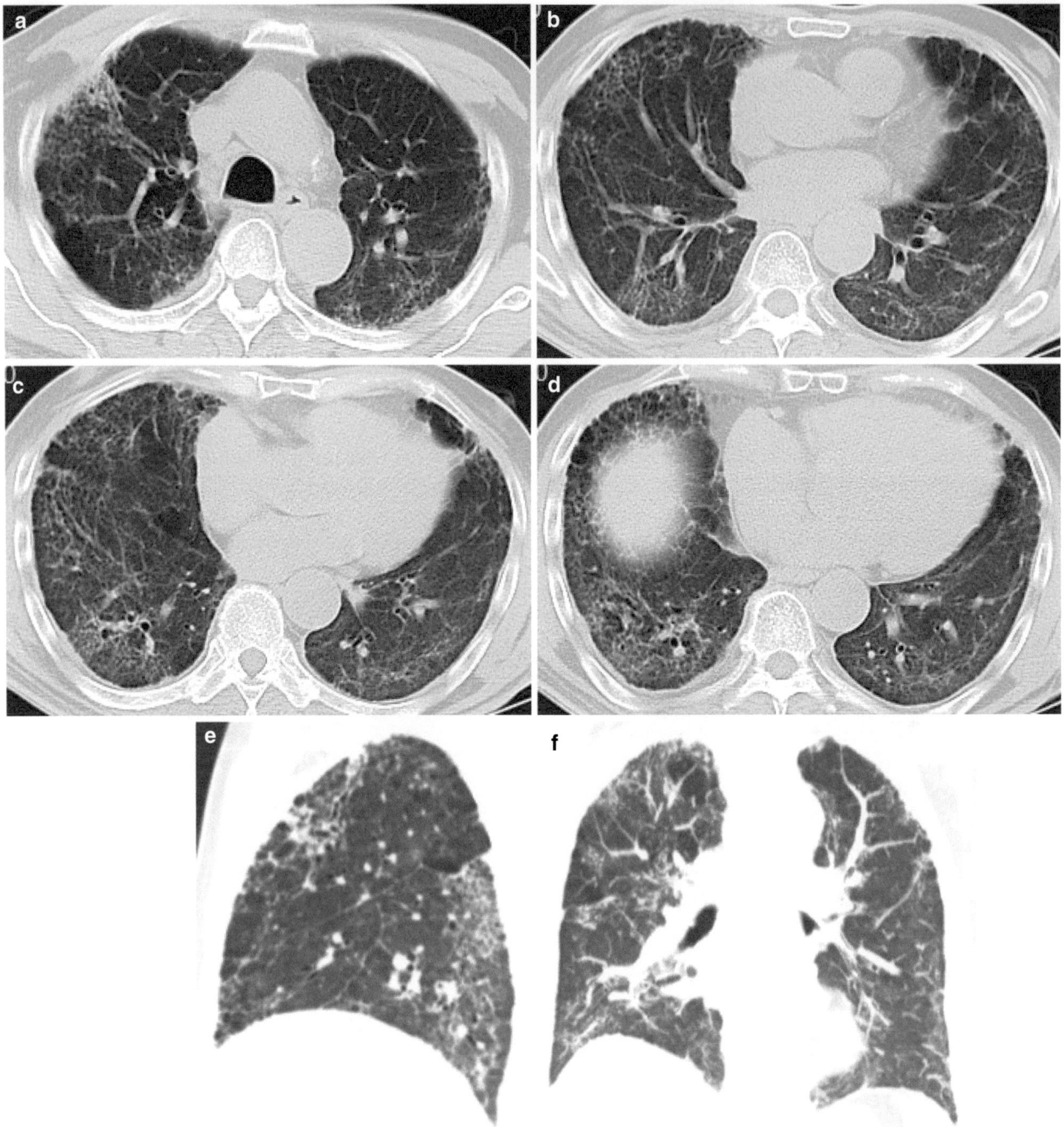

Fig. 10.1 On 213 days after onset of symptoms, chest CT images (**a**–**f**) showed patchy ground-glass opacities with thickening of the interlobular septa and linear opacities in bilateral lung

10.3 Case 2 (Fig. 10.2a–f)

A 54-year-old female was admitted with fever for 6 days. He had exposed to confirmed cases with novel coronavirus pneumonia. The body temperature at admission was 39.9 °C. White blood cell count, neutrophil count, lymphocyte count, and the C-reactive protein were 5.4×10^9/L, 3.64×10^9/L, 1.49×10^9/L, and 36.12 mg/L, respectively. The patient was laboratory confirmed by novel coronavirus nucleic acid throat swab test in Guangzhou CDC. Chest CT examination was performed on 194 days after onset of symptoms (Fig. 10.2a–f).

On 194 days after onset of symptoms, chest CT images (Fig. 10.2a–f) showed linear opacities in the middle lobe of right lung.

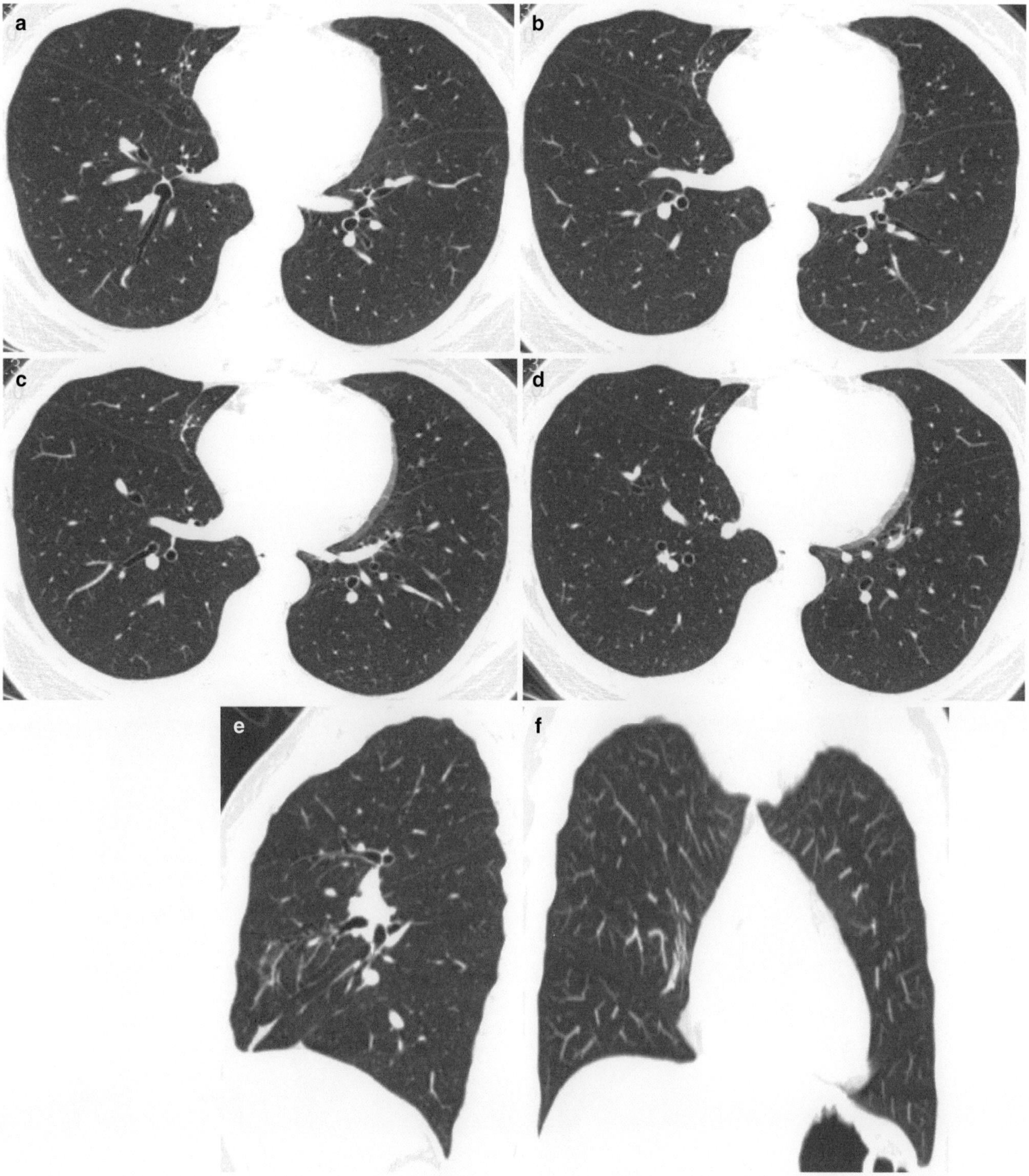

Fig. 10.2 On 194 days after onset of symptoms, chest CT images (**a**–**f**) showed linear opacities in the middle lobe of right lung

10.4 Case 3 (Fig. 10.3a–f)

A 48-year-old male was admitted with fever for 4 days, accompanied by cough and expectoration. He had exposed to confirmed cases with novel coronavirus pneumonia. The body temperature at admission was 37.8 °C. White blood cell count, neutrophil count, lymphocyte count, and the C-reactive protein were 4.59×10^9/L, 1.99×10^9/L, 2.1×10^9/L, and <10 mg/L, respectively. The patient was laboratory confirmed by novel coronavirus nucleic acid throat swab test in Guangzhou CDC. Chest CT examination was performed on 198 days after onset of symptoms (Fig. 10.3a–f).

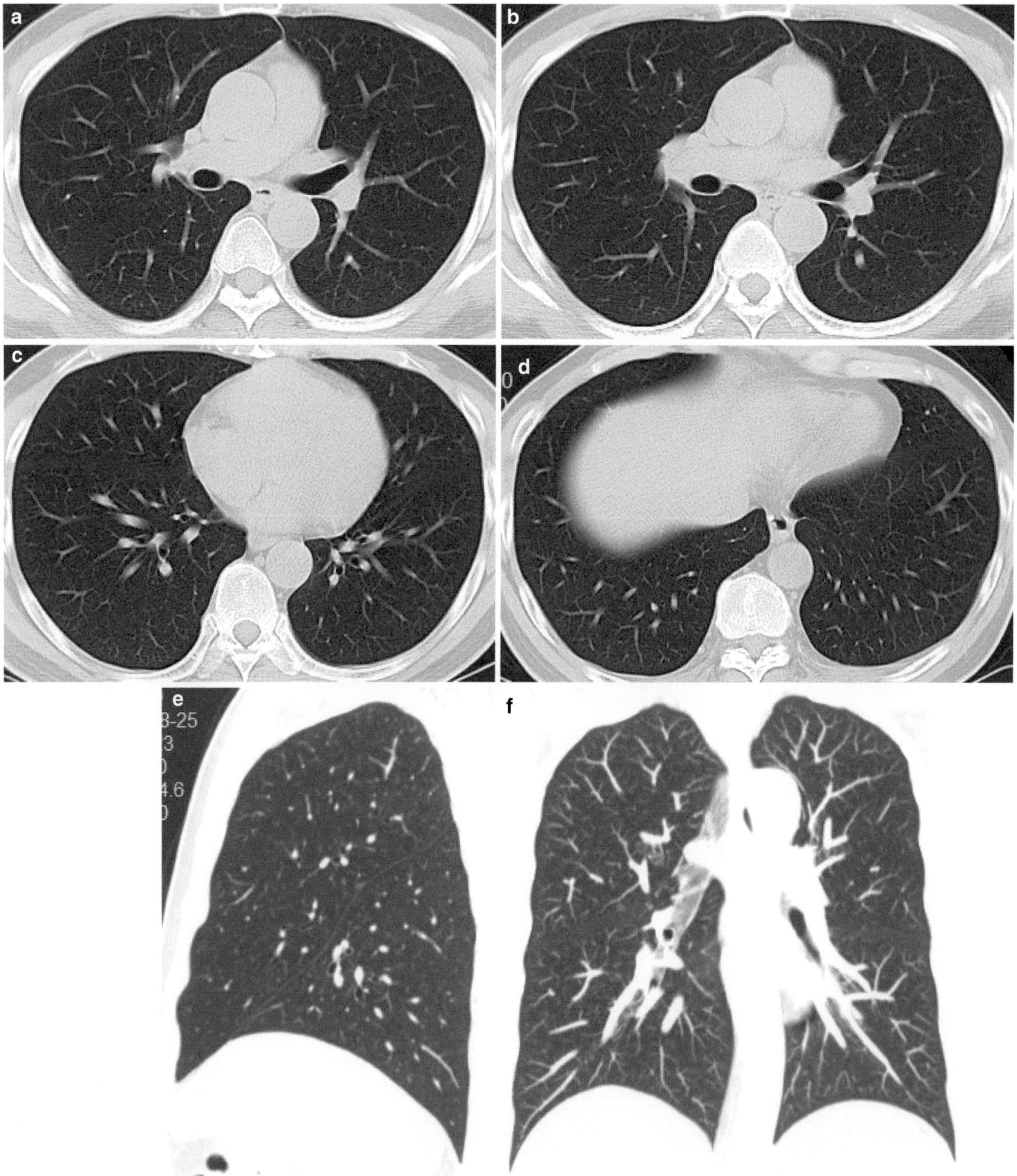

Fig. 10.3 On 198 days after onset of symptoms, chest CT images (**a**–**f**) showed patchy ground-glass opacities in the upper lobe of right lung (**b**, **e**, **f**)

On 198 days after onset of symptoms, chest CT images (Fig. 10.3a–f) showed patchy ground-glass opacities in the upper lobe of right lung (Fig. 10.3b, e, f).

10.5 Case 4 (Fig. 10.4a–f)

A 65-year-old male was admitted with fever for 8 days. He had no exposure to infected patient or epidemic area. The body temperature at admission was 37.9 °C. White blood cell count, neutrophil count, lymphocyte count, and the C-reactive protein were 5.56×10^9/L, 3.50×10^9/L, 1.75×10^9/L, and 35.36 mg/L, respectively. The patient was laboratory confirmed by novel coronavirus nucleic acid throat swab test in Guangzhou CDC. Chest CT examination was performed on 195 days after onset of symptoms (Fig. 10.4a–f).

On 195 days after onset of symptoms, chest CT images (Fig. 10.4a–f) showed normal in bilateral lung.

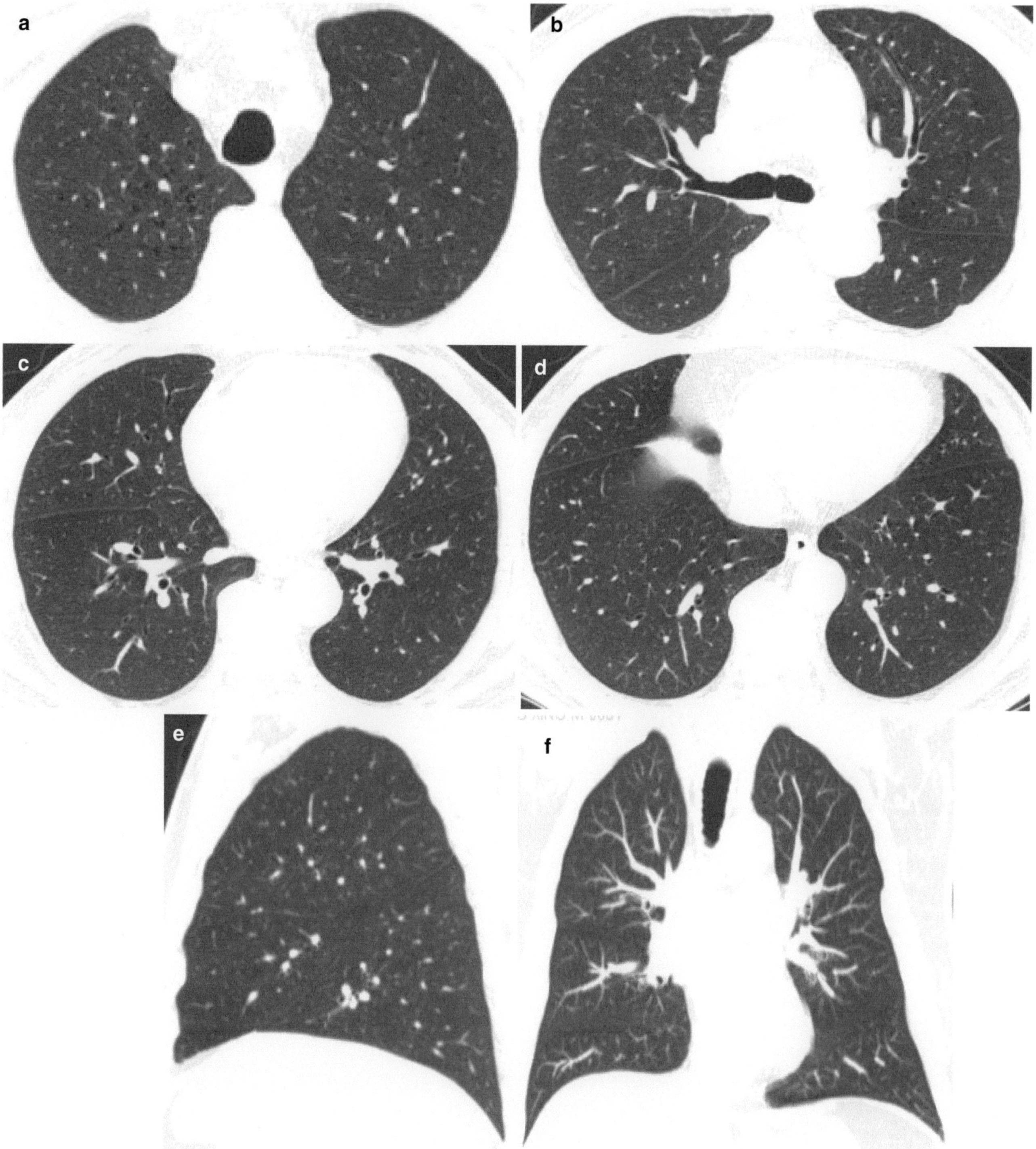

Fig. 10.4 On 195 days after onset of symptoms, chest CT images (**a**–**f**) showed normal in bilateral lung

10.6 Case 5 (Fig. 10.5a–e)

An 81-year-old male was admitted with recurrent fever for 10 days, accompanied by chills, headache, dizziness, and muscle soreness. He had exposed to confirmed cases with novel coronavirus pneumonia. The body temperature at admission was 39 °C. White blood cell count, neutrophil count, lymphocyte count, and the C-reactive protein were 6.28×10^9/L, 5.35×10^9/L, 0.77×10^9/L, and 60.5 mg/L, respectively. The patient was laboratory confirmed by novel coronavirus nucleic acid throat swab test in Guangzhou CDC. Chest CT examination was performed on 21 days after onset of symptoms (Fig. 10.5a–e).

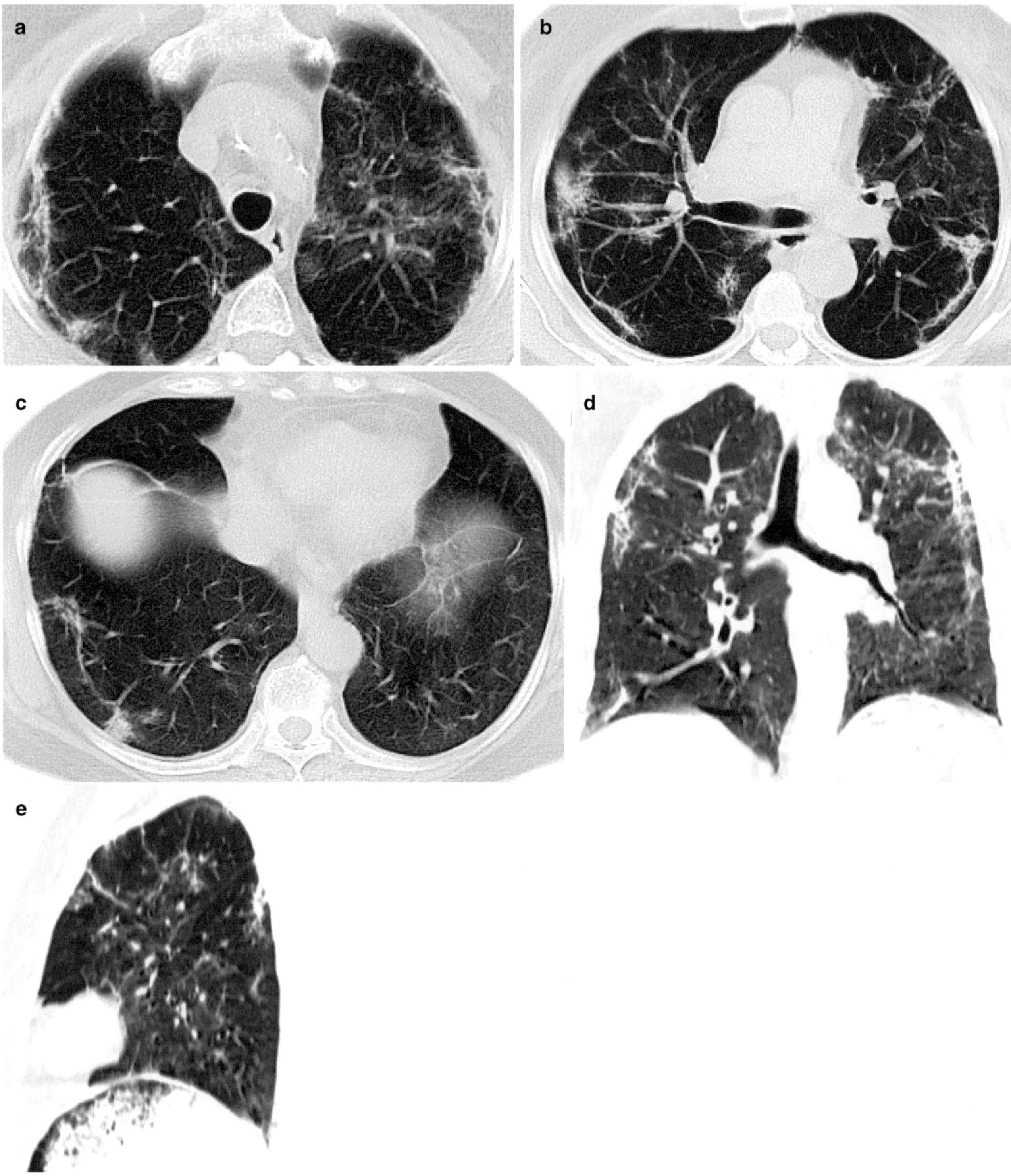

Fig. 10.5 On 21 days after onset of symptoms, chest CT images (**a**–**e**) showed linear opacities in bilateral lung

On 21 days after onset of symptoms, chest CT images (Fig. 10.4a–e) showed linear opacities in bilateral lung.

10.7 **Case 6** (Fig. 10.6a–e)

A 62-year-old male was admitted with fever for 5 days, accompanied by chills and muscle soreness. He had exposed to confirmed cases with novel coronavirus pneumonia. The body temperature at admission was 38.6 °C. White blood cell count, neutrophil count, lymphocyte count, and the C-reactive protein were 3.05×10^9/L, 2.16×10^9/L, 0.56×10^9/L, and <10 mg/L. The patient was laboratory confirmed by novel coronavirus nucleic acid throat swab test in Guangzhou CDC. Chest CT examination was performed on 29 days after onset of symptoms (Fig. 10.6a–e).

On 29 days after onset of symptoms, chest CT images (Fig. 10.4a–e) showed linear opacities in bilateral lung.

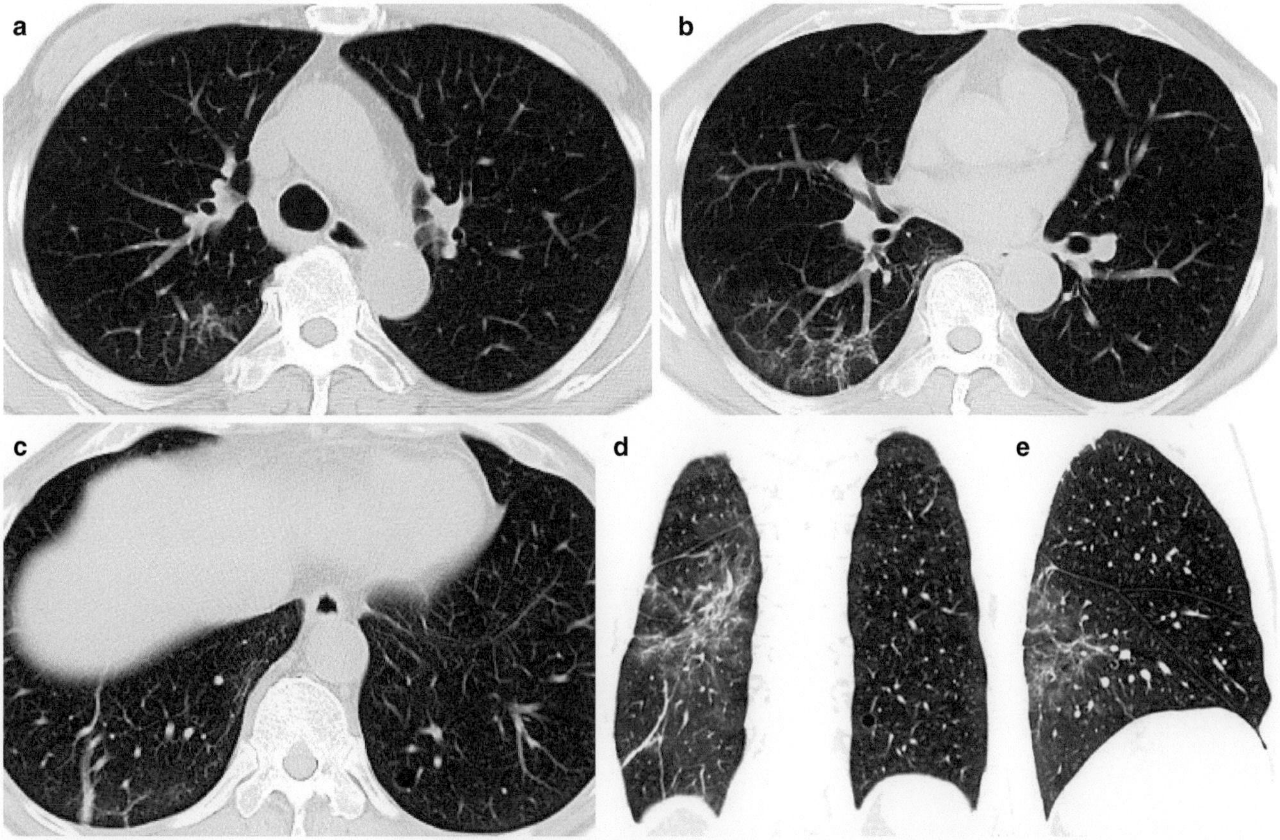

Fig. 10.6 On 29 days after onset of symptoms, chest CT images (**a**–**e**) showed linear opacities in bilateral lung

References

1. Rubin GD, Ryerson CJ, Haramati LB, et al. The role of chest imaging in patient management during the COVID-19 pandemic: a multinational consensus statement from the Fleischner Society. Chest. 2020;158:106–16. https://doi.org/10.1016/j.chest.2020.04.003.
2. Tabatabaei SMH, Talari H, Moghaddas F, Rajebi H. Computed tomographic features and short-term prognosis of coronavirus disease 2019 (COVID-19) pneumonia: a single-center study from Kashan, Iran. Radiol Cardiothor Imaging. 2020;2(2):e200130. https://doi.org/10.1148/ryct.2020200130.
3. Francone M, Iafrate F, Masci GM, et al. Chest CT score in COVID-19 patients: correlation with disease severity and short-term prognosis. Eur Radiol. 2020;4:1–6817. https://doi.org/10.1007/s00330-020-07033-y.
4. Lu X, Gong W, Peng Z, et al. High resolution CT imaging dynamic follow-up study of novel coronavirus pneumonia. Front Med. 2020;7:168. https://doi.org/10.3389/fmed.2020.00168.
5. Vernuccio F, Giambelluca D, Cannella R, et al. Radiographic and chest CT imaging presentation and follow-up of COVID-19 pneumonia: a multicenter experience from an endemic area. Emerg Radiol. 2020;11:1–10.
6. Liu N, He G, Yang X, et al. Dynamic changes of chest CT follow-up in coronavirus disease-19 (COVID-19) pneumonia: relationship to clinical typing. BMC Med Imaging. 2020;20(1):92. https://doi.org/10.1186/s12880-020-00491-2.
7. Li M, Lei P, Zeng B, et al. Coronavirus disease (COVID-19): spectrum of CT findings and temporal progression of the disease. Acad Radiol. 2020;27:603–8. https://doi.org/10.1016/j.acra.2020.03.003.
8. Huang Y, Yan Tan C, Wu J, et al. Impact of coronavirus disease 2019 on pulmonary function in early convalescence phase. Respir Res. 2020;21(1):163. https://doi.org/10.1186/s12931-020-01429-6.

CT Features and Pathological Analysis of COVID-19 Death

11

Jing Qu, Li Liang, Meiyan Liao, and Ying Liu

11.1 Introduction

SARS-CoV-2 has claimed the lives of 1 million people. The main cause of death is due to multiple organ failure, diffuse intravascular hemorrhage, septic shock, and other serious complications. There was only one death case in Guangzhou Eighth People's Hospital. To show the typical imaging features of death cases, we also include another death case in Central South University Hospital of Wuhan University.

The hyaline membrane is the end-stage manifestation of COVID-19, which is formed by diffuse alveolar injury with fibromyxoid exudate in both lungs, with significant alveolar epithelial cell detachment. It does not occur in all critically ill or dead patients. However, pulmonary edema, protein exudation, pulmonary interstitial thickening, and inflammatory cell infiltration in the alveolar cavity are the common basic pathological changes [1–3].

11.2 Case 1 (Fig. 11.1a–l)

An 82-year-old male was admitted to the hospital with fever for 5 days. The body temperature at admission was 37.4 °C. Laboratory examination: white blood cell count in peripheral blood was 4.57×10^9/L, lymphocyte count was 0.45×10^9/L, C-reactive protein was 36.7 mg/L, and oxygenation index was 245 mmHg. The patient was laboratory confirmed by novel coronavirus nucleic acid throat swab test in Guangzhou CDC. Chest CT examination was performed on day 1 (6 days after the onset of symptoms) of admission. Bedside chest radiographs were successively taken on day 8 (13 days after the onset of symptoms), day 15 (20 days after the onset of symptoms), and day 19 (24 days after the onset of symptoms) of admission. Postmortem pathology was performed on day 33 (38 days after the onset of symptoms) of admission, as shown in Fig. 11.1a–l. (Thanks to Professor Ding Yanqing and Professor Liang Li, Department of Pathology, Southern Hospital, Southern Medical University, for providing the pathological pictures of this case.)

On day 1 of admission, chest CT images showed that multiple ground-glass opacities with thickened interlobular septum were found in the bilateral lung, which showed a "crazy-paving pattern" (Fig. 11.1a–d).

Bedside chest radiographs were successively taken on day 8, day 15, and day 19 of admission, which showed that the lesions in bilateral lungs of the patient were gradually aggravated and showed "white lung" at last (Fig. 11.1e–h).

On day 33 of admission, the patient died due to multiple organ dysfunction syndrome (MODS) and dessiminated intravascular coagulation (DIC). At low magnification (Fig. 11.1i, j), consolidation and interstitial fibrosis were evidently present. Alveolar septum widened and fibrous tissue proliferated, and a small amount of fibrin-like exudate was present between alveoli. The type II alveolar epithelium was proliferated and detached in the alveolar cavity, which was intermixed with the proliferated macrophages some alveolar tissues were organized. There was a small amount of chronic inflammatory cell infiltrated in the pulmonary interstitium with focal hemorrhage. And no clear bacterial, fungal, or viral inclusions were observed.

At high magnification (Fig. 11.1k, l), alveolar septum significantly widened, and fibrous tissue proliferated. The type II alveolar epithelium was proliferated and detached in the alveolar cavity, which was intermixed with the proliferated macrophages. There was a small amount of chronic inflammatory cell infiltrated in the pulmonary interstitium.

J. Qu (✉) · Y. Liu
Guangzhou Eighth People's Hospital, Guangzhou Medical University, Guangzhou, China

L. Liang
Nanfang Hospital, Southern Medical University, Guangzhou, China

M. Liao
Zhongnan Hospital of Wuhan University, Wuhan, China

J. Liu et al. (eds.), *Atlas of Chest Imaging in COVID-19 Patients*, https://doi.org/10.1007/978-981-16-1082-0_11

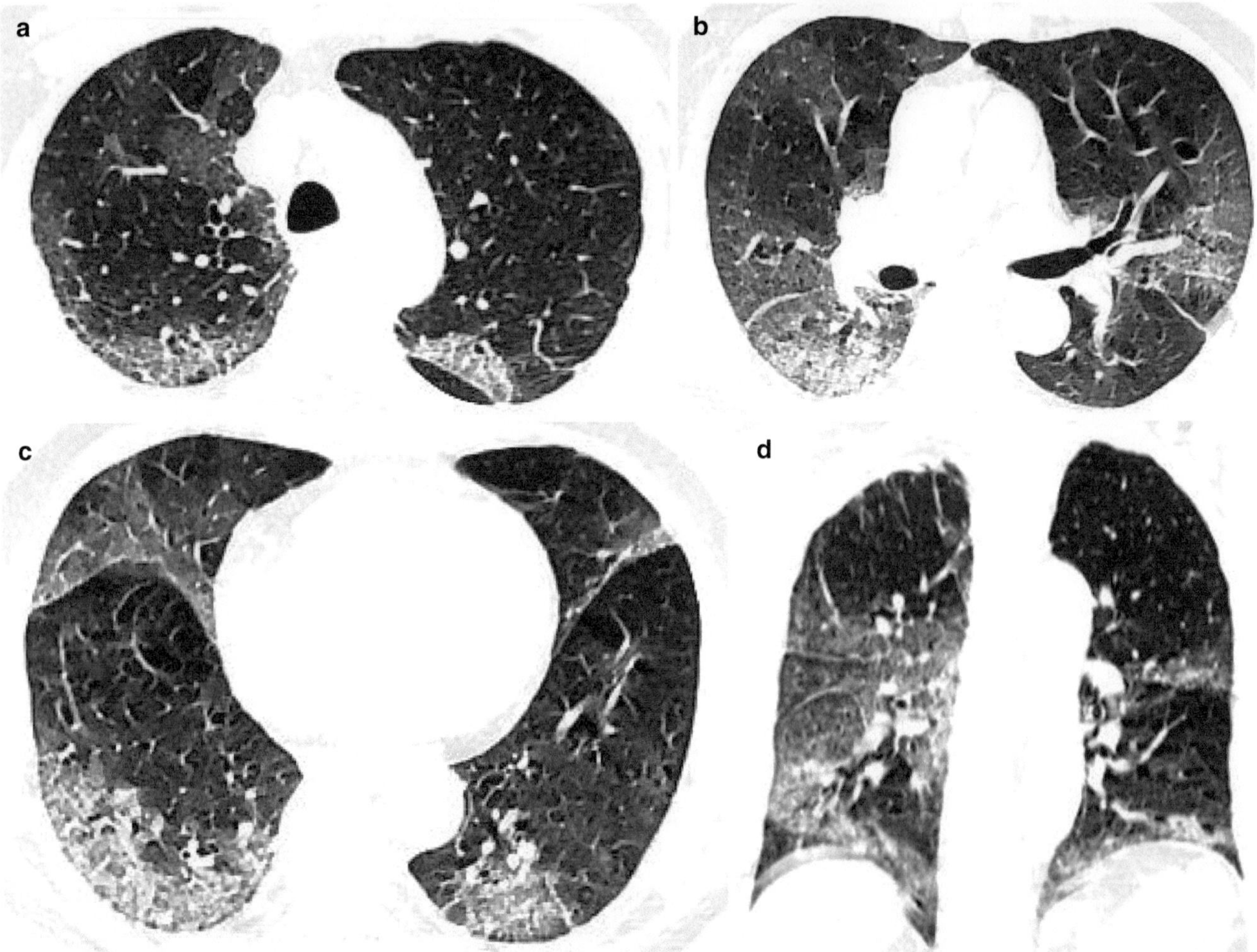

Fig. 11.1 On day 1 of admission, chest CT images showed that multiple ground-glass opacities with thickened interlobular septum were found in the bilateral lung, which showed a "crazy-paving pattern" (**a**–**d**). Bedside chest radiographs were successively taken on day 8, day 15, and day 19 of admission, which showed that the lesions in bilateral lungs of the patient were gradually aggravated and showed "white lung" at last (**e**–**h**). On day 33 of admission, the patient died due to MODS and DIC. At low magnification (**i**, **j**), consolidation and interstitial fibrosis were evidently present. Alveolar septum widened and fibrous tissue proliferated, and a small amount of fibrin-like exudate was present between alveoli. The type II alveolar epithelium was proliferated and detached in the alveolar cavity, which was intermixed with the proliferated macrophages. And partial alveolar was organized. There was a small amount of chronic inflammatory cell infiltrated in the pulmonary interstitium with focal hemorrhage. And no clear bacterial, fungal, or viral inclusions were observed. At high magnification (**k**, **l**), alveolar septum significantly widened and fibrous tissue proliferated. The type II alveolar epithelium was proliferated and detached in the alveolar cavity, which was intermixed with the proliferated macrophages. There was a small amount of chronic inflammatory cell infiltrated in the pulmonary interstitium

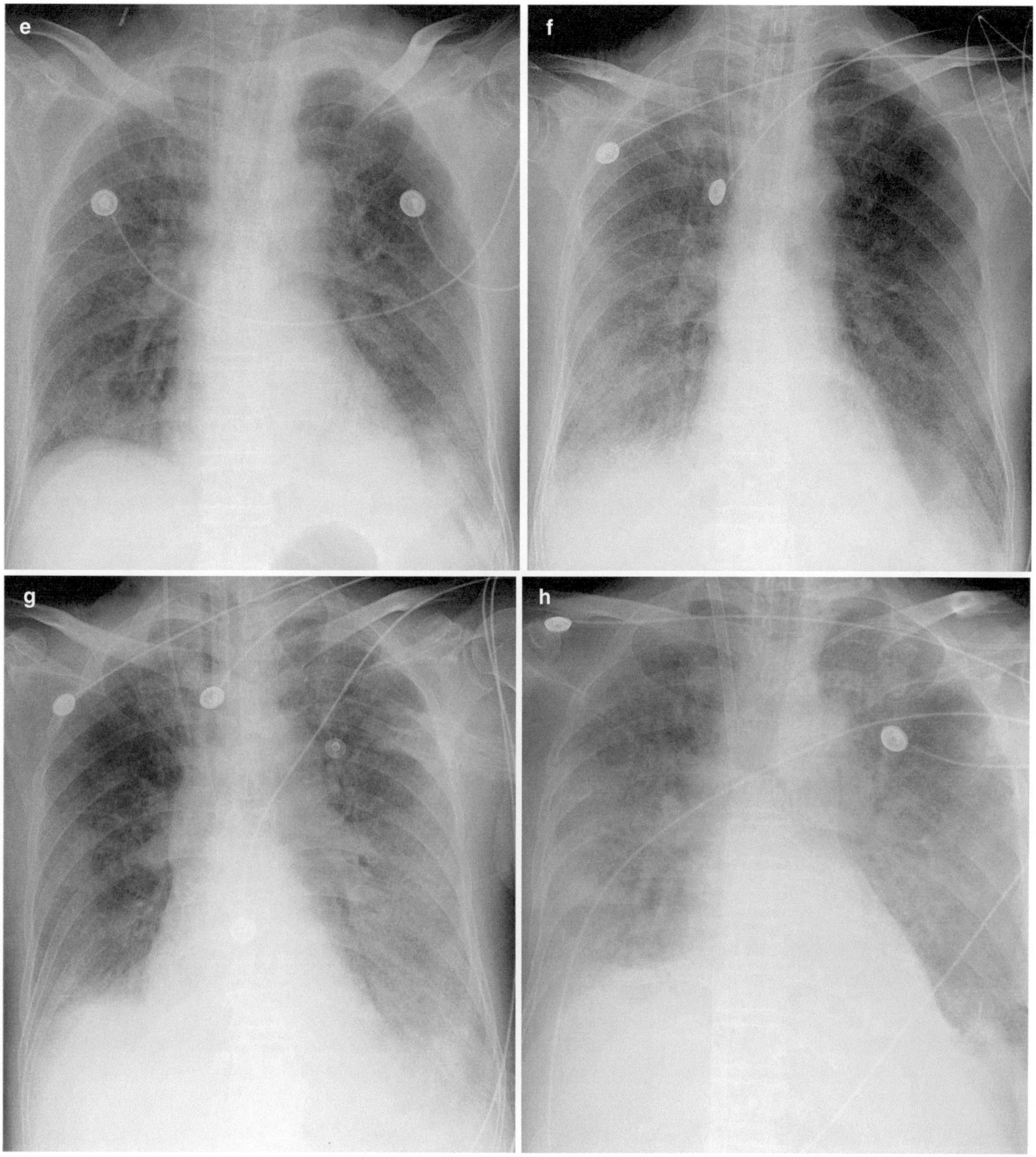

Fig. 11.1 (continued)

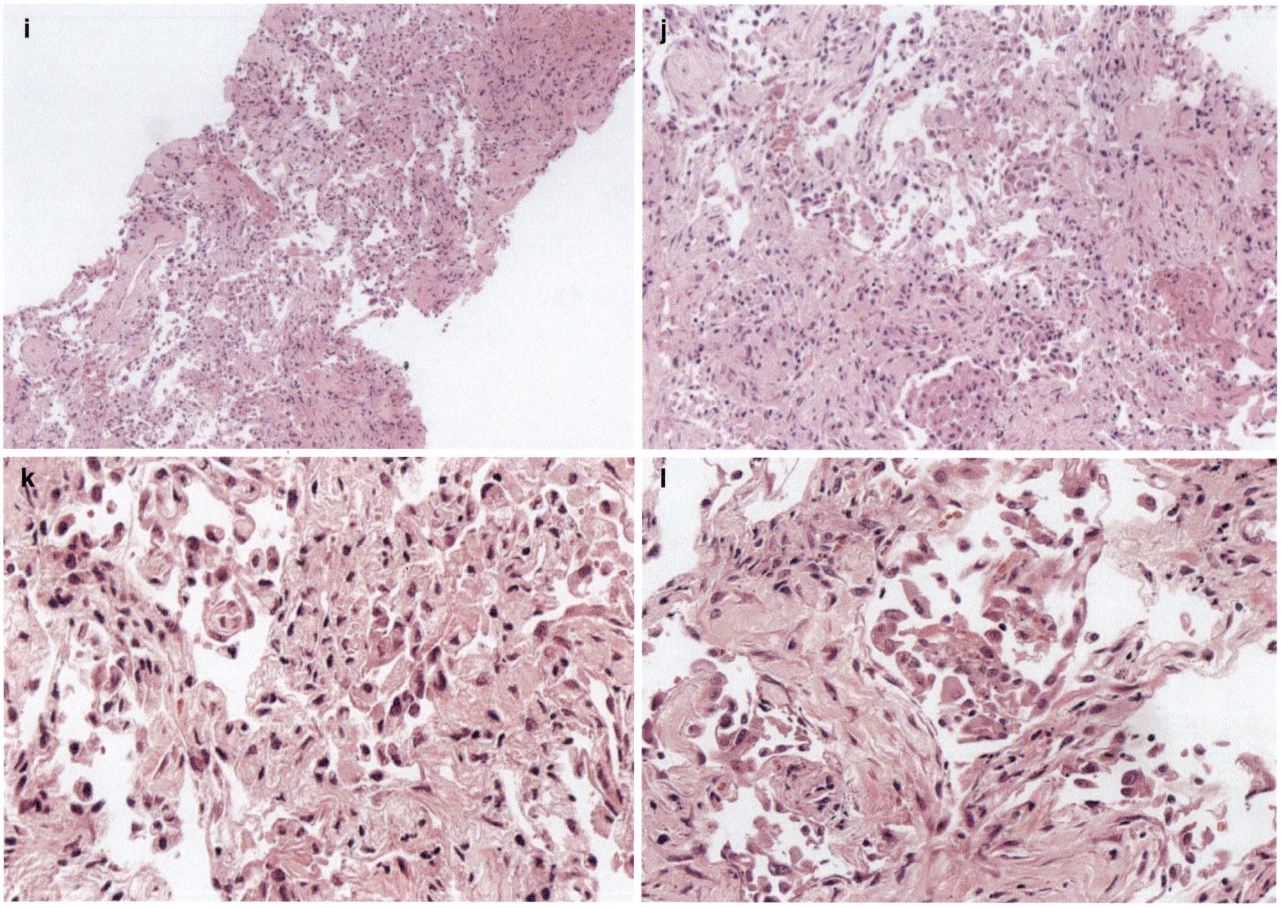

Fig. 11.1 (continued)

11.3 **Case 2** (Fig. 11.2a–h)

A 74-year-old male was laboratory confirmed by novel coronavirus nucleic acid throat swab test in Wuhan CDC. The highest temperature in the course of the disease was 38.2 °C. The patient was diagnosed as severe on day 3 and died on day 7 of admission. (Thanks to Professor Liao Meiyan of the Department of Radiology and Professor Tian Sufang of the Department of Pathology, Central South Hospital, Wuhan University, for their case.)

Chest CT images showed multiple ground-glass opacities in both lungs, especially in the right lung, which, with local consolidation and thickening of interlobular and intralobular septa, formed a "crazy-paving pattern" (Fig. 11.2a). There was a little pleural effusion (Fig. 11.2a–f).

The pathological images showed a pink hyaline membrane attached to the alveolar wall (Fig. 11.2g). The pathological images showed alveolar injury: some alveolar epithelium was detached, some type II alveolar epithelium was proliferated, and cellulose exudate was present in the upper right corner. A few inflammatory cells infiltrated the pulmonary interstitium (Fig. 11.2h).

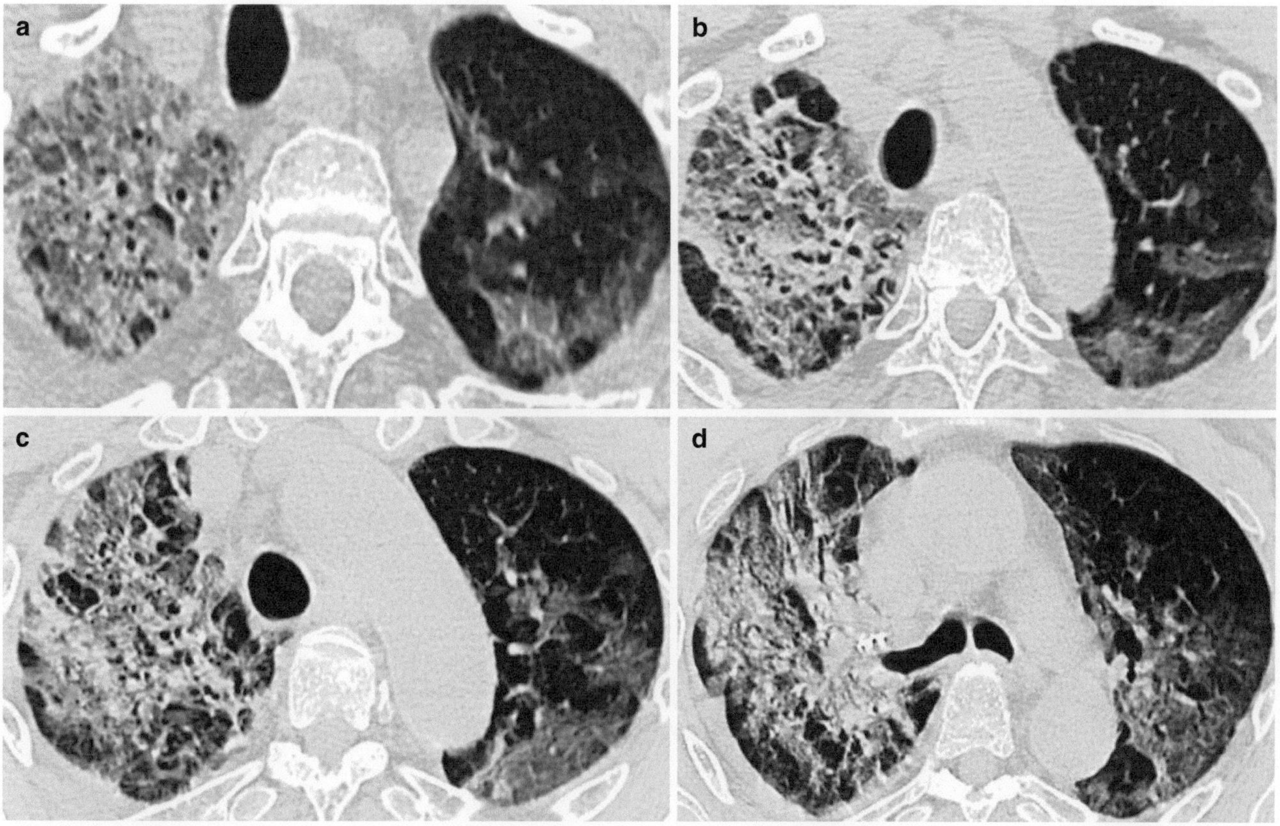

Fig. 11.2 Chest CT images showed multiple ground-glass opacities in both lungs, especially in the right lung, which, with local consolidation and thickening of interlobular and intralobular septa, formed a "crazy-paving pattern" (**a**). There was a little pleural effusion (**a**–**f**). The pathological images showed a pink hyaline membrane attached to the alveolar wall (**g**). The pathological images showed alveolar injury: some alveolar epithelium was detached, some type II alveolar epithelium was proliferated, and cellulose exudate was present in the upper right corner. A few inflammatory cells infiltrated the pulmonary interstitium (**h**)

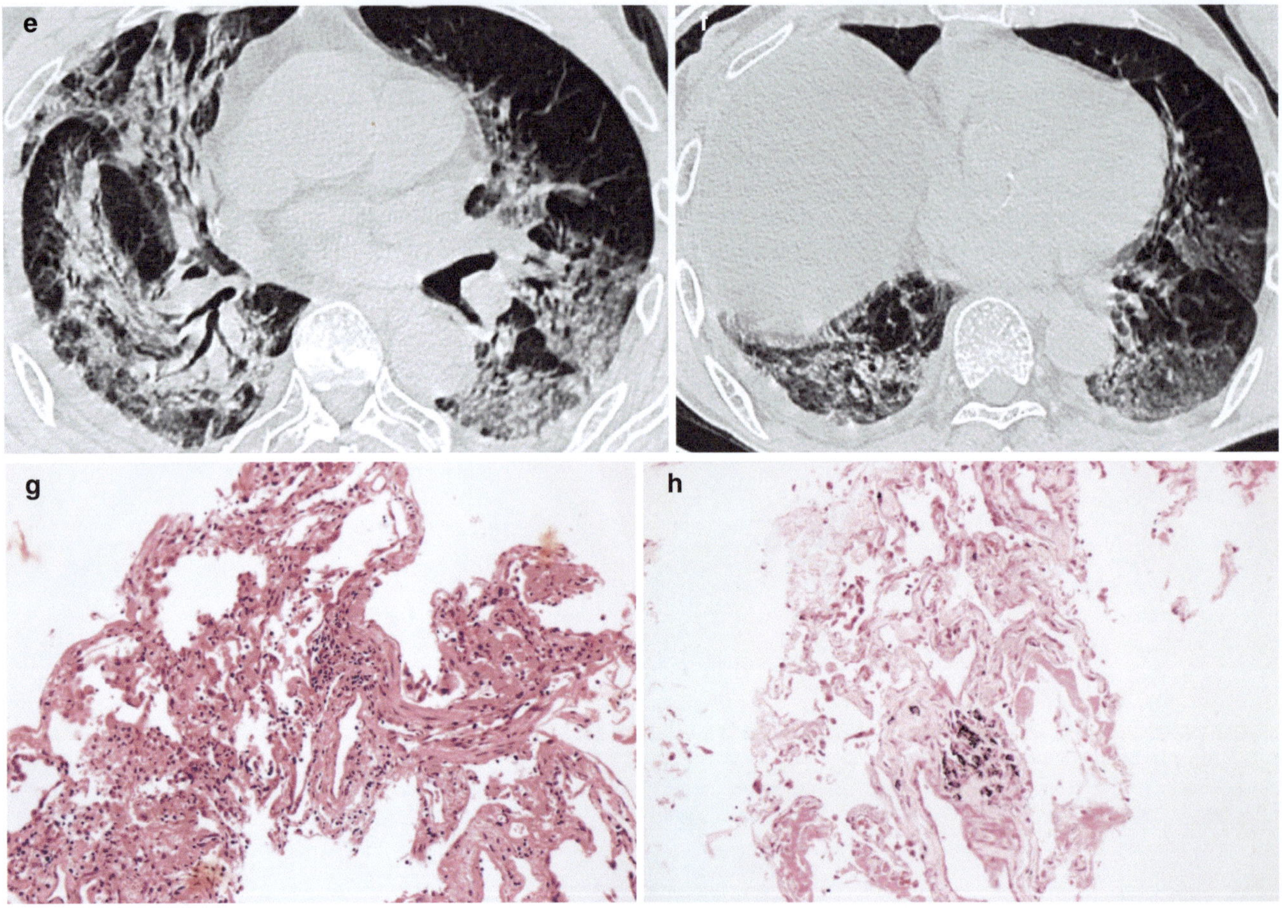

Fig. 11.2 (continued)

References

1. Tian S, Hu W, Niu L, et al. Pulmonary pathology of early-phase 2019 novel coronavirus (COVID-19) pneumonia in two patients with lung cancer. J Thorac Oncol. 2020; https://doi.org/10.1016/j.jtho.2020.02.010.
2. Xu Z, Shi L, Wang Y, et al. Pathological findings of COVID-19 associated with acute respiratory distress syndrome. Lancet Respir Med. 2020; https://doi.org/10.1016/S2213-2600(20)30076-X.
3. Joob B, Wiwanitkit V. Pulmonary pathology of early phase 2019 novel coronavirus pneumonia. J Thorac Oncol. 2020;15(5):e67. https://doi.org/10.1016/j.jtho.2020.03.013.

MIX
Papier aus verantwortungsvollen Quellen
Paper from responsible sources
FSC® C105338

If you have any concerns about our products,
you can contact us on
ProductSafety@springernature.com

In case Publisher is established outside the EU,
the EU authorized representative is:
Springer Nature Customer Service Center GmbH
Europaplatz 3, 69115 Heidelberg, Germany

Printed by Libri Plureos GmbH
in Hamburg, Germany